Homeopathy and
Mental Health Care

Homeopathy and
Mental Health Care
Integrative Practice, Principles and Research

Compiled and Edited by: Christopher K. Johannes, Phd & Harry E. van der Zee, MD Hom

Homeolinks Publishers

© 2010 Homeolinks Publishers
Postbus 68, 9750 AB Haren, The Netherlands
E-mail: office@homeolinks.nl

Our website: www.homeolinks.nl

editors: Christopher Johannes, PhD & Harry van der Zee, MD
copy correction: John Fox, Betty Wood & Gill Zukovskis
cover design: Christopher Johannes, Maurits Peerbolte & Harry van der Zee
layout: Maurits Peerbolte, Xsample
printed by B. Jain, New Delhi, India

ISBN/EAN 978-94-90453-00-8

Disclaimer

Important notice: Medicine, like every other science, is subject to continuous development. Research and clinical experience broaden our knowledge, particularly as far as treatment and medical therapy are concerned. Whenever there are dosages or applications mentioned in this book, the reader may rest assured that the authors, editors and publishers have taken great care to ensure that the information given represents **standard of knowledge at the time of completion of this book.**

However, the publishers cannot assume responsibility as far as the information on dosage and form of application of the remedies is concerned. **Each user of this book is asked to please check,** by carefully studying the patient information data and where necessary consulting a specialist, whether the indicated recommendation for dosage or possible contraindications in this book harmonise with the information given in the patient information data or by the specialist. This kind of verification is particularly important in cases of rarely used medicines or in the case of newly introduced items. **Every dosage or application is made at the user's own risk.** The authors and the publishers appeal to each user to please pass on possible inaccuracies that come to his or her notice.

Foreword by Dana Ullman, MPH

The most famous dictum of Hippocrates, the father of medicine, was "First, do no harm". These wise words were directed at physicians, but this wise advice is also meant for patients. And yet, sadly, few doctors and equally few patients honour this sound recommendation. Doctors and patients often rush to the use of powerful and risky medical treatments before exploring safer methods.

Homeopathic medicine is certainly one of those safer methods that are often ignored, except by a select group of usually educated or simply informed or just lucky individuals whose friends or family members have had experiences with these medicinal agents. It is therefore not surprising that so many of the most respected cultural heroes of the past 200 years used and/or advocated for homeopathy. World leaders (ranging from Mahatma Gandhi to 11 U.S. Presidents, 2 U.K. Prime Ministers, and heads of state from France, Germany, Norway, Mexico, and India), clergy and spiritual leaders (seven popes, leading rabbis and Muslim clerics, and the vast majority of Eastern gurus), high profile physicians and scientists (Charles Darwin, Sir William Osler, August Bier), corporate leaders (J.D. Rockefeller, Charles Kettering, Robert Bosch), literary greats (Goethe, Chekhov, Tennyson, Dickens, Tagore), musicians (Beethoven, Chopin, Wagner), artists (van Gogh, Pissarro, Gaudi), and hundreds of other world renowned individuals expressed publicly their use or advocacy of homeopathic medicines.

Homeopathic medicine may be over 200 years old, but it is still on the cutting edge of the art and science of healing. Homeopathy and homeopaths have had a long history of providing safe and effective treatment for people with a wide variety of mental health ailments.

For instance, the Menninger Clinic, initially in Topeka, Kansas, is world-renowned as one of the leading mental health centres for research and treatment. Most people don't know it, but the founder of the Menninger Clinic, Charles Frederick Menninger, MD, was a homeopathic physician. He was also the head of his local homeopathic medical society, and he was so impressed with his results from homeopathic treatment, he once asserted, "Homeopathy is wholly capable of satisfying the therapeutic demands of this age better than any other system or school of medicine" (Menninger, 1897).

Before Samuel Hahnemann, MD, discovered homeopathy, he was a highly respected German physician and chemist. German royalty sought his medical care, and medical historians note that he showed sound balance and good judgment in his advocacy for proper diet, fresh air, and exercise as a method of treatment. Further, famed medical historian William Rothstein asserted that his promotion of hygienic measures during epidemics won him praise as a public health advocate, and his kind treatment of the insane, rather than cruel and harsh care, granted him "a place in the history of psychiatry" (Rothstein, 1972, 152).

As this anthology confirms, homeopathy is sophisticated system of applying safe and effective medicinal agents to sick people in order to initiate the healing process. Homeopaths prescribe these medicinal agents based on the totality of the patient's symptoms, their overall body-mind syndrome. Homeopathy and homeopaths do not treat physical symptoms of the patient separate from the mental symptoms, or visa versa. In fact, homeopaths understand that disease is not localized.

Just as a headache is not just a local disease, nor is heart disease, nor is any mental illness. All disease is systemic and has impacts on the entire body and mind. The "head bone" is indeed connected to the "neck bone" which is connected to the shoulder bone...and on and on.

Concepts of interconnectedness are at once ancient and futuristic. Ultimately, homeopathic medicine revives and expands upon ancient knowledge of nature, of the human body, and of medicinal agents, creating an art and science of medicine and of healing.

This book verifies the links between ancient healing traditions and ancient systems of knowledge with modern understandings of the healing arts. Just as the modern-day physicist Fritjof Capra uncovered in his seminal book, *The Tao of Physics*, that ancient Buddhist and Hindu teachings of nature are accurate descriptions of nature today according to the latest understandings from quantum physics, this book substantiates the homeopathic perspective on health and healing and shows that this viewpoint is not only "modern" but that it is futuristic.

Ultimately, this book is not just for homeopaths or for homeopathic patients. This book provides insights into understanding what "deep healing" is all about. "Deep healing" is distinct from drug treatment that is effective in eliminating or palliating symptoms because such treatment tends to provide short-term benefits and too often works by suppressing the body's defences, thereby creating more serious physical illness or mental disease. "Deep healing" refers to a real overall and systemic improvement in a person's health, and this subject is of interest to anyone who has a desire for quality of life.

Anyone who is interested in deep healing will appreciate and benefit from this book. The diversity of the subjects covered by each author in this book is intellectually enriching. The international participation of its authors gives us all a more broad perspective of what homeopathy and homeopathic medicines bring to mental health care worldwide. The variety of historical, philosophical, spiritual, clinical, scientific, and ethical viewpoints weaves a beautifully complex and textured cloth of the homeopathic experience in mental health care.

By reading this book, health and medical professionals as well as patients will begin to insist upon providing or receiving safer treatments for mental health ailments FIRST before resorting to more risky medical treatment modalities. Any book that helps us all move towards incorporating Hippocrates' wise words, "First, do no harm", into our lives is indeed a book that heals. As such, this book heals. Read it, use it, and let the healing begin.

Dana Ullman, MPH
Berkeley October 2009

References

[1] Menninger, C. F. (1897) Some Reflections Relative to the Symptomatology and Materia Medica of Typhoid Fever, *Transactions of the American Institute of Homeopathy*, 1897:427–431.

[2] Rothstein, W. (1972) *Physicians in the Nineteenth Century*. Baltimore: Johns Hopkins University Press.

About Dana Ullman *(see page 328)*

Dedication

Preface

Starting some two centuries ago with its founder, Dr. Samuel Hahnemann, homeopathy has been successfully applied in mental health care. Homeopathic journals and conferences around the world are full of case reports detailing homeopathy's holistic, gentle, safe, and effective approach to mental health. Increasing numbers of health professionals who have become aware of homeopathy's utility and healing benefits have undergone additional training to fruitfully integrate homeopathy into their practices, often choosing to respecialise in it. Yet homeopathy's role, application and potential in mental health care remains largely untapped and underused. The enormous global burden of mental health suffering continues to outstrip the availability, access and affordability of conventional capacities to respond. With these capacities falling short, and with the effectiveness of some conventional mental health treatments in question, the reported successes and underexploited potential of homeopathy in mental health care surely merit our attention.

Homeopathy belongs to everyone, not to a single profession. The "right to health" is a human right everyone should be able to enjoy. The United Nations Committee on Economic, Social, and Cultural Rights spells out the obligations of states to respect, protect, and fulfil this right by, inter alia, promoting, and preventing the hindrance of equal access to, the full spectrum of conventional and non-conventional healing practices, medicines, and preventive care. One way for us to promote access and prevent hindrance to homeopathy in mental health care (or any other form of healthcare) is to take it beyond the field-specific journals and conferences that only homeopaths can understand and into an open, coherent, and integrated mainstream discourse of health research, development, and application that other professionals can examine, study, and integrate so that its full promise for everyone may be realized.

The integrative advantages of using homeopathy in mental health care are clear to those of us successfully using this approach, and certainly to our patients who tell us how much they wished more professionals would practise this integration. But how many mental health professionals do we know who are keen to consider some training in homeopathy or who would feel confident to refer to and collaborate with a homeopath? How many doctors do we know who would immediately think of homeopathy's applications in mental health? Probably not many. Homeopathy is still "popularly" thought of as useful for scrapes, bruises, allergies, infectious diseases, 'skin things', and chronic or intractable physical complaints conventional medicine doesn't have a better answer for. The existing evidence base of empirical research that homeopathy has amassed to date tends to follow along these popular grooves, which understandably, in the absence of any other guidance, does not make for a very solid basis the conventional health professional has to go on to recommend homeopathy in mental health care.

So what other guidance is there? Those books we do have dealing with homeopathy in mental health care tend to be specialist handbooks of detailed case approaches or applied homeopathic philosophy intended only for the practising homeopath. They do not really offer the larger, contextualized, and integrative picture of how homeopathy applies to mental health care, and they do not offer the greater snapshot of the issues we need to deal with to take homeopathy in mental health care further.

This anthology was born out of a desire to start positively addressing some of these issues and concerns. We were motivated by a wish to create a useful text for both homeopaths and mental and allied health professionals that touches base with as many relevant issues pertinent to homeopathy in mental health care as possible from as large and international a perspective as possible.

Besides case examples in practice for a variety of mental health conditions throughout, we are grateful to our contributing team and their richness of experience for including coverage and contextualization of issues pertinent to meaningful areas of integration and integrative process, research, theory, ethics, and possible future directions. We hope this work, convenient to dip into as a single volume, will be useful not only to those already applying homeopathy in mental health care, but also to those who intend to and to those seeking some knowledge of the implications. Beyond that, our hope is that it will stimulate further dialogue and work by others in order to advance the kind of development, research and additional integrative applications that will promote a greater realisation of homeopathy's healing capacities in mental health.

We invited an international team of leading health professionals, researchers, theoreticians, and practitioners to help us with our intention. We have been impressed and grateful at their immediate and enthusiastic response and together offer you our united voice in this anthology. With this book, we invite you to join in the delight, the challenge and the privilege of carrying this work forward.

Christopher K. Johannes
Kyoto, September, 2009

Harry E. van der Zee
Norg, September, 2009

Acknowledgements

We would like, first of all, to express our sincerest gratitude to the international team of 22 collaborating authors originating from 10 countries whose shared vision and keen participation made this work possible. The quality of their contributions is outstanding and we have really enjoyed working with them.

John Fox helped enormously in the proof reading of most of these chapters. His love for language is admirable; his work on the text encompassed so much more than ensuring correct spelling and grammar. When John, due to a fierce attack of malaria, could not complete the proof reading of the last chapters we were very happy in finding Betty Wood prepared to take over from him. Gill Zukovskis had the courage and skill to accomplish corrections for the challenging last chapter.

We thank Maurits Peerbolte of Xsample for creating the user-friendly layout for this book, for selecting fonts that are easy on the eye, and for his additional help on an attractive cover design.

And certainly, we will not neglect to thank the generations of homeopathic masters, starting over two centuries ago with Dr. Samuel Christian Hahnemann, without whom the wonderful science and art of homeopathy would not have come to blossom as it does in the work of the authors in this book, and the tens of thousands of homeopaths world-wide that on a daily basis offer safe and effective healing to those in need of it.

Table of Contents

SECTION 2: INTEGRATION, CASE APPLICATIONS, AND THERAPEUTIC PROCESS 96

⬭ Section 3: Research, Ethics, and Theory

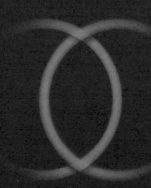

Section 1: Introduction

Chapter 1
Exploring the Role of Homeopathy in Reducing the Global Mental Health Burden

Dr. Manish Bhatia, India

Dr. Manish Bhatia
D-6, Prem Nagar
Khatipura Rd, Jhotwara
Jaipur 302012
Rajasthan, India
E-mail: manish@hpathy.com
Website: www.doctorbhatia.com

Abstract

The level of mental disorders is rising at an alarming rate in our society. Modern psychiatric drug-based therapeutic intervention has failed to reduce the global mental health burden. A large part of the world's population depends upon complementary and alternative medicine (CAM) for their health needs but policy-makers around the world have neglected the possible role of CAM therapies in helping patients with mental disorders. Homeopathy is one of the most popular CAM therapies and has a strong focus on the mental health of individuals. This paper tries to evaluate the historical, epidemiological, clinical and research data supporting the efficacy of homeopathy in mental disorders and strives to provide guidelines for the integration of homeopathy in global mental health care policies and primary mental health care.

We regard man as a fundamentally healthy organism in which there may be a temporary malfunctioning. Nature is always trying to re-establish harmony, and within the psyche the principle of synthesis is dominant.
Roberto Assagioli

1   Introduction

Mental health is defined as a state of well-being in which every individual realizes his or her own potential, can cope with the normal stresses of life, can work productively and fruitfully, and is able to make a contribution to the community[1]. A mentally healthy person can manage relationships with self and others and shows characteristics of hardiness, resilience, and freedom within ranges of experience and functioning. The concept of mental health is very broad and it is not restricted to the mere absence of mental illness. It is also related to the promotion of well-being, the prevention of mental disorders, and the treatment and rehabilitation of people affected by mental disorders.

Medicine has recognised the importance of the mind and mental health from the beginning. Even *Hippocrates* (460-370 BC), the father of medicine, had discussed the concepts related to mental health and mental sickness in his various works. Medicine has undergone radical changes and advances since the time of Hippocrates, but in spite of all the modern medical advancements the global burden of mental illness continues to rise and has now reached epidemic proportions in most parts of the world. To meet this challenge international health organizations and national governments have initiated many mental health care projects around the world. But the availability of psychiatric therapeutic aid is still restricted to a very small percentage of the world's population. Even those who do receive the modern medical aid for mental disorders often remain chronically ill and dependent upon chemical intervention for very long periods [2,3]. Since a significant percentage of people 'under treatment' always remain 'under treatment' or relapse frequently, and with new cases increasing continuously, the global mental health burden continues to rise exponentially. Researchers have even raised concerns about the possible role of psychiatric drugs in increasing the mental health burden of society [4]. If existing psychiatric and mental health policies and drugs fall short or fail in making people healthy again, we need to reflect on current practices and look for viable alternatives.

In most countries, mental health services are chronically short of resources - both human and financial. Of the health care resources available, most are currently spent on the specialized treatment and care of the mentally ill, to the detriment of expenditure on an integrated mental health system [5].

A very large percentage of the world's population depends upon various forms of Complementary and Alternative Medicine (CAM) for therapeutic aid [6]. However, most international health organizations and governments have failed to include various CAM therapies in their mental health programmes and policies.

Homeopathy is one of the most popular CAM therapies [7], and is used extensively in many parts of the world. Homeopathy is believed and reported to be effective in treating not just physical ailments but also many forms of mental illnesses. However, its clinical utility and potential in mental health remains largely untapped. It is essential to examine the existing evidence base for its efficacy and to explore the role of homeopathy in reducing the global mental health burden. A systematic analysis of the historical, epidemiological, clinical and research data available can help in finding effective ways of integrating homeopathic treatment in primary health care (where most mental health prescriptions are made) as well as mental health care.

2   Status of global mental health

Mental disorders account for nearly 12% of the global burden of disease. The burden of mental disorders is at its greatest in young adults, the most productive section of the population. According to the World Health Report 2001 [5], there are about 450 million people who suffer at one time or another from a neurological, psychiatric or behaviour-related disease and about 25% of all the inhabitants in the world suffer a psychiatric or behavioural disorder at a certain moment in their life. About 20% of all patients who consult the primary health sector have a psychiatric disorder but a considerable number of them are never diagnosed or treated properly. Four out of the ten most important diseases measured by YLD (Years of Life lived with Disability) are psychiatric conditions, namely unipolar depression, alcohol abuse, schizophrenia and Bi-Polar Disorder [5].

Worldwide, 121 million people suffer with depression, 70 million with alcohol-related problems, 24 million with schizophrenia and 37 million with dementia. According to estimates made in 2000, mental and neurological disorders accounted for 12.3% of disability-adjusted life-years, 31% of years lived with disability and 6 of the 20 leading causes of disability worldwide [8].

The National Alliance of Mental Health (2008) estimates that in the USA alone one in four adults - approximately 57.7 million Americans - experiences a mental health disorder in a given year. One in seventeen lives with a serious mental illness such as schizophrenia, major depression or Bi-Polar Disorder, and about one in ten children has a serious mental or emotional disorder. About 2.4 million Americans, or 1.1 percent of the adult population, live with schizophrenia. Approximately 20.9 million American adults, or about 9.5 percent of the U.S. population aged 18 and older in a given year, have a mood disorder. Bi-Polar Disorder affects 5.7 million American adults, approximately 2.6 percent of the adult population per year. Major depressive disorder affects 6.7 percent of adults, or about 14.8 million American adults. According to the 2004 World Health Report, this is the leading cause of disability in the U.S. and Canada between the ages of 15 and 44. Anxiety Disorders affect about 18.1 percent of adults, an estimated 40 million individuals. Anxiety Disorders frequently co-occur with depression or addiction disorders. An estimated 5.2 million adults have co-occurring mental health and addiction disorders. Alzheimer's Disease (AD) affects an estimated 4.5 million Americans. The number of Americans with Alzheimer's Disease has more than doubled since 1980 [9]. A recent study reported the prevalence of Autism in 3-10 year-olds to be about 3.4 cases per 1000 children [10].

The situation in Europe is equally grim. Today almost 50 million European citizens (about 11% of the population) are estimated to experience mental disorders [11]. In the European Union, psychiatric conditions constitute 25% of the total burden of disease [12]. Neuropsychiatric disorders are the second leading cause of disability-adjusted life-years (DALYs) in the WHO European Region, accounting for 19.5% of all DALYs. According to the most recent available data (2002), neuropsychiatric disorders are the first-ranked cause of years lived with disability (YLD) in Europe, accounting for 39.7% of those attributable to all causes. Unipolar depressive disorder alone is responsible for 13.7% of YLD, making it by far the leading cause of chronic conditions in Europe [13]. Alzheimer's disease and other forms of dementia are the seventh leading cause of chronic conditions in Europe and account for 3.8% of all YLD. Schizophrenia and Bi-Polar Disorders are each responsible for 2.3% of all YLD. Suicide rates are high in the European Region. In the EU, there are about 58,000 suicides per year and the average suicide prevalence rate in Europe is 15.1 per 100,000 of the population.

It is estimated that the burden of mental disorders will grow in the coming decades. By 2020 mental disorders are likely to account for 15% of disability-adjusted life-years lost. Depression is expected to become the second leading cause of disability in the world [14].

Developing countries with poorly developed mental health care systems are likely to see the most substantial increases in the burden attributable to mental disorders. The increasing life expectancy, especially in developing countries, will result in greater numbers of people reaching the age of vulnerability to mental disorders. The gradual gains in life expectancy can be expected to result in increasing numbers of older people affected by depression and dementia. Other possible reasons for the increase in the burden of mental disorders in developing countries include rapid urbanization, conflicts (civil unrest, political conflagrations), environmental and man-made disasters, social, technological, cultural and macroeconomic changes [15].

The financial loss and burden caused by mental disorders can be measured but the pain and suffering caused by mental disorders is not as easy to quantify. In addition to the obvious suffering caused by mental disorders there is a hidden burden of stigma and discrimination that manifests as bias, stereotyping, fear, embarrassment, anger, rejection or avoidance, further diminishing the mental health status of the affected people.

Despite the increasingly compromised mental health status of our society, the modern medical system is very inadequately equipped to provide support to the target population. Recent data (2005) shows that the median distribution of psychiatrists per 100 000 population in the world is 1.2 (SD 6.07) with a variance of 0.04/100,000 population in Africa to 9.8/100,000 population in Europe [16]. Resources are especially scarce in low and middle-income countries [17]. Researchers have also identified a huge gap in the need for psychiatric care [18]. The median treatment gap (percentage of affected population that remains untreated), as evident from a review of 37 studies across regions of the world, was estimated to be 32.2% for schizophrenia and other non-affective psychotic disorders, 56.3% for major depression, 50.2% for Bi-Polar Disorder, 78.1% for alcohol abuse and dependence, etc. The WHO World Mental Health Survey Consortium19 found that treatment was received by 0.8% to 15.3% of those affected with a mental disorder; the proportion of treatment was higher for severe cases (14.6% – 64.5%) compared to mild cases (0.5% – 35.2%). The chances of getting treated for any type of disorder were much less in developing countries.

3   Where the elixir did not work!

There seems to be an assumption that any advance in modern medicine in the treatment of a particular illness is marked by a corresponding decline in the related illness. The advent of antibiotics is considered a cornerstone in controlling bacterial diseases and the use of vaccines against childhood infections is related to reduced childhood mortality. But, surprisingly, in spite of all the advances in psychiatric medicine over the last 50 years, the level of mental disorders continues to rise at an alarming rate.

Not only have modern chemical drugs failed to reduce the global mental disease burden but there is also a lot of research that indicates that currently used psychiatric drugs might actually be contributing to it. Whitaker mentions that psychiatric drugs perturb normal neurotransmitter functioning, and while that perturbation may curb symptoms in the short term, over the long run it increases the likelihood that a person will become chronically ill, or ill with new and more severe symptoms [4]. A review of the scientific literature also indicates that the modern drug-based paradigm of mental health care might actually be contributing to the ever-increasing mental health problems.

This paradox - that a psychiatric drug may curb symptoms over the short term but worsen the long-term course of the disorder - has been found to hold true for most classes of psychiatric drugs, including antidepressants, antipsychotics, benzodiazepines and SSRI's. Some relevant studies and statistics on each of these classes of drugs are shared below in brief. There is a much larger volume of similar studies available and the reader is encouraged to search online medical research databases and other relevant literature to explore the issue in more depth. The stark statistics discussed here should compel policy-makers around the world to question the legitimacy of current mental health care policies and programmes.

3.1 Antidepressants

Antidepressants came into wide use in 1960s when monoamine oxidase inhibitors (MAOIs) and tricyclics appeared on the market. But both types soon fell out of common use because the investigators at the National Institute of Mental Health (NIMH), USA soon determined that in "well-designed studies, the differences between the effectiveness of the antidepressant drugs and placebo are not impressive" [20].

This finding led some investigators to wonder whether the placebo response was the mechanism that was helping people feel better. To test this hypothesis, investigators conducted at least eight studies in which they compared a tricyclic to an "active" placebo. In seven of the eight, there was no difference in outcomes, leading investigators at New York Medical College to conclude "there is practical value in viewing [psychotropics] as mere amplifiers or inhibitors of the placebo effects" [21].

In the early 1980s NIMH launched a long-term study of depression treatments to verify the efficacy of tricyclics. Two hundred and thirty-nine patients were randomized into four treatment groups - cognitive behaviour therapy, interpersonal therapy, the tricyclic imipramine, and placebo. The results were unexpected by the medical fraternity. At the end of sixteen weeks, "there were no significant differences among treatments, including placebo plus clinical management, for the less severely depressed and functionally impaired patients." Only the severely depressed patients fared better on a tricyclic than on placebo. However, at the end of eighteen months, even this minimal benefit disappeared. Stay-well rates were best for the cognitive behaviour group (30%) and poorest for the imipramine group (19%) [22]. Patients treated with an antidepressant were the most likely group to seek treatment following termination of the initial treatment period; they had the highest incidence of relapse [23].

In 1985, Blackburn et al reported that in a two-year study comparing drug therapy to cognitive therapy, relapse "was significantly higher in the pharmacotherapy group" [24]. In 1994, Italian researcher Giovanni Fava reviewed the outcomes literature and concluded that "long-term use of antidepressants may increase the (patient's) biochemical vulnerability to depression," and thus "worsen the course of affective disorders" [25]. In 2003, Fava revisited the issue and, from an analysis of 27 studies, he concluded that "A statistical trend suggests that the longer the drug treatment, the higher the likelihood of relapse " [26].

3.2 Selective serotonin reuptake inhibitors

Selective serotonin reuptake inhibitors or serotonin-specific reuptake inhibitors (SSRIs) are a class of compounds typically used as antidepressants in the treatment of depression, anxiety disorders, and some personality disorders. The best-known SSRI is Prozac, which was introduced in 1987.

Prozac quickly occupied the top position as America's most complained-about drug, and by 1997, 39,000 adverse-event reports about it had been sent to Medwatch. These reports are thought to represent only 1% of the actual number of such events, suggesting that nearly 4 million people in the US alone had suffered such problems, which included mania, psychotic depression, nervousness, anxiety, agitation, hostility, hallucinations, memory loss, tremors, impotence, convulsions, insomnia, and nausea. The other SSRIs brought to market caused a similar range of problems.

Studies have found a very high rate of SSRI-induced mania. In 1996, Howland reported that 6% of 184 depressed patients treated with an SSRI suffered manic episodes that were "generally quite severe." A year later, Ebert reported that 8.5% of patients had a severe psychological reaction to Luvox (fluvoxamine) [27]. Robert Bourguignon, after surveying doctors in Belgium, estimated that Prozac induced psychotic episodes in 5% to 7% of patients [28]. By 2004 the links between SSRI use and juvenile suicide became apparent and this led the American Psychiatric Association to warn that manic or hypomanic episodes are "estimated to occur in 5% to 20% of patients treated with antidepressants". The FDA's currently required packaging insert for SSRIs includes a warning that a pooled analysis of placebo-controlled trials of nine antidepressant drugs (including multiple SSRIs) resulted in a risk of suicide that was twice that of placebo.

In 2003 Fava noted, "Antidepressant-induced mania is not simply a temporary and reversible phenomenon, but a complex biochemical mechanism of illness deterioration" [29]. The best available evidence suggests that this is now happening to more than 500,000 Americans a year. Global data is not available but the statistics are clear indicators that globally the scale of problems induced by these drugs is even larger. In 2001, *Preda* and other Yale researchers reported that 8.1% of all admissions to a psychiatric hospital they studied were due to SSRI-induced mania or psychosis [30]. The US Federal Government reported that there were 10,741,000 "patient care episodes" in 2000; if 8% were SSRI-induced manic or psychotic episodes that would mean that 860,000 people suffered this type of adverse reaction in 2000 in the USA alone [16]. In the past nine years, the use of SSRI's has increased further and there is little doubt that the associated morbidity induced by them must have increased significantly.

In April 2006, the drug maker GlaxoSmithKline disclosed that adults with major depression were almost seven times more likely to attempt suicide after taking the SSRI Paxil than after taking a placebo. A 2004 Food and Drug Administration (FDA) analysis of clinical trials on children with major depressive disorder found statistically significant increases in the risks of "possible suicidal ideation and suicidal behaviour" by about 80%, and of agitation and hostility by about 130% [31]. An additional analysis by the FDA also indicated a1.5-fold increase in suicidality in the 18–24 age group [32,33].

Thus, the SSRI path to a disabling mental illness can be easily seen. A depressed patient treated with an antidepressant suffers a manic or psychotic episode, at which time his or her diagnosis is changed to Bi-Polar Disorder. The person is then prescribed an antipsychotic drug to go along with the antidepressant, and, once on a drug cocktail, the person is well along on the road to permanent disability. Since Prozac was introduced in 1987, the number of disabled mentally ill people in the US has risen by 2.4 million.

In 2005, Moncrieff and Kirsch reviewed the efficacy of antidepressants [34] and came to the following conclusions:

1. recent meta-analyses show that selective serotonin reuptake inhibitors (SSRIs) have no clinically significant superiority over placebo;
2. claims that antidepressants are more effective in more severe conditions have little evidence to support them;
3. methodological artifacts may account for the very small (and clinically insignificant) statistical margin by which SSRI efficacy exceeds that of placebos;
4. antidepressants have not been convincingly shown to affect the long-term outcome of depression or suicide rates;
5. given the significant doubts about their benefits and concerns about their risks, current recommendations for prescribing antidepressants should be reconsidered.

With such clear indicators of the apparent failure of modern medicine in controlling the mental health problems, one has to question the legitimacy of channelling all the global funds and resources in search of an elusive panacea!

3.3 Antipsychotics

Antipsychotics (also called Neuroleptics) are a group of psychoactive drugs commonly but not exclusively used to treat psychosis, which is typified by schizophrenia. The study that is still cited today as proving the efficacy of antipsychotics for curbing acute episodes of schizophrenia was a nine-hospital trial of 344 patients conducted by the NIMH in the early 1960s. At the end of six weeks, 75% of the drug-treated patients were "much improved" or "very much improved" compared to 23% of the placebo patients [35].

However, three years later, the NIMH reported on one-year outcomes for the patients. Much to their surprise, they found that "patients who received placebo treatment were less likely to be rehospitalized than those who received any of the three active phenothiazines" [36]. In the wake of that disturbing report, the NIMH conducted two medication-withdrawal studies. In each one, relapse rates rose in correlation with neuroleptic dosage before withdrawal [37].

To investigate the merits of neuroleptic drugs, NIMH funded three studies during the 1970s. In each instance, the newly admitted patients treated without drugs did better than those treated in a conventional manner [38,39]. The final study came from Mosher, head of schizophrenia research at the NIMH. As in the other studies, Mosher reported that the patients treated without drugs were the better functioning group as well [40].

Together, the various studies painted a compelling picture of how antipsychotics shifted outcomes away from recovery. Bockoven's retrospective and the other experiments all suggested that with minimal or no exposure to antipsychotics, at least 40% of people who suffered a psychotic break and were diagnosed with schizophrenia would not relapse after leaving the hospital, and perhaps as many as 65% would function fairly well over the long term. However, once first-episode patients were treated with antipsychotics, their brains would undergo drug-induced changes that would increase their biological vulnerability to psychosis, and this would increase the likelihood that they would become chronically ill.

The World Health Organization twice compared schizophrenia outcomes in the rich countries of the world with outcomes in poor countries, and each time the patients in the poor countries - where drug usage was much less - were doing dramatically better at two-year and five-year follow-ups. In India, Nigeria and Colombia, where only 16% of patients were maintained continuously on antipsychotics, roughly two-thirds were doing fairly well at the end of the follow-up period and only one third had become chronically ill. In the US and other rich countries, where 61% of the patients were kept on antipsychotic drugs, the ratio of good-to-bad outcomes was almost precisely the reverse. Only about one third had good outcomes, and the remaining two thirds became chronically ill [41,42].

More recently, MRI studies have shown the same link between drug usage and chronic illness. In the mid 1990s, several research teams reported that the drugs cause atrophy of the cerebral cortex and an enlargement of the basal ganglia [43,44,45]. These findings clearly showed that the drugs were causing structural changes in the brain. Then in 1998 researchers at the University of Pennsylvania reported that the drug-induced enlargement of the basal ganglia was "associated with greater severity of both negative and positive symptoms" [46]. In simple words, they found that over the long term the drugs cause changes in the brain associated with a worsening of the very symptoms the drugs are supposed to alleviate.

3.4 Benzodiazepines

The benzodiazepines are a commonly prescribed class of sedative hypnotic psychoactive drugs with varying sedative, hypnotic, antianxiety, anticonvulsant, muscle relaxant and amnesic properties. In 1988, researchers who led a large Cross-National Collaborative Panic Study, which involved 1,700 patients in fourteen countries, reported that at the end of four weeks 82% of the patients treated with Alprazolam were "moderately improved" or "better," versus 42% of the placebo patients. However, by the end of eight weeks there was no difference between the groups [47].

As a follow-up to that study, researchers in Canada and the UK studied benzodiazepine-treated patients over a period of six months. They reported that the Alprazolam patients got better during the first four weeks of treatment, that they did not improve any more in weeks four to eight, and that their symptoms began to worsen after that. As patients were weaned from the drugs, a high percentage relapsed, and by the end of 23 weeks, they were worse off than patients treated without drugs on five different outcomes measures [48]. Pecknold (1988) also found that as patients were tapered off Alprazolam they suffered nearly four times as many panic attacks as the non-drug patients, and that 25% of the Alprazolam patients suffered from rebound anxiety more severe than when they began the study. The Alprazolam patients were also significantly worse off than non-drug patients on a global assessment scale by the end of the study [49].

It is now well known that all of the major classes of psychiatric drugs - antipsychotics, antidepressants, benzodiazepines, and stimulants for ADHD - can trigger new and more severe psychiatric symptoms in a significant percentage of patients. Many researchers believe it to be an important factor in causing a rapid rise in the number of disabled mentally ill. Research by David Healy, an eminent U.K. psychiatrist, concluded that today's drug-treated patients spend much more time in hospital beds and are far more likely to die from their mental illness than they were in 1896. "Modern treatments," he said, "have set up a revolving door" and appear to be a "leading cause of injury and death" [50].

There is much more literature and research available on the inadequacies of many other drugs of this class and other psychiatric drugs. The side effects of all the drugs are also well documented. The data provided here is merely an indicator of the limited use of modern drug-based therapeutic intervention in reducing mental diseases and lessening the global mental health burden. The limitations of existing conventional treatment point to a need to revise national and global mental health policies. It is not possible to analyze the topic in further detail here and the reader is encouraged to make further enquiry through a search of the literature.

4   Homeopathy - a different approach

4.1 Use and prevalence

Homeopathy was developed by a German physician, *Dr. Samuel Hahnemann*, more than 200 years ago. Homeopathy became very popular in the 19th century owing to the remarkable results that homeopathic physicians procured in treating infectious epidemic disease. Epidemics of cholera, scarlet fever, typhoid, and yellow fever were frequent and had a very high mortality associated with them. But death rates in homeopathic hospitals were commonly a half or even an eighth of the death rates in conventional medical hospitals [51]. By 1900, homeopathy came into common use in large parts of Europe, America and India. In the USA alone there were 22 homeopathic medical schools, more than 100 hospitals, and approximately 15,000 practitioners [52]. In the 1920s, with the introduction of modern pharmacotherapies and the standardization of conventional physician training programmes using funding guidelines favouring American Medical Association (AMA)-approved institutions, homeopathic hospitals and schools disappeared from the USA or were converted to allopathic medicine. But homeopathy survived in some parts of the world like Britain, France, Brazil, Argentina and India.

The practice of homeopathy again increased around the world after the 1950s. Homeopathic medicines are sold over the counter in the United States and since 2002 the U.S. homeopathic remedy market has increased by 89 percent to an estimated $830 million in 2008 [53]. In U.S., the FDA (Food and Drug Administration) has recognized the Homeopathic Pharmacopeia of the United States (HPUS) since 1983. Today 30-40% of French doctors and 20% of German doctors prescribe homeopathic medicines. Over 40% of British doctors refer patients to homeopathic doctors, and 45% of Dutch physicians consider these natural medicines to be effective [54]. Homeopathy is being practised in 41 out of 42 European countries. According to a report from the government of Norway, homeopathy is the most frequently used complementary and alternative medicine therapy in five out of fourteen European countries: France, Belgium, Netherlands, Norway, and Switzerland. Homeopathic medicines are used by between 20 and 25% of European Union citizens. In several countries like India, Mexico, Cuba and Brazil, homeopathy is integrated in the national system of health care. In India, there are over 183 five-year homeopathic colleges and more than 200,000 homeopathic doctors [55]. It is estimated that globally over 300 million patients take homeopathic treatment annually.

4.2 Underlying philosophy

Homeopathy, as a system of medicine, believes in testing non-toxic doses of drugs on healthy human volunteers to identify their sphere of action and pathological affinity. The test on healthy human beings is called a 'remedy-proving'. During a remedy proving, the subjects are administered non-toxic doses of a remedy and the symptoms appearing in different parts of the body are recorded to identify its therapeutic sphere. The medicines thus proved are used to treat varied forms of disease conditions on the basis of symptom similarity, i.e., a medicine in which the maximum numbers of patient symptoms match with the proving symptoms is administered to the patient.

These homeopathic remedies are usually given in very dilute doses. The doses can be physiological or sub-physiological (below Avogadro's limit). Homeopathy has received criticism for its use of sub-physiological doses but the clinical experience of homeopaths over the past two centuries indicates that the sub-physiological homeopathic remedies are effective. Some recent research now supports the fact that the so-called high-potency homeopathic remedies – remedies that are highly diluted and dynamised (shaken with force) in subsequent steps – are not inert and still have healing properties. One of the proposed mechanisms for this observed activity is the ability of the vehicle (usually water) to retain the *information* about the initial solute through subsequent dilutions and the changes in the solvent due to the process of dynamisation. (Please see Section 4.5.5 for relevant research studies). There are many positive research studies that provide evidence for this proposed mechanism of activity of homeopathic remedies diluted and dynamised below the Avogadro Limit [56-65].

Homeopathy is considered to be a holistic system of medicine. It does not treat a symptom, pathology or disease in isolation. It believes that any sickness affects an individual as a whole and accordingly the focus of a homeopath is to find a remedy that covers the totality of the individual (or "case"). The totality of a case combines the current symptoms including any deviations on the mental and emotional plane, possible causative modalities, past medical history and family history. The past medical history and the family history are often used to identify the underlying susceptibility and predisposition of an individual case. Homeopathic remedy-provings have revealed a rich array of mental symptoms and accordingly homeopathic medicines are often used by homeopaths in treating mental disorders.

Homeopathy teaches that the aim of a physician should be to 'cure' and the cure is defined as:

"The highest ideal of cure is rapid, gentle and permanent restoration of the health, or removal and annihilation of the disease in its whole extent, in the shortest, most reliable, and most harmless way." [66]

It does not consider a disease as an isolated 'entity'. Every disease is nothing but a nosological name given to a group of symptoms and phenomena. Every disease is considered a 'process' and the symptoms are considered the end result of that process. So the focus is not on suppressing the symptoms but on reversing the process that has led to the pathological changes and abnormal signs and symptoms. The focus is on restoring health!

4.3 Studying the psychological effect of medicines
To treat mental disorders, conventional medicine looks for molecules that have an effect on the brain or have an influence over mental symptoms. Homeopathy, on the other hand, does not look for remedies specifically for mental conditions; it explores the mental symptoms produced by every remedy tested on healthy human beings. Homeopaths realized long ago that the mind and body

are not two distinct entities. There are hardly any physical conditions that do not affect the patient mentally and there are very few mental disorders that do not have their associated symptoms on the somatic plane. Acknowledging this fundamental difference in approaching mental diseases as a whole, homeopaths began recording the psychological effect of each medicine as early as 1790. This makes homeopathy the first medical modality to systematically study the psychological effects of medicines. The collection of data has continued since then and homeopaths have been able to differentiate minute psychological characteristics and symptoms of their patients through careful observation and meticulous data gathering.

Today science recognises that even the food that we eat can have an impact on our mind. Hahnemann realized this more than two centuries ago, when he wrote:

> "...there is no powerful medicinal substance in the world which does not very notably alter the state of the disposition and mind in the healthy individual who tests it, and every medicine does so in a different manner." [67]

He further states:

> "We shall, therefore, never be able to cure conformably to nature - that is to say, homoeopathically -
> if we do not, in every case of disease, even in such as are acute, observe, along with the other symptoms,
> those relating to the changes in the state of the mind and disposition, and if we do not select, for the patient's
> relief, from among the medicines a disease-force which, in addition to the similarity of its other symptoms to
> those of the disease, is also capable of producing a similar state of the disposition and mind." [68]

The homeopathic Materia Medica and Repertories list the mental symptoms (along with other symptoms) that were found during the homeopathic remedy provings. The symptoms are minutely classified. If depression is recorded in a medicine, then further details are sought as to what caused the depression, what makes the person feels better or worse and what other associated symptoms, physical or mental, the patient experiences. Similarly other psychological symptoms like anxiety, anger, mania, mood, attention deficit, hyperactivity, dullness, delusions, illusions, hallucinations, memory problems and dreams etc are recorded in minute detail with fine differentiation that makes it possible to differentiate one remedy from another.

A conventional psychiatrist will most likely prescribe the same antidepressant if you have depression after your mother passed away or if you have depression after losing your job or failing a test. Homeopaths on the other hand will differentiate their remedies based on what led the patient to depression, how the individual copes with it and what aggravates or ameliorates the patient. Such individualization is possible because of systematic data-gathering during remedy provings. This individualised focus on the whole patient is what distinguishes the homeopathic approach to mental disorders.

Another very specific homeopathic methodology that makes it more suitable for the treatment of mental disorders is the method of patient-interview used by homeopaths, which is called 'case taking'. Homeopaths delve deep into the mental and emotional aspects of most cases, are taught to listen to patients carefully and with empathy and provide longer consultation time to chronically ill patients. The approach to discover the mental characteristics and causative modalities can often be similar to psychoanalysis and counselling techniques used in the modern medicine (see related chapters discussing this theme in this anthology). Research has already proved that the therapeutic relationship can play a significant role in patient recovery. The therapeutic relationship depends to a large extent upon the patient's perception of empathy, of 'being listened to' and 'of being cared for'. Research has also shown that most patients find the physician-patient encounter more satisfactory during homeopathic treatment, thus amplifying the role of the therapeutic relationship in treatment.

Today even modern medical science is realizing that tissues and systems do not work in isolation; many ailments that until recently were classified as 'physical' or 'mental' are now classified as 'psychosomatic'. The classification has been modified, there are newer drugs available on the market but the therapeutic approach has not changed. The focus is still on suppressing isolated symptoms. This explains the failure of conventional medicine to reduce the global mental health burden – it is making more and more people drug-dependent and has failed to make them 'healthy', to restore their health!

4.4 Tracing the importance of mental health in homeopathy
Dr. Hahnemann was a leading conventional doctor who, dismayed by the barbaric treatments (leeching, blood-letting, purging, diaphoretics, massive use of Mercury etc) available in his time, left the profession in search of a better approach. But even while he was practising as a conventional physician, Hahnemann had a very good understanding of mental disorders and was among the first doctors who advocated more humane treatment of the mentally ill [69].

Hahnemann mentions the importance of mental symptoms in 'The Organon of Medicine', the core text he wrote on homeopathic philosophy and treatment:

> "Mental diseases ... do not, however, constitute a class of disease. The condition of the disposition and mind is always altered; and in all cases of disease we are called on to cure, the state of the patient's disposition is to be particularly noted, along with the totality of the symptoms, if we would trace an accurate picture of the disease, in order to be able to treat it homoeopathically with success." [67]

He also states:

> "Almost all the so-called mental and emotional diseases are nothing more than corporeal diseases in which the symptom of derangement of the mind and disposition peculiar to each of them is increased, while the corporeal symptoms decline (more or less rapidly), till it attains the most striking one-sidedness, almost as though it were a local disease in the invisible subtle organ of the mind or disposition.

> ...There are, however, as has just been stated, certainly a few emotional diseases which have not merely been developed into that form out of corporeal diseases, but which, in an inverse manner, the body being but slightly indisposed, originate and are kept up by emotional causes, such as continued anxiety, worry, vexation, wrongs and the frequent occurrence of great fear and fright. This kind of emotional diseases in time destroys the corporeal health, often to a great degree.

It is only such emotional diseases as these, which were first engendered and subsequently kept up by the mind itself, that, while they are yet recent and before they have made very great inroads on the corporeal state, may, by means of psychical remedies, such as a display of confidence, friendly exhortations, sensible advice, and often by a well-disguised deception, be rapidly changed into a healthy state of the mind (and with appropriate diet and regimen, seemingly into a healthy state of the body also.)" [70]

The above quotes represent only a small sample of the many insights from the founder of homeopathy. Readers interested in exploring the guidelines for homeopathic treatment of mental disorders are urged to read Aphorisms 210 to 230 from the Organon of Medicine, which will show how far ahead Hahnemann was of his contemporaries and how relevant his words still are.

Homeopaths from the time of Hahnemann have given due importance to psychological ailments and the case records available in various professional homeopathic journals have recorded numerous cases of mental disorders treated with homeopathic remedies. Such a long tradition of awareness of mental diseases and clinical records indicating the efficacy of homeopathic medicines in mental disorders should encourage systematic research to scientifically evaluate the efficacy of homeopathic medicines in the treatment of mental disorders.

4.5 The research evidence

In spite of its large-scale use, homeopathy has continued to attract criticism for its use of very high dilution "drugs" and the relative lack of robust scientific evidence. However, particularly in the last 25 years, there has been a steadily growing interest in the plausible action and clinical effects of homeopathic potencies resulting in a large and growing body of research studies that have started providing valuable insights into the action and efficacy of homeopathic medicines, an accessible evidence base, and guidelines for advancing further research. That said, despite this positive trend, clinical research in homeopathy remains very limited when compared to that of conventional allopathic medicine. Besides the formidable challenges involved in designing metho-dologically appropriate trials, one of the major reasons has been a dire lack of funds. The scale for funding of medical research is disproportionately tipped to favour conventional medicine over alternative medicine. According to Global Forum estimates, the worldwide spending on medical research was at least US$ 160 billion by 2005 with more than $90 billion spent in the USA alone [71]. In comparison, in the USA the National Center for Complementary and Alternative Medicine spent approximately US$ 33 million on herbal medicines (not just homeopathy) in the fiscal year 2005 [72]. Another example of this may be seen in the 0.08 percent of the British National Health Service research budget set aside for alternative medicine research. Also, out of $12 billion allocated every year in the USA by Congress to the National Institutes of Health, a mere $5.4 million goes to the Office of Alternative Medicine to investigate the claims of approximately 50 therapies. Considering this, the funds for researching the clinical efficacy of homeopathy are nearly non-existent.

Kaplan believes that many alternative medicine systems are in the early stage of research-based evaluation:

"The treatment methods have not been developed through Western research methods but do have complex theoretical bases and centuries of reported experience with clinical applications. Modern medicine and psychiatry evolved out of a similar accumulation of empirically based knowledge, much of which has been, or is now being, subjected to modern research examination. For example, the origin of psychotherapy was based on nonsystematic case study reports, followed in the 1920s and 1930s by surveys of reports on improvement rates, then by studies that included control groups in their design, and from the 1950s to today, there has been exponential growth in research studies on psychological therapies with greater research rigor. It appears that alternative and complementary health practices are on a similar trajectory but, one hopes, at an accelerated rate, given the availability of contemporary research methodology and analyses." [73]

Kaplan has rightly pointed out that research in complementary medicine is in an early phase. Over the past 20 years there have been many small-scale clinical studies and some large-scale retrospective studies that have provided valuable data on the action and efficacy of homeopathic remedies. There seems to be an equal proportion of trials with positive and negative outcomes and the debate about the validity of many trials is long and on-going. Trials with a positive outcome are often claimed by sceptics to be of low methodological quality while most trials with negative outcomes are criticised by homeopathic supporters for having used research methodologies unsuitable for homeopathy. The ongoing dialogue has resulted in identification of research methodologies more suitable for testing homeopathic treatment and future research might prove to be more conclusive. Such research issues are dealt with in greater detail below.

The available research data is still impressive enough to warrant serious consideration by global health policy makers. There is a substantial and growing body of published research in good-quality peer-reviewed journals showing that homeopathy has a positive effect. Between 1950 and 2008, 138 randomised controlled trials (RCTs) in homeopathy have been reported. This represents research into 71 different medical conditions. Of these 138 trials, only ten had negative outcomes. The rest were either positive (60 trials) or inconclusive (68 trials). The sections below list some of the research data that can help policy makers and professionals in judging the merit of using homeopathy as one of the primary therapeutic modalities in the global mental health care programme.

4.5.1 *General research evidence for homeopathy*

1991: A meta-analysis carried out by Kleinen et al reported that of 105 trials with interpretable results, 81 trials indicated positive results. Most studies showed results in favour of homeopathy, even among those randomized controlled trials that received high-quality ratings for randomization, blinding, sample size, and other methodological criteria. They came to the following conclusion: "The amount of positive evidence even among the best studies came as a surprise to us. Based on this evidence we would readily accept that homeopathy could be efficacious, if only the mechanism of action were more plausible. The evidence presented in this review would probably be sufficient for establishing homeopathy as a regular treatment for certain indications" [74].

1994: Another meta-analysis of three trials on homeopathic immunotherapy, conducted by Reilly et al, found a significant a effect in favour of homeopathic treatment [75].

1994: Meta-analysis of 105 articles on laboratory research was carried out by Linde et al. Result: positive effect 50% more frequently than negative effect among trials of highest methodological quality [76].

1996: HMRG report with overview of clinical research in homeopathy identified 184 controlled clinical trials. They selected the highest quality randomized control trials, which included a total of 2617 patients for a meta-analysis. This meta-analysis resulted in a p-value of 0.000036 (which means that results are highly significant) indicating that homeopathy is more effective than placebo. The researchers concluded that the "hypothesis that homeopathy has no effect can be rejected with certainty" [77].

1997: Linde et al conducted a meta-analysis of 89 trials of homeopathic medicine versus placebo. Results were significantly in favour of homeopathy (OR 2,45 (95% CI 2,05-2,93)). This meta-analysis included 186 placebo-controlled studies of homeopathy published until mid-1996, of which data for analysis could be extracted from 89. The overall odds ratio was 2.45 (95% confidence intervals 2.05-2.93) in favour of homeopathy, which means that the chances that homeopathy would benefit the patient were 2.45 times greater than placebo. Even after correction for publication bias the results remained significant. The main conclusion was that the results "were not compatible with the hypothesis that the effects of homeopathy are completely due to placebo" [78].

2000: A systematic review and meta-analysis by Cucherat et al showed highly significant results for surveys adding up to a total of 2617 patients (P=0.000036). Results were not that significant for high quality surveys (P=0.08). The author concludes that further high quality studies are needed to confirm results [79].

2001: M.E. Dean conducted an exhaustive review of homeopathic research trials carried out between 1940 and 1998 [51]. Out of the total 205 trials included, 163 showed positive results in favour of homeopathy. The trials were divided into 4 groups: Classical Homeopathy, Clinical Homeopathy, Complex Homeopathy and Isopathy. 67% of the negative trials were reported in a single category: clinical homeopathy. The results of the analysis indicated that homeopathy was equivalent or superior to orthodox treatment in most cases where it was compared. Homeopathic medicines appeared to be relatively risk-free in terms of adverse reactions and unwanted effects.

2003: A systematic review of results from 93 substantive RCTs was carried out by Robert Mathie. It concludes that of the 35 different medical conditions covered by these trials the weight of evidence favours a positive treatment effect in eight: childhood diarrhoea, fibrositosis, hay fever, influenza, pain (miscellaneous), side-effects of chemotherapy or radiotherapy, sprains and upper-respiratory tract infections. [80]

2003: In a review of homeopathy research conducted by Jonas et al, the authors found three independent systematic reviews of placebo-controlled trials on homeopathy that reported effects that seem to be more than placebo, and one review that found its effects consistent with placebo [81].

2003: A review of placebo-controlled clinical trials using homeopathic medicines to treat people who have AIDS or are HIV-positive identified five controlled clinical trials. Results showed statistically significant results in subjects with stage III AIDS, and specific physical, immunologic, neurologic, metabolic, and quality-of-life benefits, including improvements in lymphocyte counts and functions and reductions in HIV viral loads in patients receiving homeopathic treatment [82].

2006: A health technology assessment report on effectiveness, cost-effectiveness and appropriateness of homeopathy was compiled on behalf of the Swiss Federal Office for Public Health. Results showed a positive overall result in favour of homeopathy in 29 studies on upper respiratory tract infections and allergic reactions. Results also showed many high-quality investigations of pre-clinical basic research proved homeopathic high potencies inducing regulative and specific changes in cells or living organisms. 20 of 22 systematic reviews detected at least a trend in favour of homeopathy. The authors of this article concluded that the effectiveness of homeopathy can be supported by clinical evidence and treatment is safe [83].

4.5.2 Efficacy in various diseases

4.5.2.1 Anxiety and depression

1981: Stanton reported a placebo-controlled trial of a homeopathic preparation (Argentum nitricum D12) for test anxiety in 40 subjects. Test anxiety as measured by the Test Anxiety Scale (TAS) was reported to be significantly reduced with the homeopathic preparation compared with placebo [84].

1985: Heulluy reported a non-blinded RCT that compared L72 homeopathic complex with Diazepam. The study was carried out on 60 patients under treatment for depression, postmenopausal involution or thymo-effective dystonia. The outcome measure was the ratio of pre and post scores on the Hamilton Rating Scale for Depression. The results indicated that L72 was as effective as diazepam on all measures. One patient taking L72 and two patients taking Diazepam reported drowsiness as a negative outcome [85].

1990: Alibeu & Jobert [86] reported a randomised controlled trial of a single homeopathic medicine, *Aconitum*, for post-operative agitation in children with '95% good results'.

1991: Hariveau et al reported a randomised controlled trial of proprietary homeopathic complex Lithium Microsol using Benzodiazepines (Loraepam) as the comparator. The homeopathic complex was reported to be as effective as the benzodiazepine [87].

1995: Clover and colleagues reported an uncontrolled study of 50 cancer patients in whom response to homeopathy treatment was assessed using the Hospital Anxiety and Depression Scale (HADS) and Rotterdam Symptom Checklist. Improvements were seen on the HADS Anxiety subscale when comparing scores on initial and later (3rd) visits and the percentage with normal HADS anxiety scores increased from 48% to 75% by the 4th visit [88].

1996: McCutchenon reported a double-blind placebo-controlled trial conducted in France with patients suffering from anxiety in which half were given a homeopathic "Anti-anxiety" formula and the other half were given Diazepam. The study was conducted on 77 adults with above-average anxiety scores (mean Spielberger State-Trait Anxiety Inventory [STAI] scores between 40 and 50 for state and trait anxiety). No significant differences between the groups were found either at pre- or post-test on STAI but there were differences in sleep loss with those in the homeopathy group reporting significantly less loss of sleep. Mean sleep loss in the subjects who received 'Antianxiety' improved by 1.3 hours compared with a mean improvement of only 0.5 hour in the placebo group. The author concluded that the homeopathic 'Antianxiety' complex, may be useful for this aspect of anxiety although it appeared to have little value in the reduction of either state or trait anxiety [89].

1997: Davidson et al reported an uncontrolled study in which individually selected homeopathic remedies were used on an outpatient basis to treat twelve adults who had major depression, social phobia, or panic disorder. The patients either requested homeopathic treatment or received it on a physician's recommendation after partial or poor response to conventional therapies. The duration of treatment was 7 to 80 weeks. Response was monitored by using a clinical global scale (n = 12), the self-rated SCL-90 scale (n = 8), and the Brief Social Phobia Scale (n = 4). Seven (58%) patients were reported to have responded to homeopathic treatment, on the basis of the Clinical Global Improvement (CGI) scale including two of the patients with social phobia, two cases of social phobia combined with panic disorder and one with social phobia combined with major depression. The study concluded that homeopathy may be useful in the treatment of affective disorders and Anxiety Disorders in patients with mildly to severely symptomatic conditions [90].

1999: Zenner & Weiser [91] reported a prospective study of homeopathic treatment in 269 women with gynaecological disorders, 38% of whom were assessed as having mood disorders. On the basis of the physician and patient assessment, the treatment was rated on a 5-point scale and for 67% of women in the study a 'very good' or 'good' improvement in the mood disorder symptoms was reported.

2002: Thompson & Reilly [92] reported a well-designed uncontrolled study of individualized homeopathy for symptom relief in 100 cancer patients; 63% of the patients completing the study were found to have some improvement in anxiety scores at the end of the study period. Up to three symptoms perceived by the patient as problematic were rated on a self-rating scale while anxiety was assessed using the Hospital Anxiety and Depression Scale (HADS). At the beginning of the study, 59 patients were found to be anxious with 30 having anxiety (scores above 10), 29 borderline anxiety (scores 8–10), and a greater percentage of those with metastatic disease being anxious (67% compared with 52%). The mean overall improvement in anxiety scores was 1.6 (95% CI 0.4–2.9) but the attrition rate was high. Seventeen patients suffered an aggravation of symptoms or a return of old symptoms considered to be previously described remedy reactions but no adverse reactions resulted in withdrawal of treatment. Satisfaction with treatment was measured by a self-completion questionnaire and was high among those who completed the study; 75% regarded homeopathic treatment as having been at least helpful.

2003: Baker and colleagues [93] attempted a replication of the 1981 Stanton study. The study was conducted in an Australian university with 70 test-anxious student volunteers and the methodology used was rigorous with adequate randomisation to one of three arms, traditional homeopathy, radionics or placebo. Concealment of allocation and blinding of students and assessors were also acceptable and a positive check on power at the end of the study was obtained (62 completed the study) with the study adequately powered to demonstrate a 5% difference between groups. A revised version of the TAS was used, and comparison with Stanton's data suggested that anxiety scores pre-treatment might have been slightly higher in the earlier study but analysis of the data revealed no significant difference between the groups for reduction in test anxiety.

2003: Bonne and colleagues [94] reported no significant difference between adults with generalized anxiety disorder treated with individualized remedies and those treated with placebo for ten weeks. A significant improvement was observed in both the active and placebo groups, including reduction in Hamilton Rating Scale for Anxiety (HAM-A) scores, over the period of the study. However, this study may have been underpowered, as a power calculation had demonstrated that a minimum of 60 participants was required but only 44 were recruited and of these only 39 completed the study.

2003: In a further uncontrolled study by Thompson & Reily [95], individualized homeopathy was used to treat symptoms of oestrogen withdrawal in 45 breast cancer patients. A significant improvement in anxiety scores was reported with mean change being 2.1 (95% CI 0.7–3.4). Twenty-six of the patients had also been included in the 2002 study. Eighty-nine per cent of patients completed this study and again satisfaction with treatment was high; 67% regarded homeopathic treatment as having been helpful, very helpful or extremely helpful for their symptoms.

2007: Meerschaut & Sunder [96] reported an open-label, prospective non-randomized cohort study, the effectiveness and tolerability profiles of the homeopathic combination remedy, Nervoheel N2, with those of the benzodiazepine, lorazepam, in 248 patients with insomnia, distress, anxieties, restlessness or burnout and similar nervous conditions ('mild nervous disorders'). Patients were treated with Nervoheel N or lorazepam at the recommended doses for a maximum of four weeks. Dose variations were allowed if in the patient's best interest. Treatment effects were evaluated by the practitioner in a dialogue with the patient at the start of treatment, after two weeks and after maximally four weeks of treatment. Tolerability data were recorded as adverse events. Both treatment groups reported significant symptomatic improvements of similar magnitude during the course of the study. A total of 72.1% in the homeopathic group rated the results as "excellent" or "good," while 73.7% reported similar results from lorazepam. The sum of symptom scores improved by 4.4 points with Nervoheel N and by 4.2 points with lorazepam. The differences between the treatment groups were not significant. The researchers also found that the use of additional medications was low in both groups: 6.8% in the homeopathic group and 8.1% in the lorazepam group. All differences between treatments were within 10% of the maximum score ranges, demonstrating non-inferiority of Nervoheel N. Both treatments were well tolerated, with few adverse events and very good self-assessed tolerability ratings by the patients. However, 81.9% of patients using the homeopathic medicine rate the tolerability as "excellent, while only 45.5% in the lorazepam group gave it this rating (P<0.001). The researchers concluded that the effects of Nervoheel N are non-inferior to those of lorazepam in the treatment of mild nervous disorders. Since the long-term use of benzodiazepine drugs is known to have serious side effects, the use of this safer homeopathic medicine may make sense.

Apart from these studies, outcome studies done by Clover, Richardson, Van Wassenhoven & Ives and Mathie & Robinson have reported positive results in patients with a range of conditions including anxiety and depression [97].

4.5.2.2 ADHD
1997: John Lamont [98], a psychologist in Southern California, conducted a placebo-controlled, double-blind, randomized trial of 43 children with Attention Deficit Hyperactivity Disorder (ADHD). The evaluations of improvement were based on parent or caretaker ratings of ADHD be-

haviours. A 5-point scale was used: much worse (-2); a little worse (-1); no change (0); a little better (+1); much better (+2). Parents or caretakers were contacted by telephone 10 days after the remedy/placebo was taken and again after two months.

Half of the children were given an individualized homeopathic medicine and half were given a placebo that resembled a homeopathic medicine for ten days. After this, the half that was given a placebo was given an individualized homeopathic medicine. The mean improvement scores after ten days were .35 for the placebo group and 1.00 for the homeopathically treated group (p=.05). The greatest improvements were noticed by the third day, while a smaller number showed improvement after ten days.

Children who were initially given a placebo were given a homeopathic prescription after ten days and then compared with their earlier score. The mean improvement scores were .35 for the placebo group and 1.13 after a homeopathic medicine was given (p=.02). When parents reported that improvement from the treatment was not obvious, the homeopath prescribed a second or a third remedy. When comparing the results after these remedies, improvement from the homeopathic group was 1.63 and from the placebo group. 35 (p=.01).

Follow-up interviews conducted ten days after the homeopathic medicine observed that the majority of children who were treated homeopathically experienced sustained and increased improvement in their condition. After two months, 57% of children experienced continued improvement; 24% showed improvement for several days or weeks following homeopathic treatment, but relapsed by the two-month interview. 19% said that they only observed improvement while taking homeopathic treatment (one could guess that this improvement was primarily from the placebo effect). This study indicates that the effects of the homeopathic medicine were relatively rapid and a significant proportion (57%) of children experienced sustained and increased improvement at two months follow-up.

2001: Frei & Thurneysen [99] report a trial to assess the efficacy of homeopathy in 115 hyperactive patients (mean age 8.3 years, range 3-17 y) compared to the use of methylphenidate. 75% of the children responded to homeopathy, reaching a clinical improvement rating of 73%. Children who did not respond to homeopathic treatment were prescribed methylphenidate (after an average period of 22 months of homeopathic treatment). The children were also evaluated according to the Conner's Global Index (CGI), a scale that measures the degree of hyperactivity and attention deficit symptoms. The children who responded to the homeopathic medicine experienced a 55% amelioration of their scores CGI, while the children who responded to Ritalin experienced a 48% lowering of their CGI scores.

2005: Frei et al [100] reported a randomized double-blind placebo controlled crossover trial of 62 children, aged 6-16 years, with ADHD diagnosed using the Diagnostic and Statistical Manual of Mental Disorders-IV criteria, showed significant improvement in visual global perception, impulsivity and divided attention. The responders received either verum for six weeks followed by placebo for six weeks (arm A), or vice versa (arm B). At the beginning of the trial and after each crossover period, parents reported the CGI and patients underwent neuropsychological testing. The CGI rating was evaluated again at the end of each crossover period and twice in long-term follow-up. At entry to the crossover trial, cognitive performance such as visual global perception, impulsivity and divided attention had improved significantly under open label treatment. During the crossover trial, CGI parent-ratings were significantly lower under homeopathic treatment (average 1.67 points) than under placebo (P =0.0479). Long-term (defined as fourteen weeks) CGI improvement reached 12 points (63%, P <0.0001). This indicates significant improvement under homeopathic treatment. The trial suggests scientific evidence for the effectiveness of homeopathy in the treatment of ADHD, particularly in the areas of behavioural and cognitive functions.

2007: A Swiss randomised, placebo-controlled, crossover trial in ADHD patients was designed with an open-label screening phase prior to the randomised controlled phase [101]. During the screening phase, the response of each child to successive homeopathic medications was observed until the optimal medication was identified. Only children who reached a predefined level of improvement participated in the randomised, crossover phase. Although the randomised phase revealed a significant beneficial effect of homeopathy, the crossover caused a strong carryover effect diminishing the apparent difference between placebo and verum treatment. During the screening phase, 84% (70/83) of the children responded to treatment and reached eligibility for the randomised trial after a median time of five months (range 1-18), with a median of three different medications (range 1-9). Five months after the start of treatment the difference in Conner's Global Index (CGI) rating between responders and non-responders became highly significant (p = 0.0006). Improvement in CGI was much greater following the identification of the optimal medication than in the preceding suboptimal treatment period (p< 0.0001).

4.5.2.3 Drug abuse

1990: The Government of India conducted a double-blind study of 60 heroin addicts, of whom 30 were given individualized homeopathic medicines and 30 were given placebo. The number and intensity of the symptoms during withdrawal were significantly less in patients given an individualized homeopathic medicine than those given a placebo. The number of days for the resolution of complaints was also fewer in the homeopathically treated group. There was a difference in the adherence too - 35% of patients on the placebo left the study prior to its completion due to lack of therapeutic benefit, while only 5% of those taking the homeopathic medicine left the study [102].

1993: A double-blind, placebo-controlled trial [103] applying homeopathy to chemical dependency was conducted by the Hahnemann College of Homeopathy, Albany, California. The results showed a reduced relapse rate among recovering alcoholics and drug addicts undergoing homeopathic treatment.

1994: A study was carried out by Central Council for Research in Homoeopathy (CCRH) at its Clinical Research Unit, Varanasi, India [104]. Out of 261 drug dependent patients referred from a Drug De-addiction Centre at Varanasi, 20 cases dropped out and the remaining 241 were followed up from September 1988 to March 1994. All the cases were in the age group of 12-52 years and all except one were male. The medicines were administered usually 8-12 hours after abstinence of drug substance abuse, where withdrawal symptoms became obvious. Prescription was made on the basis of totality of symptoms of the individual case.

Out of 241 cases followed up regularly, 209 cases showed improvement in withdrawal symptoms against 32 cases which did not improve. *Rhus toxicodendron* (n=85) was found to be the most effective medicine. Other medicines found effective were *Avena sativa* (n=43), *Nux vomica* (n=34), *Arsenicum album* (n=26), *Bryonia alba* (n=8) and *Chamomilla* (n=7).

The outcome of the study shows that homeopathic medicines are efficacious in the management of withdrawal symptoms of drug dependent people and can check the menace of chemical dependency. The results have prompted CCRH to take up this study in collaboration with the Society for Promotion of Youth and Masses (SPYM) from April 2008.

4.5.2.4 Insomnia

1985: A double-blind placebo-controlled trial was conducted in France with patients suffering from anxiety, in which half were given a homeopathic formula marketed as "L72" in France and "Anti-anxiety" in the USA [75]. The study is interesting because it did not find that this homeopathic formula product was effective in treating anxiety, but it was found to have statistically significant beneficial effects in the treatment of insomnia (p=0.05).

2007: In a prospective, non-randomized cohort study, the effectiveness and tolerability profiles of the homeopathic combination remedy, Nervoheel N3, were compared with those of the benzodiazepine lorazepam, in 248 patients with insomnia, distress, anxieties, restlessness or burnout and similar nervous conditions ('mild nervous disorders') [86]. Both treatment groups reported significant symptomatic improvements of similar magnitude during the course of the study. A total of 72.1% in the homeopathic group rated the results as "excellent" or "good," while 73.7% reported similar results from lorazepam. The sum of symptom scores improved by 4.4 points with Nervoheel N3 and by 4.2 points with lorazepam. Both treatments were well tolerated, with few adverse events and very good self-assessed tolerability ratings by the patients. However, 81.9% of patients using the homeopathic medicine rated the tolerability as "excellent, while only 45.5% in the lorazepam group gave it this rating (P<0.001). The researchers concluded that the effects of Nervoheel N3 are non-inferior to those of lorazepam in the treatment of mild nervous disorders. Finally, because the long-term use of benzodiazepine drugs is known to have serious side effects, the use of this safer homeopathic medicine may make sense.

2008: An open-label, prospective cohort study in 89 German centres offering both conventional and complementary therapies tested a homeopathic formula product, Neurexan, with a herbal product, valerian, for 28 days [105]. Doses were at physicians' judgments. Sleep duration and latency were evaluated based on patients' sleep diaries over fourteen days; sleep quality was evaluated at 28 +/- 1 days. A total of 409 subjects were enrolled. Differences between the groups in improvement on sleep duration were significantly in favour of Neurexan therapy on Days 8, 12, and 14. On Day 28, the quality of sleep was improved in both groups with no significant differences between the treatments. Significantly more patients reported lack of daytime fatigue with Neurexan than with valerian therapies (49% vs. 32%; p < 0.05 for the comparison). The researchers concluded that for patients favourable towards a CAM-based therapy, Neurexan might be an effective and well-tolerated alternative to conventional valerian-based therapies for the treatment of mild to moderate insomnia.

4.5.2.7 Stress

One study [106] sought to evaluate the use of homeopathic doses of a herb to determine its efficacy in preventing handling stress in bovines. Sixty Nelore calves were randomly distributed into two equal groups. One group was administered *Chamomilla* 12CH (aka 12C) in their food and the control group was not. Animals in both groups were maintained unstressed for 30 days to allow them to adjust to the feeding system and pasture, and were then stressed by constraint on the

31st, 38th, 45th and 60th experimental days. Blood samples were taken on these days after animals had been immobilised in a trunk contention for five minutes. Stress was followed by analyzing serum cortisol levels. These peaked on the 45th day and then fell, but not to baseline, on the 60th day. On the 45th day cortisol levels were significantly lower in animals fed Chamomilla 12CH, suggesting that this medicine reduces stress. These effects may be a consequence of its inhibiting cortisol production and its calming and anxiolytic effects.

4.5.3 Improvement in co-morbidity

Apart from these studies directly related to the psychological sphere, there have been many other positive clinical studies documenting the efficacy of homeopathic remedies in a variety of psycho-somatic and somatic conditions with known correlation with mental state, like Chronic Fatigue Syndrome, Fibromyalgia, Pre-Menstrual Syndrome, Menopause, Allergic Conditions, Asthma, Dermatitis etc [107].

It is now widely acknowledged that the relationship between mental disorders and physical disorders is complex and reciprocal and that it acts through multiple pathways. Mental disorders lead to poor physical outcomes, as illustrated by the significantly reduced life expectancies of persons with schizophrenia. Persons with mental disorders are less likely than other people to pay attention to symptoms of physical illness. Consequently, they delay seeking treatment for co-morbid conditions such as diabetes and hypertension. They face significant barriers to receiving treatment for physical disorders because of stigma and discrimination. Mental disorders also increase the likelihood of non-adherence to treatment regimens for physical conditions, and this leads to poorer outcomes. Among people with mental disorders there is an increased biological vulnerability to suffering from physical disorders. Depression, for example, is associated with reduced levels of functioning of the immune system and consequently with an increased risk of other physical disorders. The reverse relationship also holds true: people suffering from chronic physical conditions have a higher likelihood of developing mental disorders such as depression.

Effective use of homeopathic medicines for the treatment of any disease has the potential to bring about therapeutic relief in associated mental and emotional symptoms as well. The reverse also holds true. Treatment for any mental disorder with homeopathy will bring about positive therapeutic outcome in associated physical disorders.

4.5.4 Improvement in general well-being, quality of life and patient satisfaction

1987: A randomized trial of classical homeopathy for migraine measured the global outcome. Patients were asked to rate their own general wellbeing on a 10-point visual analogue scale (VAS) on three occasions. The verum group showed significant improvement, unlike the placebo group [108].

1994: A British prospective survey of homeopathic treatment of 160 patients found 'very positive effect' in 73% patients and 'some effect' in the rest 27% [109].

1995: In a retrospective survey of homeopathic treatment, Danmarks Farmaceutiske Højskole, 1995, 73% of patients stated they improved after homeopathic treatment [110].

1996: A British prospective survey of homeopathic treatment of 223 patients, 1996, found: 90% improvement or more: 32%. 60% improvement or more: 65% 50% improvement or more: 72% [111].

1996: Richardson conducted a quasi-randomised trial to assess the effect of homeopathy, acupuncture and osteopathy. Result: 89% of patients stated they experienced positive effect from the treatment. The effect was particularly clear on reduction of pain, increased vitality, ability to function socially and with regard to limitations at work and in daily activities influenced by physical problems. Homeopathy was generally effective and particularly for patients suffering from arthritis, hay fever, asthma and skin complaints [112].

1998: British prospective survey of homeopathic treatment of 37 patients suffering from psychological complaints, 1998. Very satisfied: 81%. Satisfied: 16%. Not satisfied at all: 3% [113].

1998: In an innovative study, Kuzeff [114] asked whether homeopathy causes a greater improvement in sensation of well-being than placebo and whether it changes immune function as evidenced by CD4 levels. A number of patients were admitted to a prospective, double-blind, randomized, placebo-controlled crossover study. Data was analyzed on an intention-to-treat basis. Visual analogue scales (VAS) of "sensation of well-being" and CD4 levels were the variables which were measured. It was concluded that the study provided evidence for the ability of homeopathic prescribing to improve "sensation of well-being", and provided evidence in support of ultra-high dilution effects. The study also suggests that homeopathic medicines may affect CD4 levels.

2000: In a study carried out by Attena et al [115], one year after their first visit to a homeopathic clinic, 609 patients were asked to rate their general health compared with a year previously. 73.5% reported a marked or moderate improvement in their health status.

2000: In a study of 829 patients treated with homeopathic medicines, where conventional treatment had been unsatisfactory or contraindicated, 61% had a substantial improvement with homeopathy [116].

2004: A survey of more than 900 patients treated homeopathically showed substantial improvement in quality of life over the first six months after treatment and this effect remained more or less stable over the following years [117].

2005: In an observational study of 6,544 patients during a six-year period, and over 23,000 consultations, results showed that 70.7% reported positive health changes, with 50.7% recording their improvement as better (+2) or much better (+3). Of the 1270 children that were treated 80.5% had some improvement, and 65.8% were better (+2) or much better (+3) [118].

2005: Seven out of ten patients visiting Norwegian homeopaths reported a meaningful improvement in their main complaint six months after the initial consultation [119].

2005: In a prospective, multi-centre cohort study [120] with 103 primary care practices treating 3,981 patients, disease severity decreased significantly (p<0.001) over a two-year period. Major improvements were observed in quality of life for adults and young children. 28% (1,130) of the patients were children and 97% of all diagnoses were chronic with an average duration of 8.8 years. The most frequent diagnoses were allergic rhinitis in men, headache in women, and atopic dermatitis in children.

2009: In a survey carried out in New Zealand [121], researchers surveyed 124 patients in GP surgeries and found that 65% had used homeopathic products. More than 92% of those who had used homeopathy believed that homeopathy helped at least sometimes and 65% of users believed that it helped most times or every time.

4.5.5 Research on microdilutions

1997: The effect of high dilutions was documented in an experiment showing the effect of highly diluted *Belladonna* on acetylcholine-induced contraction of the rat ileum [122].

2001: Neuroprotection from glutamates toxicity with ultra-low dose glutamates [123]. Jonas et al showed that exposure of nerve cells to ultra-low doses of glutamate has a protective effect during subsequent exposure to toxic doses of glutamate (a chemical compound). Growth and recovery of cells was stimulated.

2003: In an experimental study of ultra-high dilutions of lithium chloride and sodium chloride, researchers found emission of light even in dilutions beyond Avogadro's number (10-30 g cm-3). The solutions were irradiated by x- and gamma-rays at 77 K, then progressively rewarmed to room temperature. Thermoluminescence was studied during the process [124].

2003: In an experimental study on the effect of histamine on basophile granulocytes, researchers found an effect of histamine diluted beyond Avogadro's number [125].

2004: Dutta, Biswas and Khuda-buksh tested two potencies of *Mercurius solubilis* (Merc Sol-30 and Merc Sol-200), for their possible efficacy in ameliorating mercuric chloride-induced genotoxicity in mice. Healthy mice, Mus musculus, were intraperitoneally injected with a 0.06% solution of mercuric chloride at the rate of 1 ml/100g of body weight, and assessed for genotoxic effects through conventional endpoints. i.e. chromosome aberrations, micronuclei, mitotic index and sperm head abnormality, keeping suitable controls. It was observed that the chromosome aberrations, micronuclei and sperm head anomaly were generally reduced in the drug-fed series, and the mitotic index showed an apparent increase. The amelioration by Merc Sol-200 appeared to be slightly more pronounced. The authors concluded that the potentised homeopathic drugs could serve as possible anti-genotoxic agents against specific environmental mutagens, including toxic heavy metals [126].

2004: In a multi-centre study including four research centres in Europe the effect of high dilutions of histamine (10-30 – 10-38 M) was confirmed. Researchers were able to document that high dilutions of histamine inhibit human basophil degranulation. Results cannot be explained through molecular theories [127].

2006: A placebo-controlled homeopathic pathogenic trial, more commonly known as a proving, clearly demonstrated that provers who took the substances in C30 potency experienced significantly more symptoms than a placebo group (P<0.001). Provers were given either *Etna Lava* C30,

Hydrogenium peroxidatum C30, or placebo. Where the placebo group experienced some symptoms, they were more short-lived compared to the verum group, which experienced persistent symptoms for the first 30 days. Provers in the verum group also experienced more 'old symptoms' returning. A weakness of the survey is that it only included 21 provers. The original researchers have now called for more data from more provers [128].

2009: Researchers at Amala Cancer Research Institute in India evaluated the cytotoxic activity of 30C and 200C potencies of ten dynamised medicines against Dalton's Lymphoma Ascites, Ehrlich's Ascites Carcinoma, lung fibroblast (L929) and Chinese Hamster Ovary (CHO) cell lines and compared activity with their mother tinctures during short-term and long-term cell culture [129]. The effect of dynamised medicines to induce apoptosis was also evaluated and the researchers studied how dynamised medicines affected genes expressed during apoptosis. Mother tinctures, as well as some dynamised medicines showed significant cytotoxicity to cells during short and long-term incubation. Potentiated alcohol control did not produce any cytotoxicity at concentrations studied. The dynamised medicines were found to inhibit CHO cell colony formation and thymidine uptake in L929 cells and those of *Thuja*, *Hydrastis* and *Carcinosinum* were found to induce apoptosis in DLA cells. Moreover, dynamised Carcinosinum was found to induce the expression of p53 while dynamised Thuja produced characteristic laddering pattern in agarose gel electrophoresis of DNA. These results indicate that dynamised medicines possess cytotoxic as well as apoptosis-inducing properties.

4.5.6 The safe choice
2000: Doctors at the Royal London Homeopathic Hospital carried out a worldwide literature review of homeopathic studies published between 1970 and 1995 in which they looked for adverse effects of homeopathic treatment. While they found that ten clinical trials, nineteen case studies and eighteen provings reported possible adverse effects, in only three reports were these adverse effects deemed to be due to homeopathic medicine. Of these three reports, two were 'proving' symptoms (a temporary induction of symptoms foreign to the patient, consistent with symptoms induced by the homeopathic medicine when tested on healthy patients and that cease when the homeopathic medicine is stopped). The third report concerned a compound medicine, which also contained herbs [130].

2009: A review looked at whether homeopathic medicines could help patients with problems caused by cancer treatments. Eight studies with a total of 664 participants were included in this review. This review found preliminary data in support of the efficacy of topical calendula for prophylaxis of acute dermatitis during radiotherapy and Traumeel S mouthwash in the treatment of chemotherapy-induced stomatitis. One of the findings of the review was that the homeopathic medicines used in all eight studies did not seem to cause any serious adverse effects or interact with conventional treatment [131].

4.5.7 Cost-effectiveness
1992: A study of the cost and effectiveness of homeopathy suggested that doctors practising homeopathy issue fewer prescriptions and at a lower cost than their colleagues. The main costs for homeopathic treatment are for consultations with each individual patient. Costs for the actual medications used are low when compared with conventional drugs [132].

1996: In a survey of 223 patients in an NHS General Practice, the number of consultations with general practitioners was reduced by 70% in a 1-year period. Expenses for medication were reduced by 50% when homeopathic treatment was made available [112].

2002: In a study of 351 adults suffering from allergies, 35.3% received homeopathic treatment. The study assessed the results of alternative medicine as very good (28.6%) or rather good (53.8%). The researchers also concluded that alternative medicine is used widely for allergies by the general population. This has freedom of choice and cost-benefit implications for the healthcare system and health policy [133].

2002: A retrospective outcome study designed as a before-after trial was conducted to assess the effects of homeopathic intervention on medication consumption in atopic and allergic disorders [134]. Patients were studied in a complementary medicine clinic affiliated with an Israeli health maintenance organization. 48 patients were treated for allergic diseases with homeopathic remedies and conventional medications. 56% of patients in this study reduced their use of conventional medication following the homeopathic intervention. Patients who used conventional medications for their allergic disorders reduced their medication expense by an average of 60%, with an average savings of $24 per patient in the three-month period following the homeopathic intervention.

2003: A four-year study of 84 patients treated homeopathically showed average cost savings for drugs per patient of £60.40 (range £12.48 to £703.95 – average duration of treatment was 4.2 months). 64 patients were cured, sixteen showed significant improvement, five moderate improvement affecting daily living, five showed no change or were unsure, and ten are still under treatment. No side-effects of treatment were reported [135].

2005: In a comparative cohort study of 493 patients with chronic diagnoses results indicated greater improvement in patients' assessments after homeopathic versus conventional treatment (adults: homeopathy from 5.7 to 3.2; conventional 5.9 to 4.4, p = 0.002; children: from 5.1 to 2.6, and 3.9 to 2.7, p < 0.001). Physician assessments were also more favourable for children who had received homeopathic treatment. There were no significant differences in costs between the two treatment groups [136].

2005: A comparative study was conducted to evaluate the efficacy of homeopathic and allopathic systems of medicine in the management of clinical mastitis of Indian dairy cows [137]. 96 mastitic quarters (non-fibrosed 67 and fibrosed 29) were treated with a homeopathic combination medicine. Another 96 quarters with acute mastitis (non-fibrosed) treated with different antibiotics were included in the study. The overall effectiveness of homeopathic combination medicine in the treatment of acute non-fibrosed mastitis was 86.6% with a mean recovery period of 7.7 days (range 3-28), and a total cost of therapy as Indian Rupees 21.4 (.39 Euros, US$ .47). The corresponding cure rate for the antibiotic group was 59.2% with a mean recovery period of 4.5 days (range 2-15) and an average treatment cost of Rs.149.20 (2.69 Euros, US$ 3.28). The authors concluded that the combination of *Phytolacca, Calcarea fluorica, Silica, Belladonna, Bryonia, Arnica, Conium* and *Ipecacuanha* (Healwell VT-6) was effective and economical in the management of mastitis in lactating dairy cows.

2005: The data pertaining to homeopathic clinics of one year (1999-2000, 24,943 patients) with respect to patient turnover, morbidity profile and expenditure incurred was compared to that of the allopathic clinics (27,508 patients) functional at the same centre [138]. 1.25 million patients visited these clinics and their morbidity profile included respiratory diseases (26%), gastro-intestinal diseases (20%), skin diseases (20%), gynaecological diseases (9%), viral diseases and injuries (4% each) and other miscellaneous diseases (14%). The expenditure incurred per patient per visit in allopathic clinic was Rupees 76.90 compared to Rupees 15.43 (20%) in homeopathic clinics. The study concluded that homeopathy is quite popular, very cost-effective and can be used widely at primary health care level for common diseases. Its adoption at primary health care level can serve as a model for promoting homeopathy in developing countries.

2009: A retrospective observational study [139] was conducted on 105 out of 233 patients suffe-ring from chronic respiratory disease attending the Homeopathic Clinic of the Campo di Marte Hospital in Lucca (Tuscany, Italy) between October 1998 and May 2003. The cost of conventional medicinal products using the Anatomic Therapeutic Chemical (ATC) classification, specific for the pathology in question, and the general costs in the year preceding the first appointment at the Homeopathic Clinic vs. the first and second year subsequent to homeopathic treatment was as-sessed. The costs of conventional drugs for a group of patients affected by asthma (eight patients) and recurrent respiratory infections (sixteen patients) with previous long-term use of conventional medicine treated by homeopathy were compared with the expenses of conventional drugs of a matched group of 16 and 32 patients, respectively. Results indicate that the costs of pharmacologi-cal therapy specific for respiratory diseases were reduced by 46.3% (n = 105) in the first year (P<0.01); and by 47.5% (n = 72) in the second year (P<0.01) of homeopathic treatment. Reduction in general drug costs during homeopathic therapy was 42.4% in the first year (P<0.01), and 49.8 in the second year (N.S.). The costs for patients affected by chronic asthma showed a reduction in expenses of 71.1% for specific medicines relative to the group in homeopathic treatment vs. an in-crease of 12.3% in the group treated only with conventional drugs after the first year of follow-up and, respectively, a reduction of 54.4% for homeopathic treatment vs. an increase of 45.2% after the second year. The study concluded that homeopathic treatment for respiratory diseases (asthma, allergic complaints, acute recurrent respiratory infections) was associated with a significant reduc-tion in the use and costs of conventional drugs. Costs for homeopathic therapy are significantly lower than those for conventional pharmacological therapy.

4.6 Challenges in homeopathic research and the road ahead
Research in all forms of complementary medicine, including homeopathy, suffers from two signifi-cant drawbacks. One is negative research bias and the other is the use of unsuitable methodology. There is also a publication bias. In 2005, Caulfield & Debow carried out a systematic review of how homeopathy is represented in conventional and CAM peer-reviewed journals. The results sug-gested that a publication bias against homeopathy exists in mainstream journals [140].

4.6.1 The research bias
Many research studies in CAM are carried out with the intention of disproving CAM therapies, where the researcher already believes in the negative outcome of the research. Research has shown that the beliefs of the researcher can affect the outcome of the research [141] and good research practice suggests that all research should start with a neutral stance towards the possible outcome. A large body of negative research in CAM suffers from this prejudiced approach.

Micozzi [142] in an editorial in The Journal of Alternative and Complementary Medicine has noted, "...*investigations of claims of complementary medicine, all too often, take on the character and tone of 'debunking' expeditions rather than scientific experiments.*" He also states "*A willingness to report negative findings far exceeds the acceptance of positive findings and there is clear evidence of bias against CAM research.*"

One of the most cited negative meta-analyses of homeopathy research trials, carried out by *Shang* et al [143], is a glaring example of such prejudiced approaches. The review, which appeared in 2005, started with 110 placebo-controlled clinical trials of homeopathy matched with 110 of conventional medicine. Twenty-one homeopathy trials and nine conventional medicine trials were of "higher quality". From that smaller set of trials, the authors then focused their attention on respectively eight and six "large trials of higher quality" in several different medical conditions. On the basis of these fourteen studies, the review concluded that there was "weak evidence for a specific effect of homeopathic remedies, but strong evidence for specific effects of conventional interventions". The publication bias was more than evident by the fact that the accompanying editorial was entitled '*The End of Homeopathy*'. Most reputed medical journals have at times published negative research trials and meta-analysis of conventional medicine but has anybody ever come across an editorial entitled '*The End of Orthodox Medicine*'?

The review was criticised at the time for its opacity, as it gave no indication of which trials were analysed nor the various assumptions made about the data. Sufficient detail to enable a reconstruction of the analysis was eventually published by the authors. Two newly published studies [144,145] show that the conclusions of this review were seriously flawed. The new studies, which reconstruct the review's analysis, cast severe doubts on its negative conclusions, showing that it was based on a series of hidden judgments unfavourable to homeopathy. A positive conclusion for homeopathy is in fact obtained if all twenty-one "higher quality" trials are included in the analysis. If fewer than twenty-one trials are analysed, a positive or negative conclusion for homeopathy is crucially dependent on the exact number of trials selected. A firm positive conclusion is found, for example, merely by omitting four trials that showed *Arnica* is ineffective for muscle soreness after long-distance running. Whether the conclusions of the analysis are positive or negative is therefore highly sensitive to the choice of which "higher quality" trials are included. Apart from this, there was selective inclusion of unpublished trials only for homeopathy. Selecting subgroups on sample size and quality caused incomplete matching of homeopathy and conventional trials. Cut-off values for larger trials differed between homeopathy and conventional medicine without plausible reason. Sensitivity analyses for the influence of heterogeneity and the cut-off value for 'larger higher quality studies' were also missing. The Shang et al review has been found to be full of such 'systematic' mistakes and omissions.

This review is just one example of how the negative *a priori* ideas about CAM affect the research as well as research outcomes. Publishers and reviewers of CAM research should be conversant with this phenomenon and should remain vigilant to exclude research trials with a negative bias against CAM.

4.6.2 The question of research methodology
The second point pertinent to research on CAM is the question of methodology. Whenever the question of research on evidence for the effectiveness of homeopathy comes up, critics and sceptics

insist on double-blind placebo-controlled trials, like those conducted in conventional medicine or other streams of modern science. These people forget that the research methodology for any proposed research is developed to suit the stream of knowledge in question. The method of action of most complementary medicines is very different from conventional medicine and that makes it necessary to develop different research methodologies suitable to test the effect and efficacy of various CAM therapies. Blindly following the same research methodology for all research pursuits is also unscientific.

There are double standards present in even the demand for such double-blind placebo-controlled (DBPC) trials or Randomized Controlled Trials (RCT). Any research or practice in CAM that is not supported by vigorous RCT is considered junk - it is considered 'unscientific'. On the other hand, only 16% of conventional medicine trials need them in their own evidence-base [146]. Many treatments used in conventional (orthodox) medicine have not been rigorously tested either.
In fact, it is estimated that as much as 60% of orthodox treatments have not been subject to scientific scrutiny [147]. Even the vast majority of surgical practices are not based on evidence but on acquired skills and experience, yet their scientific base is never questioned!

There have been many positive RCTs for homeopathy but there are many reasons why an RCT is still not considered the optimum methodology for evaluating the clinical efficacy of homeopathy [148]. RCTs are designed to isolate the drug's effect from all other effects; but homeopathy, unlike chemical drugs which target a specific tissue or symptom and so can demonstrate a specific effect, operates indirectly, through stimulating the body's healing mechanisms. Its effect is considered non-specific. Homeopathy, being a holistic intervention, examines the whole being rather than the presenting symptom; thus homeopathy's effects manifest not merely on the presenting physical complaint. Rather, homeopathy also affects secondary physical symptoms, emotional symptoms and general symptoms, such as wellbeing. These outcomes would be considered, under most study designs, as non-specific, or placebo effects. Hence, such effects would be ignored in most studies, even if their importance to the patient's quality of life is noticeable.

Apart from its generalized healing, homeopathy also induces other non-specific effects. A homeopathic consultation can have a high quotient of therapeutic relationship. It is often emotionally involved, exposing the disharmonies in patients' lives. Some suggest that, even without receiving a remedy, patients derive extra benefit from the mere consultation, over and above conventional treatment. Therefore it is very difficult to design RCT studies for a complex intervention such as homeopathy that would preclude any interference between the different arms of the study. This, again, reduces the chance of demonstrating an effect beyond placebo.

Dean has echoed similar thoughts about RCT in his review:

> "It is certainly arguable that placebos have been over-sold in clinical research, sometimes as a way of bringing new drugs to market that are less effective than those already available. It is also true that participants in randomized placebo-controlled trials, both patients and therapists, may differ systematically from those who would not give consent. And placebos are simply unethical in many contexts. In protracted trials patients cannot be denied different treatment known to be effective just to suit the interest of the researchers." [149]

In view of these limitations, research methodologies like *clinical outcome* studies (consistently gathering and analyzing outcome data in clinical settings, using appropriate valid and reliable assessment instruments), *pragmatic trials* (pragmatic trials measure effectiveness - the benefit the treatment produces in routine clinical practice) and *equivalence trials* (the aim of an equivalence trial is to show the therapeutic equivalence of two treatments) are considered more effective for research in CAM therapies. Many clinical outcome studies in homeopathy have shown very significant positive results in favour of homeopathy [118-120].

CAM research has come a long way in the last 20 years, with excellent manuals on viable research methods such as Lewith, Jonas, and Walach's 'Clinical Research in Complementary Therapies' published by Churchill, LivingStone [150]. Researchers need to be well aware of the research issues relevant to CAM research and should choose methodologies that take into account the individuality of the therapeutic modality under investigation.

5   Integration

Homeopathy and Allopathy (conventional medicine) have now coexisted for more than two centuries. Until a few decades ago, differences in ideology made the practitioners of both systems believe that there could be no common ground. But as conventional medicine has advanced, both its strengths and weaknesses have become more apparent. Complementary and alternative medicine (CAM) also realizes that it has much to gain from the scientific methods developed in conventional medicine and the old belief of 'either this or the other' is no longer tenable. There is a growing realization that conventional and CAM medicines will need to join hands for the betterment of society. Many governments and health organizations have already made a start in this direction. But a large part of the world's population is still unable to access homeopathic treatment through national health programmes. This calls for a greater integration of homeopathy within general medical practice.

True integration requires good understanding of all the modalities concerned. Integration should not be limited to using non-conventional techniques with no understanding of their philosophy and methodology e.g. using the homeopathic remedy *Arnica* for shock and bruising. Such limited and blind use of homeopathic remedies ignores the role of homeopathy as a discrete medical system. A fully qualified homeopath is competent to work in a variety of roles ranging from an independent consultant in private practice to an integrated member of a team of healthcare practitioners working in a clinical setting.

Homeopaths usually explore every chronic case in great detail. This helps them to identify psychological traits and predispositions of a patient even before they become psychologically ill. The early treatment, effective use of the therapeutic relationship and homeopathic counselling (see related chapter in this volume) can help prevent progression of many cases towards full-blown mental illness. The focus of homeopathy on 'curing the sick' (not just treating a disease in isolation) ensures that the overall health status of a patient is going to improve under homeopathic treatment, even when the patient consults for non-psychiatric chronic disorders, and thus many complex psychological disorders may be pre-empted by effective homeopathic treatment.

All of this leads us to argue that homeopathy should be made available as part of the primary health care in all countries. This can help reduce not just the global mental health burden but the overall global health burden.

Integration should allow both conventional and homeopathic physicians to work together and refer cases to each other. Patients should be allowed to choose whether they want only conventional health care or homeopathic treatment or both together. Since homeopathic medicines have shown to reduce the overall cost of treatment and continued dependency on chemical drugs, the overall financial burden due to health problems may drop significantly after such integration takes place. The integration of both systems in health care will also ensure that the patients are cared for optimally. Patients with mild disorders can be provided with homeopathic care at the onset and severe cases needing immediate symptomatic palliation may be referred for allopathic care or managed collectively. In all cases, homeopathic care can be later introduced simultaneously in an effort to wean the patient off chemical drugs and to try to bring about a restoration of health.

Effective integration will also require changes in the mindset and practices in both conventional medicine and homeopathy. There needs to be a less mutually antagonistic and adversarial attitude between practitioners of both conventional and complementary medicine. For this, the medical profession needs to be more familiar with the multifaceted aspects of complementary medicine and their therapeutic practices through education and a change in the medical curriculum. The funding agencies for research should also provide more resources than they are doing at the moment so that basic research and clinical trials can be carried out to establish a sound scientific basis for homeopathy.

In 1995, the Council of Europe published a resolution on non-conventional medicine [151], which stresses the need for such integration and makes some salient suggestions. In it, the Council stated that:

- The various forms of medicine should not compete with one another: it is possible for them to exist side by side and complement one another;
- A common European approach to non-conventional medicine based on the principle of patients' freedom of choice in healthcare should not be ruled out;
- The best guarantee for patients lies in a properly trained profession, which is aware of its limitations, has a system of ethics and self-regulation and is also subject to outside oversight;
- Member states should model their approach on their neighbours' experiments and, whenever possible, co-ordinate their position with regard to these medicines;
- Alternative or complementary forms of medicine could be practised by doctors of conventional medicine as well as by any well-trained practitioner of non-conventional medicine (a patient could consult one or the other, either upon referral by his or her family doctor or on his or her own initiative), in the context of formalized, codified and prevailing ethical principles;
- As knowledge of alternative forms of medicine and CAM in general is still relatively limited, member states should support and speed up comparative studies and research programmes currently under way in the European Union and to disseminate the findings widely.

Conventional medicine advocates and policy makers around the world need to realize that this is not a fight for supremacy between different medical systems. Every doctor, of every medical system, wants his/her patients to improve. But the tools that we have in our hands sometimes restrict us from doing the best for the patient. Bringing together the best of all medical systems can help reduce the suffering of billions of people around the world.

6   Conclusion

The human population is increasing as are the factors (like high population density, poverty, homelessness, drug abuse, war etc) which affect its mental health. Developments in the last century have created new challenges and have precipitated new forms of diseases and newer epidemics of chronic diseases. Medical science has evolved greatly over the last 50 years, but developments in psychiatric medicine have utterly failed to reduce the global mental health burden. In fact, the burden has grown enormously. Chemical drug-based intervention has failed to improve the mental health of the general population and its role appears limited to symptomatic palliation in grave cases. Many researchers believe that the excessive use of chemical drugs is itself an important factor in increasing mental disorders in the population.

Homeopathy, one of the most commonly used CAM therapies, has focused on the mental health of its patients for more than 200 years. Its holistic approach, recording of mental symptoms during drug provings, and the importance it places on the mental and emotional symptoms in every disease, make it a strong candidate for inclusion in global mental health care policies. Scientific research is continuously adding vital data which indicates that homeopathy is effective in large number of diseases, including mental disorders like anxiety, depression, ADHD, autism, stress, insomnia etc. Research has also shown that there is greater patient satisfaction during homeopathic care, that homeopathic medicines are safe, and that they reduce the overall cost of treatment.

There is a need for integration of homeopathy in the primary health care and mental health care globally. The challenge is to find ways to effectively use the strengths of both conventional medicine and homeopathy together for the benefit of the sick human population. The focus of different systems of medicine and treatment should not be directed at finding faults with one another. Rather, there should be a collective effort to learn what is good in each system and then use it effectively for the betterment of our patients. Researchers and physicians from different therapies should come together to develop better patient care protocols. To most CAM practitioners, these words may seem like a dream but as Anais Nin has said:

> *"Dreams pass into the reality of action. From the actions stems the dream again;*
> *and this interdependence produces the highest form of living."*

So let us come together to reduce the mental and emotional suffering of our fellow humans, let us work together to give our children a better tomorrow, a healthier tomorrow – a tomorrow where life is not constantly dependent on drugs!

References

[1] World Health Organization (2007) What is Mental Health? World Health Organization. Geneva. [online] Available at http://www.who.int/features/qa/62/en/index.html (accessed 26 May 2009)

[2] Kiloh LG, Andrews G, Neilson MD. The long-term outcome of depression. *Br J Psychiatry* 1988;153:7527.

[3] Üstün TB, Sartorius N. (1995) *Mental Illness in General Health Care*. Chichester: John Wiley & Sons

[4] Whitaker, R. (2005) Anatomy of an Epidemic: Psychiatric Drugs and the Astonishing Rise of Mental Illness in America. *Ethical Human Psychology and Psychiatry* 2005; 7, 1: 23-35

[5] World Health Organization (2001) *World Health Report 2001*. World Health Organization. Geneva. [online] Available at http://www.who.int/whr/2001/en/index.html (accessed 26 May 2009)

[6] World Health Organization (2005) *Traditional Medicine Strategies: 2002 – 2005*. World Health Organization. Geneva. [online] Available at http://apps.who.int/medicinedocs/fr/d/Js2297e/7.4.html (accessed 26 May 2009)

[7] World Heath Organization (2001) *Legal Status of Traditional Medicine and Complementary/Alternative Medicine*: A Worldwide Review. World Health Organization. Geneva. [online] Available at http://apps.who.int/medicinedocs/en/d/Jh2943e/3.3.html (accessed 26 May 2009)

[8] World Health Organization (2003) *The Mental Health Context*. World Health Organization. Geneva. [online] Available at http://www.who.int/mental_health/policy/services/3_context_WEB_07.pdf (accessed 26 May 2009)

[9] National Alliance on Mental Illness (2008) *The Numbers Count: Mental Disorders in America*. [online] Available at http://www.nimh.nih.gov/health/publications/the-numbers-count-mental-disorders-in-america/index.shtml (accessed 26 May 2009)

[10] Yeargin-Allsopp M, Rice C, Karapurkar T, Doernberg N, Boyle C, Murphy C. Prevalence of Autism in a US Metropolitan Area. *The Journal of the American Medical Association*. 2003; 289(1): 49-55

[11] World Health Organization (2008) *European Pact for Mental Health and Well Being*, 2008. World Health Organization. Geneva. [online] Available at http://ec.europa.eu/health/ph_determinants/life_style/mental/docs/pact_en.pdf (accessed 26 May 2009)

[12] Andlin-Sobocki P, Jönsson B, Wittchen H-U et al. (2005) Costs of disorders of the brain in Europe. *Eur J Neurol* 2005;12(suppl 1)

[13] World Health Organization (2004) *Global burden of disease estimates*. Geneva, 2004. [online] Available at http://www.who.int/healthinfo/global_burden_disease/2004_report_update/en/index.html (accessed 18 May 2009)

[14] Murray CJL, Lopez AD, eds (1996) *The global burden of disease: a comprehensive assessment of mortality and disability from diseases, injuries and risk factors in 1990 and projected to 2020*. Cambridge, MA, Harvard School of Public Health on behalf of the World Health Organization and the World Bank

[15] Desjarlais R, Eisenberg L, Good B, Kleinman A (1995) *World mental health: problems and priorities in low-income countries*. New York: Oxford University Press

[16] World Health Organization (2005) *Mental Health Atlas 2005*. World Health Organization. Geneva. [online] www.who.int/mental_health/evidence/atlas/index.htm (accessed 9 May 2009)

[17] Saxena S, Maulik P.K. (2003) Mental health services in low-and- middle income countries – an overview. *Current Opinion of Psychiatry*. 2003; 16(4): 437-442

[18] Kohn R, Saxena S, Levav I, Saraceno B (2004) The treatment gap in mental health care. *Bulletin of the World Health Organization* 2004; 82(11): 858 – 866

[19] The WHO World Mental Health Survey Consortium (2004) Prevalence, severity, and unmet need for treatment of mental disorders in the World Health Organization World Mental Health Survey. JAMA 2004; 291(21): 2581-1590

[20] Smith, A. (1969) Studies on the effectiveness of antidepressant drugs. *Pscyhopharmacology Bulletin* 1996; 5: 1-20

[21] Dinnerstein, A., Lowenthal, M., & Blitz, B. (1966) The interaction of drugs with placebos in the control of pain and anxiety. *Perspectives in Biology and Medicine* 196; 10: 103-117

[22] Elkin, I. (1990) National Institute of Mental Health treatment of depression collaborative research program: General effectiveness of treatments. *Archives of General Psychiatry* 1990; 46: 971-982

[23] Greenberg, R., & Fisher, S. (1997) *Mood-mending medicines: Probing drug, psychotherapy and placebo solutions*. New York: John Wiley & Sons

[24] Blackburn, I. M., Eunson, K., St Bishop, S. (1986) A two-year naturalistic follow-up of depressed patients treated with cognitive therapy, pharmacotherapy and a combination of both. *Journal of Affective Disorders* 1986; 10: 67-75

[25] Fava, G. (1994) Do antidepressant and antianxiety drugs increase chronicity in affective disorders? *Psychotherapy and Psychosomatics* 1994; 61: 125-131

[26] Fava, G. (2003) Can long-term treatment with antidepressant drugs worsen the course of depression? *Journal of Clinical Psychiatry,* 64, 123-133

[27] Breggin, P. (2003) Suicidality, violence, and mania caused by selective serotonin reuptake inhibitor (SSRIs): A review and analysis. *International Journal of Risk and Safety in Medicine* 2003; 16: 31-49

[28] Bourguignon, R. (1997) Dangers of fluoxetine. *The Lancet* 1997; 394: 214

[29] Fava, G. (2003) Can long-term treatment with antidepressant drugs worsen the course of depression? *Journal of Clinical Psychiatry* 2003; 64: 123-133

[30] Preda A., MacLean C., Mazure C., & Bowers M. (2001) Antidepressant-associated mania and psychosis resulting in psychiatric admission. *Journal of Clinical Psychiatry* 2001; 62: 30-33

[31] Hammad TA (2004) *Review and evaluation of clinical data. Relationship between psychiatric drugs and pediatric suicidality*. FDA. 42; 115. [online] Available at http://www.fda.gov/OHRMS/DOCKETS/ac/04/briefing/2004-4065b1-10-TAB08-Hammads-Review.pdf (accessed 18 May 2009)

[32] Stone MB, Jones ML (2006) *Clinical review: relationship between antidepressant drugs and suicidality in adults*. Overview for Dec 13 Meeting of Psychopharmacologic Drugs Advisory Committee. FDA. 11–74. [online] Available at http://www.fda.gov/ohrms/dockets/ac/06/briefing/2006-4272b1-01-FDA.pdf (accessed 18 May 2009)

[33] Levenson M, Holland C (2006) *Statistical Evaluation of Suicidality in Adults Treated with Antidepressants*. Overview for Dec 13 Meeting of Psychopharmacologic Drugs Advisory Committee. FDA. 75–140. [online] Available at http://www.fda.gov/ohrms/dockets/ac/06/briefing/2006-4272b1-01-FDA.pdf (accessed 18 May 2009)

[34] Moncrieff J, Kirsch I. (2005) Efficacy of antidepressants in adults. *British Medical Journal* 2005; 331: 155-157

[35] National Institute of Mental Health Psychopharmacology Service Center Collaborative Study Group (1964) Phenothiazine treatment in acute schizophrenia. *Archives of General Psychiatry* 1964, 10: 246-261

[36] Schooler N, Goldberg S, Boothe H, & Cole J (1967) One year after discharge: Community adjustment of schizophrenic patients. *American Journal of Psychiatry* 1967; 123: 986-995

[37] Prien R, Levine J, & Switalski R. (1971) Discontinuation of chemotherapy for chronic schizophrenics. *Hospital Community Psychiatry* 1971; 22: 20-23

[38] Carpenter WTI, McGlashan T, & Strauss J (1977) The treatment of acute schizophrenia without drugs: An investigation of some current assumption. *American Journal of Psychiatry* 1977; 134: 14-20

[39] Rappaport, M., Hopkins, H., Hall, K., Belleza, T., & Silverman, J. (1978) Are there schizophrenics for whom drugs may be unnecessary or contraindicated. *International Pharmacopsychiatry*, 1978; 13: 100-111

[40] Bola, J. & Mosher, L. (2003) Treatment of acute psychosis without neuroleptics : Two-year outcomes from the Soteria project. *Journal of Nervous and Mental Disorders* 2003; 19I: 219-29

[41] Jablensky, A., Sartorius, N., Ernberg, G., Ansker, M., Korten, A., Cooper J., et al. (1992) Schizophrenia: Manifestations, incidence and course in different cultures. A World Health Organization ten-country study. Psychological Medicine 1992; Suppl. 20: 1095

[42] Leff, J., Sartorius, N., Jablensky, A., Korten, A., & Ernberg, G. (1992) The international pilot study of schizophrenia: Five-year follow-up findings. *Psychological Medicine* 1992; 22: 131-145

[43] Chakos, M., Lieberman, J., Bilder, R., Borenstein, M., Lerner, M., Bogerts, B., et at. (1994) Increase in caudate nuclei volumes of first-episode schizophrenic patients taking antipsychotic drugs. *American Journal of Psychiatry* 1994; 151: 1430-36

[44] Gur, R., Cowell, P., Turetsky, B., Gallacher, E, Cannon, T., Bilker, W (1998) A follow-up magnetic resonance imaging study of schizophrenia. *Archives of General Psychiatry* 1998; 55: 142-152

[45] Madsen, A., Keiding, A., Karle, A., Esbjerg, S., & Hemmingsen, R. (1998) Neuroleptics in progressive structural brain abnormalities in psychiatric illness. *The Lancet* 1998; 352: 784-785

[46] Our, R., lvfaany, V., Ivlozley, D., Swanson, C., Bilker, W., & Gur, R. (1998) Subcortical MP. I volumes in neuroleptic-naïve and treated patients with schizophrenia. *American Journal of Psychianry* 1998; 55: 1711-17

[47] Ballenger, J., Burrows, G., DuPont, R., Lesser, I., Noyes, R., Pecknold, J., et a1. (1988) Alprazolam in panic disorder and agoraphobia: Results from a multi-center trial. *Archives of General Psychiatry* 1988; 45: 413-421

[48] Marks, I. (1993) Alpraolam and exposure alone and combined in panic disorder with agoraphobia. *British Journal of Psychiatry* 1993; 162: 790-794

[49] Pecknold, J. C. (1988) Alprazolam in panic disorder and agoraphobia: Results from a multicenter trial: Discontinuation effects. *Archives of General Psychiatry* 1998; 45: 429-436

[50] Healy D, Harris M, Michael P, Cattell D, Savage M, Chalasani P, et al. (2001) *Treating more patients than ever before: 1896 and 1996 compared.* Unpublished manuscript

[51] Dean ME. (2004) *The Trials of Homeopathy.* Essen, Germany: KVC Verlag

[52] Coulter H.L. (1977) *Divided Legacy.* Berkeley: North Atlantic Books

[53] Mintel Marketing Intelligence. (2008) *Complementary and Alternative Medicines* - US - July 2008. Chicago: Mintel Group.

[54] Fisher P, Ward A (1994) Complementary Medicine in Europe. *British Medical Journal* 1994; 309: 107-110

[55] AYUSH, 2007. *Summary of Infrastructure Facilities Under Ayurveda, Yoga, Naturopathy, Unani, Siddha and Homeopathy as on 1.4.2007.* [online] Available at http://indianmedicine.nic.in/summary-of-infrastructure.asp (accessed 27 May 2009)

[56] Lo, Shui-Yin (1996) Anomalous state of ice. *Modern Physics* Letters B vol 10, 19:909-919

[57] Shui-Yin Lo, Angelo Lo, Li Wen Chong, Lin Tianzhang, Li Hui Hua, Xu Geng (1996) Physical properties of water with IE structures. *Modern Physics* Letters B vol 10, 19:921-930

[58] Woutersen S, U Emmerichs, H J Bakker (1997) Femtosecond Mid-IR pump probe spectroscopy of liquid water: evidence for a two-component structure. *Science,* 278:658-660

[59] Bonavida B. (1998) 'Induction and regulation of human peripheral blood TH1-TH2 derived cytokines by IE water preparations and synergy with mitogens', in: S. Y. Lo and B. Bonavida eds, *Physical, chemical and biological properties of stable water IE clusters,* Singapore, World Scientific, p. 167-83

[60] Elia, Vittorio & Marcella Nicoli (1999) Thermodynamics of extremely diluted aqueous solutions. *Tempos in Science and Nature, Annals of the New York Academy of Sciences,* vol 879: 241-247

[61] Louis Rey (2003) Thermoluminescence of ultra-high dilutions of lithium chloride and sodium chloride. *Physica A: Statistical mechanics and its applications,* Vol 323, 67-74, DOI 10.1016/S0378-4371(03)00047-5

[62] Bell IR, Lewis DA 2nd, Brooks AJ, Lewis SE, Schwartz GE (2003) Gas discharge visualisation evaluation of ultramolecular doses of homeopathic medicines under blinded, controlled conditions. *Journal of Alternative and Complementary Medicine,* 9:25–38.

[63] Anick DJ (2004) High sensitivity 1H-NMR spectroscopy of homeopathic remedies made in water. *BMC Complementary and Alternative Medicine,* 4:15

[64] Elia V, Niccoli M (2004) New physico-chemical properties of extremely diluted aqueous solutions. *Journal of Thermal Analysis and Calorimetry,* 75: 815–836

[65] Roy R, Tiller WA, Bell IR, Hoover MR (2005) The structure of liquid water; novel insights from materials research; potential relevance to homeopathy. *Materials Research Innovations,* 9-4:577–608

[66] Hahnemann S. (1849) *The Organon of Medicine,* 5th ed: 109. Dudgeon RE (tr) London: W Davy & sons

[67] Ibid, 265

[68] Ibid, 266

[69] Bradford TL (1970), *The Life and Letters of Hahnemann,* 52-55. Calcutta: Roy Publishing House.

[70] Hahnemann S. (1849) *The Organon of Medicine,* 5th ed: 267-268. Dudgeon RE (tr) London: W Davy & sons

[71] Burke MA, Matlin SA (2008) *Monitoring Financial Flows for Health Research 2008: Prioritizing research for health equity.* [online] Available at http://www.globalforumhealth.org/en/content/download/480/3028/file/s14888e.pdf (accessed 27 May 2009)

[72] Tilburt JC, Kaptchuk TJ (2008) Herbal medicine research and global health: an ethical analysis. *Bulletin of the World Health Organization* 2008; 86: 594–599

[73] Sadock BJ, Sadock VA (Editor) 2000. *Kaplan & Sadock's Comprehensive Textbook of Psychiatry*. 7th ed. Batlimore: Lippincott Williams & Wilkins Publishers.

[74] Kleijnen J, Knipschild P, Ter Riet G (1991) Clinical trials of homoeopathy. *British Medical Journal*. 1991; 302: 316-23

[75] Reilly D, Taylor MA, Beattie NGM, Campbell JH, McSharry C, Aitchison TC, Carter R, Stevenson RD (1994) Is evidence for homoeopathy reproducible? *The Lancet*. 1994; 344: 1601-1606

[76] Linde K, Jonas WB, Melchart D, Worku F, Wagner H, Eital F (1994) Critical Review and Meta-Analysis of Serial Agitated Dilutions in Experimental Toxicology. *Human and Experimental Toxicology*. 1994; 13: 481-492

[77] European Commission (1996) *Report to the European Commission Directorate General XII: science, research and development*. Vol 1 (short version). Brussels: European Commission, 1996: 16-17

[78] Linde K, Clausius N, Ramirez G, et al (1997) Are the clinical effects of homoeopathy placebo effects? A meta-analysis of placebo-controlled trials. *The Lancet* 1997; 350: 834-43

[79] Cucherat, M., Haugh, M. C., Gooch, M., & Boissel, J. P. (2000) Evidence of clinical efficacy of homeopathy. A meta-analysis of clinical trials. HMRAG. Homeopathic Medicines Research Advisory Group, *Eur J Clin Pharmacol.*, 2003; 56,1: 27-33

[80] Mathie, R (2003) The research evidence base for homeopathy: a fresh assessment of the literature. *Homeopathy* 2003; 92: 84-91

[81] Jonas WB, Kaptchuk TJ, & Linde K. (2003), A critical overview of homeopathy, *Ann Intern Med*, 2003; 138, 5: 393-399

[82] Ullman D. (2003) Controlled Clinical Trials Evaluating the Homeopathic Treatment of People with Human Immunodeficiency Virus or Acquired Immune Deficiency Syndrome. *The Journal of Alternative and Complementary Medicine*, 2003; 9,1: 133-141

[83] Boarnhoft G, Wolf U, Ammon K, Righetti M, Maxion-Bergemann S, Baumgartner S, Thurneysen AE, Matthiessen PF. Effectiveness, safety and cost-effectiveness of homeopathy in general practice – summarized health technology assessment. *Forsch Komplementarmed*. 2006; 13 Suppl 2: 19-29

[84] Stanton HE. (1981) Test anxiety - a five-drop solution. *Educ News* 1981; 17: 12–15

[85] Heulluy B, (1985) Essai Randomise Ouvert de L.72 (specialité homeopathique) *Contre Diazepam 2 dans les Etats Anxio-Depressifs*. Metz, Laboratoires Lehning

[86] Alibeu JP, Jobert J. (1990) Aconite in homeopathic relief of postoperative pain and agitation in children. *Pediatrie* 1990; 45: 465–466

[87] Hariveau E, Rufo M, Albertini C. (1991) Lithium Microsol dans le stress de l'ecolier. *Homeopathie Française* 1991; 79: 56–58

[88] Clover A, Last P, Fisher P, Wright S, Boyle H.(1995) Complementary cancer therapy: a pilot study of patients, therapies and quality of life. *Complement Ther Med* 1995; 3: 129–133

[89] McCutcheon L.(1996) Treatment of anxiety with a homeopathic remedy. *J Appl Nutr* 1996; 48: 2–6

[90] Davidson J, Morrison R, Shore J, et al., (1997) Homeopathic Treatment of Depression and Anxiety. *Alternative Therapies* 1997; 3,1: 46-49

[91] Zenner S, Weiser M. (1999) Homeopathic treatment of gynecological disorders: results of a prospective study. *Biomed Ther* 1999; 17: 31–35

[92] Thompson EA, Reilly D.(2002) The Homeopathic Approach to Symptom Control in the Cancer Patient: A Prospective Observational Study, *Palliative Medicine* 2002; 16(3):227-33

[93] Baker DG, Myers SP, Howden I, Brooks L. (2003) The effects of homeopathic Argentum nitricum on test anxiety. *Complement Ther Med* 2003; 11: 65–71

[94] Bonne O, Shemer Y, Gorali Y, Katz M, Shalev YA (2003) A Randomized, Double-blind, Placebo-controlled Study of Classical Homeopathy in Generalized Anxiety Disorder. *J Clin Psychiatry* 2003; 64(3): 282-7

[95] Thompson EA, Reilly D. (2003) The homeopathic approach to the treatment of symptoms of oestrogen withdrawal in breast cancer patients. A prospective observational study. *Homeopathy* 2003; 92: 131–134

[96] van den Meerschaut L, Sunder A. (2007) The Homeopathic Preparation Nervoheel N can Offer an Alternative to Lorazepam Therapy for Mild Nervous Disorders. *eCAM*, October 25, 2007. coi:10.1093/ecam/nem144

[97] Pilkington et al. (2006) Homeopathy for anxiety and anxiety disorders: A systematic review of the research. *Homeopathy* 2006; 95: 151-162

[98] Lamont, J. (1997) Homeopathic Treatment of Attention Deficit Hyperactivity Disorder. *British Homeopathic Journal* 1997; 86: 196-200

[99] Frei H, Thurneysen A. (2001) Treatment for hyperactive children: homeopathy and methylphenidate compared in a family setting. *British Homeopathic Journal*, 2001; 90:183-188

[100] Frei H, Everts R, von Ammon K, Kaufmann F, Walther D, Hsu-Schmitz SF, Collenberg M, Fuhrer K, Hassink R, Steinlin M, Thurneysen A. (2005) Homeopathic treatment of children with attention deficit hyperactivity disorder: a randomised, double-blind, placebo controlled crossover trial. *Eur J Pediatr.*, 2005;164: 758-767

[101] Frei H, Everts R, von Ammon K, Kaufmann F, Walther D, Schmitz SF, Collenberg M, Steinlin M, Lim C, Thurneysen A. (2007) Randomised controlled trials of homeopathy in hyperactive children: treatment procedure leads to an unconventional study design. Experience with open-label homeopathic treatment preceding the Swiss ADHD placebo-controlled, randomised, double-blind, crossover trial. *Homeopathy* 2007; 96(1): 35-41

[102] Bakshi, JPS. (1990) Homoeopathy - A New Approach to Detoxification. *Proceedings of the National Congress on Homoeopathy and Drug Abuse*, p-20-28. New Delhi, India

[103] Garcia-Swain S, (1993) *A Double-Blind, Placebo-Controlled Trial Applying Homeopathy to Chemical Dependency.* Hahnemann College of Homeopathy, Albany, California: Hahnemann etc.

[104] CCRH. (1994) *Clinical evaluation of homoeopathic medicines in the management of withdrawal symptoms of drug dependents.* [online] Available at http://www.ccrhindia.org/abstracts/cr/drugdependents.htm. (accessed 27 May 2009)

[105] Waldschütz R, Klein P (2008) The homeopathic preparation Neurexan vs. valerian for the treatment of insomnia: an observational study. *Scientific World Journal* 2008; 8:411-20

[106] Reis LS, Pardo PE, Oba E, Kronka SN, Frazatti-Gallina NM (2006). Matricaria chamomilla CH(12) decreases handling stress in Nelore calves. *J Vet Sci.* 2006; 7(2): 189-92

[107] ECCH (2007) *Positive Homeopathy Research and Surveys.* [online]
Available at http://www.homeopathy-ecch.org/content/view/33/49/ (accessed 9 May 2009)

[108] Brigo B, Serpelloni G (1991) Homeopathic treatment of migraine: a randomized double-blind controlled study of sixty cases. *Berlin Journal of Research in Homeopathy.* 1(2):98-106

[109] Christie EA, Ward AT (1994) *Report on a Homoeopathy Project in an NHS Practice. Covering 18 month period from February 1993 to August 1994.* Northampton: The Society of Homeopaths

[110] Andersen HE, Eldov P. (1995) *En undersøgelse af Klassisk Homøpati - teorier, praksis og brugererfaringer.* Forskningsrapport udgivet på anbefaling af sundhedsstyrelsens Råd vedrørende Alternativ behandling, København 1999

[111] Christie EA, Ward AT (1996) *Report on NHS practice-based homoeopathy project. Analysis of effectiveness and cost of homoeopathic treatment within a GP practice at St. Margaret's Surgery, Bradford on Avon, Wilts.* Northampton: The Society of Homeopaths

[112] Richardson J. (1996) *Quasi-randomised control trial to assess the outcome of acupuncture, osteopathy and homoeopathy using the short-form 36-item health survey.* Health Services Research and Evaluation Unit, The Lewisham Hospital NHS Trust. December 1996

[113] Dempster, A (1998) *Homoeopathy within the NHS. Evaluation of homoeopathic treatment of common mental health problems. 1995 - 1997.* Rydings Hall Surgery, Brighouse, West Yorkshire. Society of Homeopaths 1998

[114] Kuzeff, RM (1998) Homeopathy, sensation of well-being and CD4 levels: a placebo-controlled, randomized trial. *Comp Therapies in Medicine.* 6(1):4-9

[115] F. Attena et al. (2000) Homeopathy in Primary Care: self-reported change in health status. *Complementary therapies in Medicine* 2000; 8,1

[116] Sevar, R. (2000) Audit of outcome in 829 consecutive patients treated with homeopathic medicine. *British Homeopathic Journal* 2004; 89,4

[117] Güthlin C, Lange O and Walach H. (2004) Measuring the effects of acupuncture and homoeopathy in general practice: An uncontrolled prospective documentation approach. *BMC Public Health* 2004; 4:6

[118] Spence DS, Thompson EA, Barron SJ. (2005) Homeopathic Treatment for Chronic Disease: A 6-Year, University-Hospital Outpatient Observational Study. *The Journal of Alternative and Complementary Medicine* 2005; 11,5:793-798

[119] Steinsbekk, A. (2005) Patients' assessments of the effectiveness of homeopathic care in Norway: A prospective observational multi-centre outcome study. *Homeopathy* 2005; 94,1:10-16

[120] Witt CM, Luedtke R, Baur R, Willich SN. (2005) Homeopathic Medical Practice: Long-term results of a Cohort Study with 3981 Patients. *BMC Public Health* 2005; 5:115

[121] Holt S, Gilbey A. (2009) Beliefs about homeopathy among patients presenting at GP surgeries, *New Zealand Medical Journal*, Vol 122 No,1295

[122] Bastide M (ed). (1997) *Signals and Images*, 161-170. Dordrecht: Kluwer Academic Publishers

[123] Jonas W., Lin Yu, Tortella F. (2001) Neuroprotection from glutamate toxicity with ultra-low dose glutamate. *NeuroReport* 12: 335-339, 2001

[124] Rey L. (2003) Thermoluminescence of ultra-high dilutions of lithium chloride and sodium chloride. *Physica A* 2003; 323: 67–74

[125] Lorenz I, Schneider EM, Stolz P, Brack A, Strube J. (2003) Sensitive flow cytometric method to test basophil activation influenced by homeopathic histamine dilutions. *Forsch Komplementarmed Klass Naturheilkd* 2003; 10(6): 316-24

[126] Datta S, Biswas SJ, Khuda-Bukhsh AR (2004) Comparative efficacy of pre-feeding, post-feeding and combined pre- and post-feeding of two microdoses of a potentized homeopathic drug, Mercurius solubilis, in ameliorating genotoxic effects produced by mercuric chloride in mice. *EvidencepBased Complementary and Alternatative Medicine*, 1:291–300

[127] Belon P, Cumps J, Ennis M, Mannaioni PF, Roberfroid M, Sainte-Laudy J, Wiegant FAC. (2004) Histamine dilutions modulate basophil activation. *Inflamm Res* 2004; 53:181-188

[128] Dominici G, Bellavite P, di Stanislao C, Gulia P, Pitari G. (2006) Double-blind, placebo-controlled homeopathic pathogenetic trials: Symptom collection and analysis. *Homeopathy*, 2006; 96:123-130

[129] Ellanzhiyil et al. (2009) Dynamized Preparations in Cell Culture. *eCAM* 2009;6(2)257–263

[130] Dantas F, Rampes H. (2000) Do homeopathic medicines provoke adverse effects? A systematic review. *Br Homeopath J* 2000; 89: S35–8

[131] Kassab S, Cummings M, Berkovitz S, van Haselen R, Fisher P. (2009) Homeopathic medicines for adverse effects of cancer treatments. *Cochrane Database of Systematic Reviews* 2009; 2. Art. No.: CD004845. DOI: 10.1002/14651858.CD004845.pub2

[132] Swayne J. (1992) The cost-effectiveness of homoeopathy. A pilot study, proposals for future research. *Br Homoeopath J* 1992; 81: 148–150

[133] Schafer T, Riehle A, Wichmann HE, Ring J. (2002) Alternative medicine in allergies - prevalence, patterns of use, and costs. *Allergy* 2002; 57: 694–700

[134] Frenkel M, Hermoni D (2002) Effects of homeopathic intervention on medication consumption in atopic and allergic disorders. *Altern Ther Health Med*. 2002; 8(1): 76-9

[135] Jain A. (2003) Does homeopathy reduce the cost of conventional drug prescribing? A study of comparative prescribing costs in General Practice. *Homeopathy* 2003; 92, 71-76

[136] Witt C, Keil T, Selim D, Roll S, Vance W, Wegscheider K, Willich SN. (2005) Outcome and costs of homoeopathic and conventional treatment strategies: A comparative cohort study in patients with chronic disorders. *Complementary Therapies in Medicine* 2005; 13, 79-86

[137] Varshney P, Naresh R (2005) Comparative efficacy of homeopathic and allopathic systems of medicine in the management of clinical mastitis of Indian dairy cows. *Homeopathy* 2005; 94, 2: 81-5

[138] Manchanda RK, Kulhashreshtha M (2005) Cost effectiveness and efficacy of homeopathy in primary health care units of the Government of Delhi - a study. Germany: LIGA 2005

[139] Rossi et al. (2009) Cost–benefit evaluation of homeopathic versus conventional therapy in respiratory diseases. *Homeopathy* 2009; 98, 1: 2-10

[140] Caulfield T, DeBow S (2005) A systematic review of how homeopathy is represented in conventional and CAM peer-reviewed journals. *BMC Complement Altern Med*. 2005; 5: 12

[141] Rosenthal, R (1998) Covert Communication in Classrooms, Clinics, and Courtrooms. *Eye on Psi Chi*. Vol. 3, No. 1, pp. 18-22

[142] Micozzi, M S. (2001) Double Standards and Double Jeopardy for CAM Research. *The Journal of Alternative and Complementary Medicine*, February 2001, 7(1): 13-14

[143] Shang A, Huwiler-Müntener K, Nartey L, et al. Are the clinical effects of homoeopathy placebo effects? Comparative study of placebo-controlled trials of homoeopathy and allopathy. *The Lancet* 2005; 366: 726–732

[144] Lüdtke R, Rutten ALB. The conclusions on the effectiveness of homeopathy highly depend on the set of analyzed trials. *J Clin Epidemiol*, Oct 2008; 61: 1197-1204

[145] Rutten ALB, Stolper CF. The 2005 meta-analysis of homeopathy: the importance of post-publication data. *Homeopathy*, Oct 2008; 97: 169-177

[146] St. George, D. (1994) Research into complementary medicine. *Advances*, 10(3): 69-92

[147] Bower H. (1998) Double standards exist in judging traditional and alternative medicine. *BMJ* 1998; 316:1694

[148] Barr, Noam. *Homeopathy and the Question of Evidence Base.* [online]
Available at http://www.noambar.co.uk/assets/research_review.pdf (accessed 16 Jun 2009)
[149] Dean ME. (2004) *The Trials of Homeopathy* P-228. Essen, Germany: KVC Verlag
[150] Lewith G, Jonas WB, and Walach H. (2003) *Clinical Research in Complementary Therapies: Principles, Problems, and Solutions,* London: Churchill-Livingston, 2003
[151] Council of Europe (1999) *A European approach to non-conventional medicines,* Resolution 1206 (1999)

Chapter 2
The Homeopathic Healing Process, Transformational Outcomes, and the Patient-Provider Relationship

Iris R. Bell MD PhD MD(H)[1 2 3 4 5] and Mary Koithan RN PhD[1 4 6]

From the Departments of Family and Community Medicine,[1] Psychiatry,[2] Psychology,[3] Medicine (Integrative Medicine)[4] at the College of Medicine; the College of Public Health;[5] and the College of Nursing,[6] The University of Arizona, Tucson, AZ USA

Iris R. Bell, MD PhD MD(H)
Mary Koithan, RN PhD
Department of Family and Community Medicine
The University of Arizona College of Medicine
1450 N. Cherry Avenue, MS 245052
Tucson, AZ 85719 USA
E-mail: ibell@u.arizona.edu

Abstract
This chapter summarizes the nature of transformational change from the broader literature and the perspective of classical homeopathy. Concepts of dynamical unstuckness and global and local transformation often emerge in the course of homeopathic treatment of chronic complex conditions. We present exemplar cases of sustained person-wide transformational change documented during successful homeopathic treatment of individuals with a variety of major psychiatric and/or psycho-physiological disorders. Finally, we propose a unique whole-person therapeutic role for the patient-provider relationship within the context of homeopathic treatment in fostering unstuckness and comprehensive transformational change.

"...Success came everywhere. I almost thought I could raise the dead."
- Constantine Hering, MD, upon discovering the effectiveness of homeopathy in his clinical practice
(quotation, p. 31)[1]

1   Overview of transformational change
As the quotation from Hering above illustrates, providers and patients often express a sense of amazement and awe when they see and/or experience the profound and comprehensive changes that homeopathic treatment can initiate. What is the human experience of this type of transformative change? How can we understand homeopathic transformation in the context of the broader literature on the change process?

The purpose of this chapter is to (a) summarize the broader literature on the nature of transformation as it overlaps and diverges with clinical reports in homeopathy; (b) present several exemplar cases of sustained person-wide transformational change that emerged during successful homeopathic treatment of individuals whose conventional medical diagnoses included major psychiatric and/or psycho-physiological disorders; and (c) use these observations to point out a unique therapeutic role for the patient-provider relationship within homeopathic treatment in fostering unstuckness and comprehensive transformational change in persons with chronic conditions.

"Transform" originates from the Latin noun trans which means across or beyond and *forma* which means "bodily form, build, shape or appearance" [2]. Transformation is currently defined as a change in form, appearance or structure; "a metamorphosis wherein condition, nature or character is wholly altered" [3]. Although the word "transformation" can apply to dramatic changes in physical structure, the term also applies to dramatic changes in function or behavioural process.

In the mainstream literature, transformation often, but not always, addresses sudden profound spiritual or mystical insights. Miller [4] identified two primary types of quantum change: insightful and mystical. With insightful change, "the person comes to a new realization, a new way of thinking or understanding that ... break upon the person's consciousness with particular clarity and forcefulness" (p. 18). Insightful change often develops from everyday life experiences but stand out as particularly memorable instances of revelation. While they can be distinguished from everyday decision-making and reasoning by their lightening bolt nature, they are not far removed from normal, everyday "aha" experiences.

Mystical transformations are more difficult to comprehend and to understand; Miller described them as intense and overwhelming, perhaps similar to the spiritual transformation that Pargament [5,6] describes. "The person knows immediately that something major has happened and that life will never be the same again. There is no question about it and ... no choice" (p. 20). Often the mystical quantum change is uninvited, but nonetheless real and pivotal. Miller [4] identified nine attributes of mystical quantum change, including (a) ineffability, (b) noetic[1] quality, (c) transiency, (d) passivity, (e) unity, (f) transcendence, (g) awe, (h) positivity, and (i) distinctiveness.

Miller's [4,7] research did not find any difference between subjects experiencing insightful and mystical quantum change. He did find that those experiencing mystical change could: (a) remember the time of day of the occurrence, (b) felt completely loved and felt themselves to be in the presence of a powerful other, (c) heard a voice associated with the timing of the change, (d) identified that prayers were being offered for them, and (e) identified the change as a religious or spiritual experience.

Outcomes associated with both types of quantum change include: (a) change that went beyond change in a particular behaviour or characteristic—"everything" changes; (b) release from emotional patterns that were negative and longstanding; (c) an enduring sense of peace, calm and hope; (d) changes in core values and priorities; (e) increased clarity of values and life's purpose; (f) sudden changes in longstanding behavioural patterns, including a release from addictions; (g)

---

1 The word "noetic" comes from the ancient Greek *nous*, for which there is no exact equivalent in English. It refers to "inner knowing," a kind of intuitive consciousness—direct and immediate access to knowledge beyond what is available to our normal senses and the power of reason (http://www.noetic.org).

profound changes in the nature of and desire for relationships with others; (h) emotional detachment from harmful and negative interpersonal interactions; (i) deep individual sense of spirituality beyond religiosity to a personal commitment; and (j) commitment to a broader purpose and to the world in general.

2   Transformation in health care and homeopathy

Although homeopathic patients may report the types of quantum changes described by Miller (e.g., increased self-actualization or sense of purpose in life [8]), their experience of the change process appears to diverge in major ways from a purely insightful or mystical event. For homeopathy, transformation would involve an all-encompassing (global and local) dynamical change that includes marked shifts out of previous spiritual, social, mental, emotional, and physical symptom ruts into comprehensively healthier patterns of function (i.e., behaviours of the person as well as of the body parts). During the process, clinicians report that patients have a peculiar lack of self-awareness of what is happening to them and inability to describe their inner shifts with language [9]. People around the patient, including the homeopath, may notice the changes taking place, but the patient may not be able to recognize and/or describe the outcome until they emerge from the change process itself and reflect retrospectively on what occurred.

Research on remarkable recoveries may hold more direct relevance to homeopathically-triggered transformation than do the insightful or mystical event types of quantum change. For example, Hirshberg and Barasch [10] described a related phenomenon as "remarkable recovery," suggesting that lasting physical change may come about gradually as well as abruptly, including in conditions such as cancer. Such individuals with remarkable medical recoveries are people with confirmed disease who have "done extraordinarily well", living beyond statistical expectation, with regression or complete absence of disease, often holding off the natural progression of disease. Attributed to the unmapped system of the body and mind, the healing system, remarkable recovery constitutes a change in form and function that manifests within the physical domain. While suggesting several potential explanatory mechanisms, Hirshberg and Barasch identified that this phenomenon was complex, often uniquely expressed, non-linear, and profound. Identified manifestations of remarkable recovery included much more than remission of the physical illness: (a) belief/faith in cure, (b) hope, (c) personal choice to recover and survive, (d) a sense of awe and wonder, (e) expected physical changes, (f) heightened sense of perception and awareness, (g) thriving and flourishing and (h) energized. Further, they describe outcomes associated with miraculous recoveries stimulated by religious experiences [11,12] that include: (a) a perception of absolute love, (b) peace of heart, (c) forgiveness, (d) transcendence of the physical to experience a mystical oneness with the powerful, and (e) certainty of self in spite of the lack of immediate physical change that would follow months after the initial "healing" experience. These findings seem to overlap the descriptions of two types of transformative experiences offered by Miller and C'deBaca and Pargament, but extend into the physical domain as well.

Koithan, et al. [13] describe a process of transformative change found in various populations of 76 patients undergoing complementary and alternative medicine (CAM) treatment, including homeopathy, integrative oncology, and mind-body interventions. They propose a process of change that includes experiences of stuckness (repetitive ruts of dysfunctional status – e.g., see Sherr [14]), "unsticking" from the ruts during treatment, a transitional period of instability or "unstuckness," and, eventually, transformation as stages of this theoretical model of change [13].

As we discuss the homeopathic features of transformation, we will present three exemplar homeopathic cases to illustrate these stages of transformative change as lived and experienced. The patients and their homeopaths were interviewed as part of a larger qualitative research study on exceptional long-term outcomes during homeopathic care [13,15,16]. Each of these cases realized significant shifts across all planes of human existence following homeopathic treatments. Their stories reflect the changes that were experienced over the time of homeopathic care and the lived experiences of undergoing transformative change. These cases are not presented in the typical manner of a homeopathic case; rather they are used to portray the process of change that the patients reported in retrospect.

2.1 Case examples

Case 1

The first person, a woman who was in her mid-forties, described herself as having long-term depression (since early adolescence). She was eventually diagnosed with Bi-Polar Disorder and had been prescribed an array of antipsychotics/antidepressants for more than 20 years. She described her life prior to homeopathic treatment as "drama, drama, drama" with nothing that was "normal". She claims that she was totally unaware that others did not live with "hysterical crying for hours", "incessant motion – couldn't stop talking, couldn't stop moving, couldn't stop thinking, reading like a nut." The repetitive pattern in her speech was indicative of the continual repetition in her life and ultimately the repetitive or **stuck** pattern or "rut" that her life had become.

Things really started to shift or **unstick** approximately three years into the treatment when she had a major reaction to the carbamazepine she had been taking for several years. Described as an "overdose-type" reaction, the homeopath/psychiatrist decided to begin to discontinue her medications and "kick the remedies into high gear". She became very involved in yoga and meditation and things began to "change dramatically".

She described the next several years of homeopathic treatment as "traumatic". "Relationships were changing; people I was dating were changing; things started to shift." She was "unsticking" in multiple planes – social, emotional/psychological, mental, and physical. "I started seeing the world not revolving around me ... I started getting out of that framework where I saw everything as affecting me personally". True to an **unstuckness** period, not all responses were perceived as positive; rather things were simply changing – an experience she described as "bizarre". She started having allergic reactions to medications that she had taken for years. She described having "shakes and tremors", at times unable to focus "because my eyes were moving too quickly." And she would have periods where "everything felt very vivid and alive. At times I was feeling everything but it wasn't overwhelming me as it had in the past. I was able to move through things".

She describes a completely **transformed** life today. "I started to learn with homeopathy ... I'm able to see now where things are ... I'm able to sit here and watch and although I might experience a little craziness, I see it as a passing stage. Like I don't get attached to it one way or the other. I see these times as things to get through and I do things to make it easier. I don't see my world as falling part. Life's easier."

She also noted that over the course of treatment she was able to look back on her life and identify places where her life took on more and more "craziness ... places where my life seemed to spin out of control … The remedy allows you to put things into perspective, things that are already there, and it helps you to deal with them." One of the "things" that she dealt with was her sexuality. Today, she has made peace with her homosexuality and is a stable relationship for the first time.

Case 2

The second case sought homeopathic treatment because of multiple physical problems – allergic reactions, repeated sinus infections, migraines, pre and peri-menstrual symptoms and insomnia with night terrors. She describes herself as "highly strung with a high stress job". When describing the **stuck** patterns prior to homeopathic treatment she stated, "my migraines were getting worse. I mean really worse. Really bad. I kept getting them and it was so bad – really awful."
Following her first simillimum dose, she recalled that she was working and by noon she became "a basket case. I became very depressed and couldn't figure out what was wrong with me … It was to the point of crying – almost hysterically. And, it all started coming back to me … how unhappy my childhood was. I hadn't remembered much of it and there it was." The next several days, the **unsticking** continued. The night terrors intensified, "It was awful. Everything looked black. I had typically been a very positive person, but everything now looked very bleak, black and gray. It took all I had to get out of bed. I'd burst into tears because the memories kept coming back. I was a 48 year old body with a 4 year old mind."

When questioned if this depth of despair had been necessary or "worth it", the patient responded that "although it was awful, I would do it all again. I had to be unprogrammed. I wanted more than what I had in life. I wanted to understand. I had to look it in the face, the fear." The six to eight months that followed – the period of **unstuckness** – was an uncertain time. She stated, "there were days and days of choices – did I face this or not? Things kept coming up so I was trying to maintain an outward life while living through the terror of my life … I was there in body but I was not there in mind. It was a miracle that the whole thing happened." Within three months, she thought that the depression started to subside, "it was still bad … rough because I was still trying to work through things, make connections, forgive my father, but I was not completely dysfunctional like in the beginning. I knew I was getting better because I was interested in my outfits". "I was excited to go to work again." She continued to have revealing or "breakthrough" dreams that helped her "let the whole thing go". Her allergies began to subside, the depression was lifting and by month eight, things really started to improve.

She discusses her **transformed** life as "not a quick fix. I chose reality. I wanted my issues or symptoms to go away permanently. After two years, I now have no headaches, have not had any infections (that's a miracle), my relationships are on track and so much more whole." Referring to her life before homeopathic treatment she described failed marriages, fights with her family members, real issues with men, and her inability to have the spiritual relationship that she really desired. "I created a whole new life. It's like I woke up from a coma. My other life was the life before and that was no life. I didn't exist before."

Case 3

In the final case, a woman whose husband's military career had taken her to many exotic places describes 30 years of progressively worsening symptoms, including gastrointestinal discomfort with distention, bloating, poor appetite and eventually uncontrollable diarrhoea; insomnia; lack of energy; hepatomegaly and splenomegaly. She described the many medications that had been tried:

Flagyl, Cipro and others, "over and over again with no resolution". Eventually, she became socially isolated and described herself as fearful of social situations – first because of her uncontrollable symptoms and altered appearance and then because she hadn't been out of the house very much. "Things were looking pretty grim and this was not the life we planned to lead at all … I could not live a normal life." Yet, she "learned to live with all of it; accepted it as something I was just going to have to live with for the rest of my life. I stopped praying for a solution to it anymore because it had gone on for so long, I just couldn't believe there could be a solution." She was **stuck** – physically with never-ending symptoms, socially by her inability and fear of social situations, and emotionally because she could not imagine a life without these issues. "In the military, you're not a complainer. You just get on with what you have."

She first sought homeopathic treatment for a degenerating hip disorder, thinking that the treatment might be able to help with pain and immobility. During the intake history, she described her gastrointestinal issues and lack of energy with the homeopath as well as her "chief" complaint. Approximately one week after beginning the remedy, the patient suddenly noticed that "my stomach wasn't so noisy. It was dramatic – 30 years of noise so loud you could hear it across the room and well it just stopped". Following this **unsticking** moment, she described the course of several months where "the gears really started to shift".

"My memory of that time is just the overwhelming sense of relief that someone really understood what was going on. I began to move easier." She had a bit of a dry cottonmouth but the diarrhoea had begun to subside a little. Suddenly one day she went into the bathroom and she "expelled a huge parasite". She described the situation as "surreal", something she never expected, particularly after so many years. But given where she had lived, it made sense since the symptoms had begun when living in the Philippines. Following this, things were on the upswing – she began to volunteer at the hospital, began working more with the church, she travelled with her husband. She even described her hair as more full and thick. She was **unstuck**.

Today, her life "is a blessing"; she is living "a whole different [**transformed**] life". During a recent bilateral hip replacement at 84 years old, she reports that she was out of the hospital in three days with no transfusion and no real problems. She is walking now and living alone. Although her husband passed away several years ago, she had the energy and strength to care for him in their home – something she could never have done prior to treatment. She is involved in organizing a military volunteer program as well as continuing her work with her church. Her exuberance and love of life clearly bubbles forth – her voice strong and clear. "Life is so much fun … I am so grateful."

2.2 The multidimensional nature of patient outcomes in homeopathic treatment: inclusion of the physical domain in transformation

Cases 2 and 3 from our qualitative study of exceptional outcomes in homeopathic patients illustrate the multidimensional quality of the transformational experience in homeopathy. Oberbaum et al. [9] highlighted the multidimensional nature of homeopathic patient outcomes in their 2005 paper "The colour of the homeopathic improvement: the multidimensional nature of the response to homeopathic therapy". These authors point out the holistic (unitary) global and comprehensive nature of the changes that individuals who respond to homeopathic treatment report. Change during homeopathic treatment is not specific to the patient's chief complaint. Rather, homeopathic treatment appears to initiate multiple global (patient-wide or general) and local changes across the patient in patterns that conventional drugs do not [13,15,17,18]. For instance, in the ideal, the changes include early global (general) improvements in energy, sleep, sense of well-being and a gradual shift in the centre of gravity of local symptoms in the case from more important to less important organs (e.g., mind, brain, nervous system, downward), in accord with Hering's Law of Cure (from above downward, from inside out, in reverse order in time of appearance of the different symptoms) [19].

Homeopaths are not the only health care providers to report an interconnectedness of changes in allopathically-defined "separate" subsystems of the person. For instance, in the fields of allergy and mental health, early clinical observers, watching the natural history of the patient rather than of a specific diagnosis, have documented an alternation process, for example, between allergic and psychiatric manifestations, in patients who carry both types of diagnoses. That is, the psychiatric manifestations recede when the physical manifestations (e.g., asthma or eczema) emerge, and vice versa [20-22].

Subsequent allergists such as Randolph [20,21] noted a bipolar pattern of acute adverse reactions to certain foods and environmental chemicals, in which the symptoms peaked with behavioural and emotional symptoms (irritability, mania), but eventually resolved through emergence of physical symptoms such as headache and rhinitis (similar to predictions from Hering's Law of Cure). In these cases, however, susceptibility to the repetitive reactive patterns persisted, simply alternating without effective homeopathic treatment, between one type of manifestation or another upon re-exposure to the offending food or chemical agent. Nonetheless, the implication of such clinical alternation or symptom "oscillation" is that the patient is an integrated whole system, not a collection of independently functioning body parts or functions. The observations also highlight the nonlinear dynamical quality of the transitional change process [18,23-26].

2.3 The role of the patient-provider relationship in homeopathic care and transformative outcomes

Although some have questioned the empirical validity of Hering's Law in homeopathy [27], most classical homeopaths agree that their treatment has a multidimensional impact, beyond merely specific local effects within a given patient [9,19]. The nature of human beings is that they are complex adaptive systems whose parts (mind, brain, body) are interconnected and interactive [18,28]. As a result, the process of healing is predicted to shift in some related manner, across the various subsystems of the person [29]. In contrast with allopathic assumptions that the parts function separately, the interconnectivity of the parts would lead to the emergence of interrelated changes over multiple subsystems of the person and the global (general) level of the patient [18]. Thus, homeopathic transformational outcomes may have two major features: (a) dramatic shifts of function across all domains; and (b) lack of awareness of the extent of changes during the process of unstuckness and/or inability to articulate them until after the change has taken hold as a persis-tent transformation [9]. In our interview study, some patients described the transitional period as a "fog" from which they later emerged into sustained health. Moreover, the transitional period of unstuckness appears to manifest with instability [30,31] and even volatility in clinical course across multiple domains [13].

A key implication of the multidimensional outcomes and lack of awareness during the change process for a homeopathic patient, however, is that time factors will play a practical role in the unfolding of the treatment response. The patient may undergo changes in many symptoms and domains other than their original chief complaint early in the course of treatment. While successful treatment eventually should address the deepest, longest-standing pathology, homeopathy may not always meet modern patients' expectation of quick suppressive relief from specific suffering associated with a particular symptom or symptoms.

At the pragmatic level, beyond the ability of the practitioner to pick the "right" remedy, the provider's capacity to educate, empathize, and support the patient through an often lengthy and challenging period of changes will determine if the treatment even occurs, let alone helps [32]. The patient-provider relationship [33] becomes as central to the patient's likelihood of staying in and completing treatment for a complex chronic condition, especially one involving psychiatric symptomatology, as does proper selection of the simillimum remedy.

Bikker et al. [32], for example, showed that patients' ratings of the homeopath's degree of empathy during the initial case taking visit led to an increased sense of patient empowerment. In turn, the increased empowerment after three months of treatment correlated with improved ratings for both global well-being and local chief complaint symptom at the twelve-month point in time.

Moreover, the length of the initial case taking session correlated significantly with empathy, enablement, and clinical outcome ratings at three and twelve months. The ratings of the patient-provider relationship did not statistically account for all of the effects of the favourable patient outcomes, but the evidence shows that they played a meaningful role. Furthermore, Frei et al. [34] showed in children with Attention Deficit Hyperactivity Disorder that even experienced homeopaths can require an average of five months and three different remedies before finding the optimal remedy choice. Consequently, patients need the therapeutic relationship with the homeopath to sustain their engagement in the care, until both the right remedy can begin acting and the transitional instability of unstuckness resolves.

A proposed precursor of transformation in whole systems of complementary and alternative medicine (CAM) such as homeopathy is "unstuckness". Outside homeopathy, many people consider unstuckness in terms of psychological state [35] or mood alone, e.g. breaking out of a chronically depressed state [36]. Within homeopathy, various clinicians [14] have described unstuckness as breaking out of repetitive patterns of dysfunction that could involve not only the spiritual and emotional realms, but also concomitantly extensive shifts across all of the domains of a person, including social, mental, and physical function.

Clarifications of the concept of unstuckness recently emerged in research from content analysis of questionnaires completed by homeopaths attending professional conferences in the U.S. [13,17]. Here unstuckness related to an increased sense of freedom, defined as "the ease or facility of mental, emotional, spiritual, or physical movement, progress, or growth [17]". For instance, a patient who gets unstuck during homeopathy might finally leave a long-term dysfunctional relationship in which the person had felt trapped, but unable to escape.

The risk of simply becoming unstuck, however, is that the individual could relapse or revert to old patterns. Persons who become unstuck could (a) continue on into a healthy new, i.e., positively transformed, pattern, or (b) revert to previous "stuck" patterns, e.g., by returning to the original dysfunctional relationship or by re-creating a similar adverse interactional process with a new partner. At the same time, however, in a successfully-treated homeopathic patient, the unstuckness (a) extends beyond spiritual or social or psychological domains to cover all aspects of the person; and (b) gradually restabilises into a permanent functional change, i.e., multidimensional transformation.

The potential advantage of a positive patient-provider relationship in homeopathic treatment is the ability of the provider to serve as a guide or anchor through the change process, a period when many patients are unable to recognize or articulate their inner shifts. During such a vulnerable period, the risk is that the patient might delay or drop out of treatment. As shown in the cases above, some patients may not be able to cope successfully with their inner instability on their own during the unstuck, transitional period. Under these circumstances, the patient would fall out of the transitional state and, presumably, be at higher risk of relapse and resumption of previous dysfunctional spiritual, social, mental, emotional, and physical health patterns.

3   Conclusions

Implicit in the current discussion is a consideration of the patient as an indivisible, dynamical system or network of interdependent, interactive parts, whose overall behaviours are emergent properties of the person as a whole, behaviours not predicted from understanding the separate capacities of the isolated parts [18,28,37-39]. Patients showing a good response to homeopathic treatment often exhibit resolution of long-standing symptoms across many subsystems of the person. Indeed, the extent of the changes is often far beyond incremental linear improvements in the chief complaint and the unexpected resolution of a few isolated symptoms. Rather, clinical changes during homeopathic treatment are often non-linear, qualitative shifts into better health at a global level and over multiple local levels of the person. Spiritual, social, mental, emotional, and physical realms all undergo profound shifts in a transformational outcome with homeopathy.

The role of the homeopath in the total treatment process is that of a unique type of "whole-person" therapist, not merely a psychotherapist. Clinical theory and practice in classical homeopathy involve evaluating and treating the person as an integrated whole system, using a single remedy at a time [19]. Mental, emotional, and physical symptoms are all interactive and inseparable elements contributing to the total pattern of clinical manifestations, i.e., the simillimum remedy picture, in the individual case. Despite the enthusiastic quotation from Constantine Hering, MD given at the beginning of this chapter, contemporary homeopaths often focus their writings more on the clinical rationale for choice of remedy than on the human experience of the treatment process. Many homeopaths mention their sense of wonder at the transformative effects of homeopathic treatment on their patients in general, but, to date, they have rarely examined in detail the person-wide process of individualized patient outcomes from the patient's perspective of the transformative experience itself [15]. As some homeopathic investigators have raised, the homeopath as a "whole-person" clinical therapist is part of the overall treatment package, together with the simillimum remedy [40-42].

In addition to the descriptions of healing and transformative change that occurred in response to homeopathy, our exemplar homeopathic patients from our three cases described the processes of care that were central to their healing. The most compelling aspect of their care was the relationship that developed with their homeopathic provider. Without exception, these three patients (as well as the 35 others included in this study), described this relationship as a "trusting alliance", something that they could "count on through everything", a place where it was "safe to explore who I was and what I was feeling", a place where "I was heard – truly, wholly heard". They felt that their suffering was validated, their experiences and feelings understood within the totality of life, not as a dis-embodied mind experiencing fear and social anxieties, but as an embodied person where the phobias might have a physical cause.

They were not "treated as a complainer" with a body full of complaints, aches, and pains but as a person whose rashes, allergies and pains might be linked to a trauma locked away in their memory. Furthermore, as "homeopathic" rather than "psychiatric" patients, they bypassed the societal stigmatizing labels of allopathic psychiatry that sometimes inhibit people from seeking treatment. And, it was within this non-judgmental relationship with the homeopath [43] that they found a trusted confidante ("I could call him day or night – he was there for me"); ready to hold the course through the ups and downs of treatment ("She never gave up on me although I had given up on myself"); and sustain them through their periods of self-discovery and "ugliness" ("No matter how bad it was, I knew I could trust that he would listen"). The provider was a diligent guide for the journey of unsticking and unstuckness, and bore witness with the patient to the transformation that continues to unfold.

Taken together, the literature on the nature of transformation and homeopathic outcomes means movement beyond current condition, form, appearance and structure. It suggests that transformative change is fundamental and irreversible; a whole person change that occurs at the spiritual core of human form and manifests system-wide across the person's way of being in the world and in local physical, social, and psychological domains of the human experience [44]. It is the capacity to trigger transformative change and the role of the homeopath in facilitating and supporting the process for the individual patient that merits further attention and study.

Acknowledgements
This work was supported in part by NIH/NCCAM grants R21 AT01319, R21 AT00315, K24 AT00057, T32 AT011287, and R13 AT005189-01, and by grants from the Lotte and John Hecht Memorial Foundation.

References
[1] Winston J. (1999) *The Faces of Homeopathy*. Tawa, Wellington, New Zealand: Great Auk Publishing

[2] *Oxford Dictionary of English*. (2005) Oxford, England UK: Oxford Press

[3] *American heritage dictionary of the English language* (4th Ed). (2005) Boston, MA: Houghton Mifflin Co.

[4] Miller WR, C'deBaca J. (2001) *Quantum Change: When Epiphanies and Sudden Insights Transform Ordinary Lives*. New York: Guilford Press

[5] Pargament KI. (2001) *The Psychology of Religion and Coping: Theory, Research, Practice*. New York: Guilford Press

[6] Pargament KI. (2006) *The meaning of spiritual transformation.* In: Koss-Chioino JD, Hefner, P., editor. Spiritual Transformation and Healing: Anthropological, Theological, Neuroscientific, and Clinical Perspectives. Walnut Creek, CA: AltaMira Press: p.10-39

[7] C'de Baca J, Miller, W. (2003) Quantum change: Sudden transformation in the tradition of James's varieties. *Streams of William James* 2003; 5: 12-15

[8] Bell IR, Lewis DAI, Brooks AJ, Schwartz GE, Lewis SE, Caspi O, Cunningham V, Baldwin CM. (2004) Individual differences in response to randomly-assigned active individualized homeopathic and placebo treatment in fibromyalgia: Implications of a double-blind optional crossover design. *J Alternative & Complementary Medicine* 2004; 10: 269-283

[9] Oberbaum M, Singer SR, Vithoulkas G. (2005) The colour of the homeopathic improvement: the multidimensional nature of the response to homeopathic therapy. *Homeopathy* 2005; 94: 196-199

[10] Hirshberg C, Barasch MI. (1996) *Remarkable Recovery. What Extraordinary Healings Tell Us about Getting Well and Staying Well.* New York: Riverhead Books

[11] Loder JE. (1989) *The Transforming Moment* 2nd edition. Colorado Springs USA: Helmers and Howard

[12] Koss-Chioino JD, Hefner, P. (2006) Spiritual transformation and healing: *Anthropological, theological, neuroscientific, and clinical perspectives.* Walnut Creek, CA: AltaMira Press

[13] Koithan M, Verhoef M, Bell IR, Ritenbaugh C, White M, Mulkins A. (2007) The process of whole person healing: "unstuckness" and beyond. *J Alternative & Complementary Medicine* 2007; 13: 659-668

[14] Sherr J. (2002) *Dynamic Materia Medica. Syphilis: A Study of Syphilitic Miasm through Remedies.* Great Malvern Worcestershire, England: Dynamis Books

[15] Bell I, Koithan, M., DeToro, D. (2004) Outcomes of homeopathic treatment: patient perceptions and experiences. *Focus on Alternative and Complementary Therapies* 2004; 9: 21

[16] Koithan M, Bell, I., Campesino, M. (2005) Holographs and jigsaw puzzles: processes of care and approaches to healing of classical homeopaths. *Focus on Alternative and Complementary Therapies* 2005; 10: 29

[17] Bell IR, Koithan M, Gorman MM, Baldwin CM. (2003) Homeopathic practitioner views of changes in patients undergoing constitutional treatment for chronic disease. *Journal of Alternative & Complementary Medicine* 2003; 9: 39-50

[18] Bell IR, Koithan M. (2006) Models for the study of whole systems. *Integrative Cancer Therapies* 2006; 5: 293-307

[19] Vithoulkas G. (1980) *The Science of Homeopathy.* New York: Grove Weidenfeld

[20] Randolph T. (1978) Specific adaptation. *Annals of Allergy* 1978; 40: 333-345

[21] Randolph TG. (1973) *The history of ecologic mental illness.* In: Frazier CA, editor. Annual Review of Allergy. Flushing, NY: Med Exam Publishing Company: p.425

[22] Savage GM. (1884) *Insanity and Allied Neuroses: Practical and Clinical.* Philadelphia USA: Henry C. Lea Son and Co.

[23] Tang TZ, DeRubeis RJ. (1999) Sudden gains and critical sessions in cognitive-behavioral therapy for depression. *Journal of Consulting & Clinical Psychology* 1999; 67: 894-904

[24] Tang TZ, Luborsky, L. Andrusyna, (2002) T. Sudden gains in recovering from depression: are they also found in psychotherapies other than cognitive-behavioral therapy? *Journal of Consulting & Clinical Psychology* 2002; 70: 444-447

[25] Tang TZ, DeRubeis, R.J. Hollon, S.D., Amsterdam, J. Shelton, R. (2007) Sudden gains in cognitive therapy of depression and depression relapse/recurrence. *Journal of Consulting & Clinical Psychology* 2007; 75: 404-408

[26] Pincus D. (2009) *Coherence, complexity, and information flow: self-organizing processes in psychotherapy.* In: Guastello SJ, Koopmans, M, Pincus, D., editor. Chaos and Complexity in Psychology The Theory of Nonlinear Dynamical Systems. Cambridge New York: University Press: p.335-369

[27] Saine A. (1991) *Seminar: Psychiatric Patients Back to the Roots. Steps in Case Taking Materia Medica Cases.* Eindhoven, Netherlands: Lutra Services BV

[28] Bell IR, Caspi O, Schwartz GE, Grant KL, Gaudet TW, Rychener D, Maizes V, Weil A. (2002) Integrative medicine and systemic outcomes research: issues in the emergence of a new model for primary health care. *Archives of Internal Medicine* 2002; 162: 133-140

[29] Bellavite P. (2003) Complexity science and homeopathy: a synthetic overview. *Homeopathy* 2003; 92: 203-212

[30] Hollenstein T. (2007) State space grids: analyzing dynamics across development. *International Journal of Behavioral Development* 2007; 31: 384-396

[31] Hyland ME, Lewith GT. (2002) Oscillatory effects in a homeopathic clinical trial: an explanation using complexity theory, and implications for clinical practice. *Homeopathy* 2002; 91: 145-149

[32] Bikker AP, Mercer SW, Reilly D. (2005) A pilot prospective study on the consultation and relational empathy, patient enablement, and health changes over 12 months in patients going to the Glasgow Homoeopathic Hospital. *Journal of Alternative & Complementary Medicine* 2005; 11: 591-600

[33] Quinn J.(1989) *Healing: The emergence of right relationship*. In: Carlson R, Shield, B., editor. Healers on Healing. Los Angeles, CA: J.P. Tarcher

[34] Frei H, Everts R, von Ammon K, Kaufmann F, Walther D, Schmitz SF, Collenberg M, Steinlin M, Lim C, Thurneysen A. (2007) Randomised controlled trials of homeopathy in hyperactive children: treatment procedure leads to an unconventional study design Experience with open-label homeopathic treatment preceding the Swiss ADHD placebo controlled, randomised, double-blind, cross-over trial. *Homeopathy* 2007; 96: 35-41

[35] Simon S. (1988) *Getting unstuck: Breaking through your barriers to change*. New York: Warner Books

[36] Gordon JS. (2008) *Unstuck: Your Guide to the Seven-Stage Journey Out of Depression*. New York: Penguin Press HC,

[37] Bell I, Koithan, M. (2009) Patient-Centered Research on Whole Systems of Complementary and Alternative Medicine: A Complex Systems Science Perspective (Part II: Applications). Submitted for publication

[38] Bell I, Koithan, M. (2009) Patient-Centered Research on Whole Systems of Complementary and Alternative Medicine: A Complex Systems Science Perspective (Part I: Concepts). Submitted for publication

[39] Bell IR. (2008) The evolution of homeopathic theory-driven research and the methodological toolbox. *The American Homeopath* 2008; 14: 56-74

[40] Milgrom LR. (2002) Patient-practitioner-remedy (PPR) entanglement: a qualitative, non-local metaphor for homeopathy based on quantum theory. *Homeopathy* 2002; 91: 239-248

[41] Milgrom LR. (2002) Vitalism, complexity, and the concept of spin. *Homeopathy* 2002; 91: 26-31

[42] Milgrom LR. (2006) Towards a new model of the homeopathic process based on quantum field theory. *Forsch Komplementarmed* 2006; 13: 174-183

[43] Rowe T. (1998) *Homeopathic Methodology. Repertory, Case Taking, and Case Analysis*. Berkeley CA: North Atlantic Books

[44] Bell IR, Lewis DAI, Lewis SE, Brooks AJ, Schwartz GE, Baldwin CM. (2004) Strength of vital force in classical homeopathy: bio-psycho-social-spiritual correlates in a complex systems context. *Journal of Alternative & Complementary Medicine* 2004; 10: 123-131

Chapter 3
Wholistic[2], Spiritual Aspects of Homeopathy

Daniel J. Benor, MD ABIHM

Daniel J. Benor, Wholistic Psychotherapist (Canada), MD ABIHM (US)
565 Victoria Road North
Guelph, Ontario N1E 7M1
Canada
E-mail: DB@WholisticHealingResearch.com

Abstract

Homeopathy in its fullest applications is a wholistic therapy – addressing body, emotions, mind, relationships and spirit. By addressing every aspect of a person's being, the whole person is harmonized within himself and within the context of his relationships with other people and the world beyond. This is the truest form of health and healing. Within this framework, a person is able to live unstressed on any level of his existence, and also has the tools with which to address any challenges in his life. Within this framework, mental health is an integrated aspect of wholistic health.

Even some homeopaths may have difficulty making the transition from prescribing remedies for symptom clusters to harmonizing the whole person, on every level of her or his being. They may be content to deal with body, emotions and mind, sometimes extending into relationships. Spirit, which is difficult to define, is often relegated to interventions of the clergy – just as it is in the practice of conventional medicine and psychotherapy.

This article explores research and clinical observations that suggest homeopathy can be a doorway into spiritual awarenesses, which then become a wonderful resource for deeper healings. Not only mental health but all of a person's health can be enhanced.

…Hahnemann stumbled upon a phenomenon that is barely beginning to be understood by modern physics, a dynamic that might be likened to spirit, information or meaning in matter…
– Edward Whitmont (1993, p. 7)

---

2 Wholistic is preferred by some authors as a spelling variant of 'holistic'. I prefer this as an indication that I am addressing all levels of a person's being: body, emotions, mind, relationships and spirit.

1   Spirituality

The difference between spiritual and non-spiritual is:
How much of reality are you ready to bite off?
- Author unknown

There are two broad ways that people connect with their spirituality. The first is through religious beliefs and ritual practices, and the second is through personal spiritual awarenesses.

Religious beliefs are based on teachings that have been filtered through many generations, following their birthing through the lives and lessons of enlightened individuals. They are articles of faith, taught by clergy and learned through family, houses of worship, and written and/or oral traditions. These modes of connecting with spirituality are outside the realms of influence of homeopathy.

Personal spiritual awarenesses may be awakened and deepened through religious practices. They may also arise spontaneously, either unbidden or as fruits of meditative, ritual or other practices.

Many have sought to explain spirituality – in religious, philosophical and psychological explorations of that which is, ultimately, beyond words. It is like wanting to describe the taste of a persimmon to people who have never had this fruit in their mouths. No words will adequately convey its taste. Only in putting it in our mouth, chewing on it, and savouring its essence directly will we know its actual taste. So it is with spirituality: we must personally experience it in order to know its nature and its effects.

Common experiences that stimulate spiritual awarenesses include: communing with nature; being touched by deep emotions; being inspired by the words and actions of others and relationships with them – including poetry, music, images, dance and other creative arts; intuitive and psychic awarenesses; synchronistic experiences; Out-of-Body Experiences (OBE); Near-Death Experiences (NDE); apparitions (ghosts); mediumistic (channelled) communications; past-life memories; transformations with bio-energy therapies and/or spiritual healing; encounters with historical religious figures (e.g. Christ, Mary, the saints), angels and nature spirits; and communications with God. Sceptics may question whether reports of such experiences are anything more than wishful thinking, fantasies, delusions or hallucinations. Those who have had these experiences often report they carry an aura or essence of truth and validity that leaves them absolutely certain of their reality.

My favourite among the above are the reports of bereavement apparitions. Apparitions come very frequently to those who have lost someone close to them. Vargas et al. (1989)[21] published a survey of bereaved people in *The American Journal of Psychiatry*, a conservative professional publication not given to featuring ghost stories. Two thirds of those surveyed reported they perceived the person who had died – either seeing them, hearing them, or intuitively sensing their 'presence.' I have made it a point to ask clients, friends and colleagues who have been bereaved whether they have had such experiences. As in the survey, more than half have responded affirmatively and favourably, often being relieved to have confirmation that their experiences are common, real, and deeply meaningful to others – just as they are to themselves.

My explorations of personal spiritual awarenesses have been even more convincing to me. They have led me to appreciate and trust my inner, intuitive knowing of the validity and rightness of my inner awareness of the Transcendent. I call this my inner 'gnowing,' which is an immediate connection with some aspect of that which is beyond myself, beyond words and beyond full conceptualization or comprehension in linear, everyday awareness – and yet an essential aspect of my being.

I will discuss spirituality in homeopathy from the definition that personal spirituality is the awareness that we are part of a world that is vaster than our physical selves. I mean this not just in the sense that we participate as individuals and in a social collective in ways that impact on ourselves and the world. Spirituality as here defined includes our interactions through biological energies and consciousness with aspects of our world that are beyond our physical body.

2   Wholistic healing

Be yourself completely. Love every part as good. Only then can you know peace...
- Ron Van Dyke

Wholistic healing addresses every level of our being: body, emotions, mind, relationships and spirit (Benor, Web reference)[9]. The first four levels are generally acknowledged in Western society as relevant to health and illness, and will not be discussed here – with the exception of the biological energies of the body, which I understand to be aspects of the level of spirit.

The body is addressed in many complementary therapies through its energy aspects, perhaps most clearly in spiritual healing. Spiritual healers can identify the state of other people's health and illness through visual, tactile or mental perceptions – without direct physical interaction with those they are examining. They can also intervene to alter the states of other people without direct physical or verbal interactions.

I used to be sceptical of healers' and intuitives' reports. I thought that their apparent interventions to influence 'healees' were no more than effects of suggestion in its many and varied manifestations. Having been trained in psychology, medicine, psychiatry and research, I kept a measure of reserve and scepticism about this, owing to the potentials for effects of suggestion. Hypnosis and other forms of suggestion have been well investigated, demonstrating that people have an enormous capacity for self-healing that can be activated by clinicians (Benor, 2004; 2005)[4,5].

Over the years, I collected clinical reports of healers and healees supporting their claims. I identified 191 controlled studies of healing – on humans, animals, plants, bacteria, yeasts, cells in laboratory culture, enzymes and DNA. Of the 52 most rigorous studies, 74% demonstrated significant effects (Benor, 2001a; 2001b)[2,3]. It was this substantial body of research on spiritual healing that has been most convincing to me - and others with whom I've discussed spiritual healing over the years – in accepting what healers have been saying.

Healers and healees often report sensations of heat, tingling and vibration when the healers hold their hands near the body without touching it. This suggests that there is an energy exchange between healers and healees during the healing. Other complementary modalities report they address various aspects of bio-energies too, including craniosacral therapy, applied kinesiology, Qigong, and acupuncture, along with its derivatives (Benor, 2004; 2006)[4,6].

While explanations that involve interactions between people on the basis of bio-energies may seem plausible, spiritual healing also demonstrates that the intention to heal, without the healer's presence near the organisms needing healing, can bring about significant effects. This suggests that there are interactions of consciousness between healers and healees. (Healers' explanatory systems are often clothed in religious garments, but non-religious healers can produce similar effects, and non-human subjects can respond to healings, so the religious explanations may add to the healings in some ways but are not requisite for them to occur.)

Meticulous research in parapsychology has confirmed the occurrence of mind-to-mind interactions (telepathy); informational transfer from inanimate objects to the minds of people (clairsentience); accurate perceptions/predictions of the future (precognition); and mind-matter interactions (psychokinesis/PK). Meta-analyses of these studies start in the millions to one against chance (Benor, 2008b; Radin, 1997)[8,19]. The results are in many cases from non-gifted subjects, confirming that most people have a measure of parapsychological ability and awareness.

The effects of consciousness in producing healing effects thus find a broad base of supporting research. The fact that these effects can be produced at some distance from the healer provides confirmation for the subjective reports of spiritual awareness that extend people's consciousness beyond their physical body.

3   Homeopathy as a wholistic practice that includes spirituality

If a living system is suffering from ill health,
the remedy is to connect it with more of itself.
- Francisco Varela

Edward Whitmont was a Jungian psychotherapist and a gifted homeopath. He was also a writer gifted with exceptional pattern recognition and eloquence in explaining the wholistic nature of homeopathy. Whitmont (1993, p., 74)[23] beautifully illustrates the blending of symptom, substance and symbol in the clinical case of a man of about 40, whom I will call "Henry," who suffered from acne.

After taking a detailed history, Whitmont prescribed a single dose of *Calcarea carbonica* (extracted from oyster shells) at a dilution of C1000. This produced temporary spasms of the finger muscles, similar to tetany. This is a typical symptom of parathyroid gland dysfunction, which would produce lower blood calcium levels. The spasms evoked memories from Henry's childhood, when his mother had taped his fingers to his bedside in a position that resembled that of the spasms he experienced from the homeopathic calcium carbonate. His mother had done this to prevent him from masturbating. During the treatment, vivid memories arose in Henry of his anger and shame connected with this experience. As a child, he had completely repressed these memories in his unconscious mind. This somehow was translated into his skin condition and a boisterous personality. With the release of these memories, the spasms in his fingers also released, and this healing process furthered his progress in psychotherapy.

> ...Shame, anger, finger spasm, parathyroid hormonal activity, calcium metabolism, the dynamic field of the oyster (in homeopathic practice the "personality of the Calcarea carbonica type can be likened to an oversensitive but heavily defended person, akin to an oyster without or with too thick a shell) and the functioning of the skin all appear here as different transduction codes of one and the same dynamic field process. (Whitmont 1993, p. 74-75)[23]

As Whitmont eloquently points out, it may be impossible to clarify many of the complexities of linked energetic and imagery components that produce these effects. Every remedy has its particular spectrum of effects – its *personality*. When a person has a cluster of symptoms and personality traits that match those of a particular remedy, then that remedy can facilitate a clearing of those symptoms, and it may also alter the accompanying personality traits. The art and challenge of the practice of homeopathy is to ask the right questions in order to identify the relevant symptom clusters. If the homeopath did not ask the patient about specific related symptoms, many of which might not be at all obvious or likely to be reported spontaneously, the best remedy could easily be missed.

Even more fascinating and also relevant to the energy aspect of wholistic healing, is a study by P.C. Endler [15] of homeopathic dilutions of thyroid hormone that produced significant effects on climbing behaviour in frogs. In this study the remedy was entirely encased in a glass tube that was simply held near the frogs. This suggests even more clearly that homeopathy is a subtle energetic intervention.

In the treatment of human health problems, a major consideration in prescribing homeopathic remedies is the personality of the subject. B. Brewitt et al. [12] used the Myers-Briggs Type Indicator (MPTI) to look for personality types that might be more prone to using and benefiting from homeopathy. In their homeopathy user sample of 125 people [29 healthy; 76 HIV+ (most of whom were homosexual)] they found significantly higher personality test scores on the intuitive vs. the sensing scales, as compared to general population norms for these tests (p < .001). Similarly, they found higher scores for feeling over thinking (p < .001), despite the predominance of males in their sample. It is unclear to what degree these findings reflect homeopathy preference and to what extent they may reflect attitudes of homosexual men.

Whitmont points out that correspondences between remedies and dis-ease or disease (in homeopathy and other therapies) may be metaphoric as well as symptomatic. He gives the example of metallic gold (*Aurum metallicum*). Part of its potency as a remedy may lie in the correspondence of gold with the sun. Intuitively, both gold and the sun are associated with the human heart. Homeopathic gold is indicated as a treatment for excesses in expressions of personality traits, as in an over-scrupulous conscience, a tendency to focus on darker sides of issues and problems, and in vulnerabilities to burnout and tendencies to black depressions. Homeopathic applications of gold include the treatment of disorders of the heart, circulation, bones and joints.

Whitmont also provides excellent discussions on the collective unconscious, pointing out that if we explore the realms of psychotherapy, in dreams and synchronistic occurrences, we will find ample evidence that the mind of man has access to all knowledge, through all time. This capacity enables us to diagnose our own illnesses and to identify the root causes of our problems.

Whitmont wisely notes that many physical problems have their origins in emotional traumas. Memories of these traumas are encoded within specific states of consciousness. Therefore, accessing and releasing these memories may require alternative states of consciousness, often achieved by invoking emotions that are similar to those that were felt during the original traumas. If the traumas were very severe or occurred during pre-verbal years, and if they have been expressed through the body in physical pathology, homeopathic remedies may be helpful in accessing and releasing them – when they may otherwise be inaccessible.

Whitmont proposes that we can best understand the human condition and homeopathic treatment as manifestations of a holographic universe, in which every living and non-living thing is interconnected with every other thing through subtle and intricate dimensions of existence.

Homeopathic remedies, whether based on animate or inanimate matter, restore the innate patterns of people whose physical, psychological or spiritual order has gone awry.

> ...Homeopathy... demonstrates that every possible illness that can affect living organisms has a corollary in some substance that is part of the earth's organism. External substances replicate psychosomatic patterns and are able to induce pathology when foisted upon the organism. However, they are also able to cure when applied in the appropriately diluted or "potentized" form. In a mosaic of unknown scale, the various states of human consciousness and the ingredients of the human drama are encoded in various mineral, plant and animal substances – the unit "particles" of our earth. They slumber in these materials waiting for their unfolding on the human level. (Whitmont 1993, p.22)[23]

Whitmont points out that within a holographic universe, everything in the cosmos may influence a given organism. Conversely, a given organism is an intimate, enfolded part of everything in the cosmos. (These observations have been echoed by others, such as Bohm 1980; Bohm and Peat 1987)[10,11]. Illness and health are therefore seen from perspectives that differ from those of allopathic medicine and the reductionist philosophies that underpin it. A holographic understanding of the universe suggests that in the unfolding of enfolded orders of reality, illness in individuals or groups (such as in epidemics) may serve as challenges that unsettle established orders and make new developments possible. The same may be true of natural disasters.

Whitmont suggests that life is characterized by *entelechy*, which is an Aristotelian term denoting an *inherent goal-directedness*. Though the ultimate goals are often beyond our appreciation, the influence of entelechy is seen in our avid pursuit of excitement and drama and in our vigorous rebellion against boredom. Illnesses are mechanisms for disrupting stultifying patterns. Death – either in miniature (as when we relinquish old patterns of being and behaving) or in major expressions (as when a physical existence on earth comes to an end), is a clearing of the way to invite new patterns and experiences to develop.

This briefest of summaries in no way does justice to the enormous range of wisdom integrated by Whitmont, nor to his style – which is erudite and frequently poetic in its metaphoric richness.

3.1   Imponderable / meditative / symbolic / metaphoric remedies

Meditative provings are not an easier way than the conventional of arriving at the symptoms of a remedy… but they are quicker as each meditation takes about three and a half hours… The remedy pictures that are elucidated by this method are as clear and as accurate as those arrived at by conventional provings, providing the meditational proving has been carried out correctly.
- Madeline Evans [16]

The intuitive, symbolic and metaphoric applications of homeopathy are being explored by other homeopaths. These are sometimes referred to as the *imponderable* remedies.

Colin Griffiths [17] describes a new intuitive approach that is called *meditative proving*. A group of thirteen homeopaths gather for the proving. Only one of them, the *Chair* for that session, knows what the remedy is. All of the participants except the Chair take the remedy and report their physical, emotional and general states. The Chair then records their observations over a 3-4-hour period of group meditation.

What became readily apparent, as Griffiths and his group explored remedies in these ways, was the way a dynamic field seemed to be set up in the group as a whole, as though the provers resonated on a deeper level, and were able to spontaneously elicit unique insights into aspects of the remedy that normally would take years of slow and meticulous research. The ensuing empathy created by a group in a state of stillness can establish a situation of direct cognition bypassing our normal rational states of awareness, thus eliciting a far more direct and dynamic identification with the actual object under consideration – the remedy in this case. Griffiths suggests: "This proving method is tentative in nature but sufficiently germane to excite new explorations in homeopathy. We would therefore request our fellow homeopaths to invoke freedom from prejudice as their first therapeutic ideal, and put these proving insights to the test of empirical experience."

Griffiths provides the example of a homeopathic remedy that was developed from a piece of concrete taken from the *Berlin Wall* when it was torn down. The wall was built of concrete, incorporating bricks and other debris that had been gathered after the bombings of World War II. The piece of the wall that was used to develop the remedy was brought to Britain by a German woman who had lived in the UK since childhood. It was given to Griffiths as a curiosity, and it lay in a drawer for about a year till he presented it to a psychic sensitive (also a homeopath) for her intuitive impressions. She instantly felt fear, panic and distress, though she was totally unaware of the source of the little piece of concrete. (This sort of intuitive reading of an inanimate object is a form of extrasensory perception called *psychometry* or *clairsentience*, which is well validated in research reviewed by Radin, 1997.)[19] This encouraged Griffiths to have a homeopathic company prepare a remedy from the stone. When the sensitive was given a dose of a 30C dilution of the Berlin wall preparation she felt that it was so extraordinarily potent that she strongly advised it should be kept separate from other remedies because it might mutate them or antidote them.

The Berlin wall was built in 1961, separating Communist-ruled East Germany from West Berlin, which was a Western enclave buried deep within East Germany. The wall was the product of Communist fears about the infiltration of Western influences, and the source of enormous tensions and conflicts between East and West. Thousands died in attempts to escape to the West, hoping for freedom and reunification with families that had been torn asunder by the war and its aftermath. With the coming of *glasnost* the wall was torn down, releasing floods of people who had been trapped and powerless to oppose the governing authorities.

Griffiths and other homeopaths have found that the remedy prepared from this highly symbolic material is helpful in treating people who are suffering in various ways from oppression, suppression, depression or repression. An example from Griffith follows.

> *A 28-year-old woman had been taking homeopathic remedies for several years to treat depression and a number of other complaints. One day, she came to the clinic in deep misery, feeling that nothing was right with her, or had ever been right before, or would ever be right thereafter. She felt deprived in her inner life and her relationships, and in particular she felt short-changed by her parents, who had separated when she was a little girl. She complained of always giving and not receiving in return, of being alienated from her loved ones, and of marking time to no purpose. She longed to be protected from the world, feeling that she had never really wished to grow up, and pining for the security of her family and the place of her birth, in Berlin.*

The woman was given a single dose of *Berlin Wall* 30C, and after 3 days she reported that she was quite changed.

> *...She had resolved a number of difficult issues with both her boyfriend and her father and, in the case of the latter, felt that she had established the first proper communication for years. She had also been offered a decent job, after years of doing indifferent work. She felt as though a wall had been broken through that had stood between herself and the rest of the world. She has not needed to come since.*

Numerous other metaphoric homeopathic remedies are being created around the world. It is unclear to what degree and how these overlap with or differ from similar metaphoric remedies produced by flower essence practitioners.

3.2   Homeopathic remedies as radionics treatments

Radionics is a form of spiritual healing that focuses the intent of the healer through a radionics device. The device usually includes:

1. a link to the healee (called a *witness*) – e.g. a drop of the healee's blood, urine or saliva on a piece of blotting paper; or a photograph of the healee; or the healee's name written on a piece of paper
2. a set of dials that are attuned to the vibration of the healee
   a. to connect with the healee
   b. to assess the condition of the healee, its severity, and remedies that will be helpful in treatment
3. a set of dials that are attuned to a remedy to be sent by distant healing to the healee
4. a place to insert a sample of the selected remedy; a drawing or abstract design that embodies the energetic pattern of the remedy; or the name of the remedy written on a piece of paper

Homeopathic remedies have been sent through radionics devices with claims for good effects. I know of no research to confirm these claims.

It is more important to know what sort of person has a disease than to know
what sort of disease a person has.
- Hippocrates

Intuitives and spiritual healers often report intuitive awarenesses of the root origins of people's problems (Benor, 2001a, b)[2,3] . Any symptom, be it psychological or physical, may have antecedent factors such as:

- Genetic predisposition;
- Stress – individual, personal or interpersonal/relationship issues, social stressors;
- Stress – collective, expressing issues of family, community and culture;
- Trauma - physical or psychological;
- Allergies;
- Environmental stressors – toxic or electromagnetic pollutants; and
- Spiritual factors – past life residues, lessons from the collective consciousness

The abilities of these sensitives and healers to connect with the care-seekers and identify their problems through their intuition are an example of collective consciousness. Healers often report that their healings involve life lessons not only for the person seeking help, but also for their families and communities. In Native American tradition, for example, a medicine man will often include family and community members in the healing ceremonies (Cohen, 2003)[13]. The healer becomes an agent for identifying and interpreting the metaphoric message of the symptoms in ways that invite healing for all who are involved with the person who manifested the information about the disharmony in the community that had resulted in the development of their symptoms or illness.

Plant remedies may have parallels with homeopathic remedies. Growing numbers of gifted intuitives are developing flower essences using intuitive approaches similar to those of Griffiths. For example, Machaela Small Wright (US)[25], Andrea Mathieson (Canada)[18], Lilja Asgeirsdottir (Iceland)[1], and others around the world who prepare flower essences report that the plants may tell them for which ailments essences from these plants can be of help. Conversely, if a healer holds a mental question in focus while walking in nature - about which plant will be helpful for a given symptom or disease – plants that can be helpful will identify themselves telepathically.

There are two ways of preparing flower essences. The original methods required the flowers or other plant parts to be placed in pure water in the sunshine over periods of several hours. The water then becomes 'charged' with the essence of the plant and can be used as a remedy. Unlike homeopathic remedies, the plant remedies are not diluted to achieve greater potencies.

Taking this a step further, various flower essence producers have found that they are able to imbue water with the essence of a remedy through mental focus and intent. Karen Cremasco [14] is one of these. Cremasco is Board-Certified in Counselling Intuition with the American Board of Scientific Medical Intuition. She received a Bachelor degree in Psychology at the University of Waterloo, and 'is' a Bachelor of Education from University of Western Ontario. She completed her PhD in

Energy Medicine at Greenwich University and a post-doctorate in Theology and Spiritual Healing at Holos University. Karin developed her own work, called Body Harmonization, which combines her counselling, intuitive and healing knowledge and clinical experience. In her clinical practice, she started using the Raven Flower Essences of Andrea Mathieson. Cremasco discovered that if she focused mentally on the essence, she was able to provide the effects of the essence by mental concentration alone. She calls this 'Vibrational Infusion.' Her clients did not need to take the actual essence orally.

Cremasco discussed this with Mathieson, who initially was intrigued and gave her blessing to this method of applying the Raven Essences. However, on reflection several months later, Mathieson found herself unhappy with this new development, because it meant that she would not be compensated financially for the essences that she had laboured to develop. Cremasco shares:

> ... in September 2005 she called me to say that it no longer felt right to her for anyone to offer the essences without some compensation to her, as the originator of the essences, for doing so. I agreed with her point of view. I was aware that Andrea had invested a great deal of time and money to develop and produce these essences. Since it was not necessary either for me or my students to purchase the essences, Andrea was not compensated. I felt awkward and embarrassed. Suddenly, the Raven Essences no longer tested as appropriate for any clients. It was like they had vanished. I felt an immense loss. (Curiously, one of my students commented to me six months later that the Raven Essences stopped testing for her in her private practice at precisely the same period!) I shared my feelings openly with Andrea and we began to dialogue. We then created a two-tiered approach that honors both the many years of work that went into creating and developing the essences, and the method of Vibrational Infusion. As soon as Andrea and I arrived at our mutual agreement, the Raven Essences tested once again. I teach students and clients the sacredness of Vibrational Infusion, and to share Andrea's story of how they were created. I trust my students will continue to practice this method for administering Raven Essences with the same level of integrity that I do my best to model and have taught them. (Cremasco 2007)[14]

Cremasco and her students now pay users' fees to Mathieson for her permission to apply them by Vibrational Infusion. This is the first licensing agreement I am aware of for the intellectual property of a vibrational remedy that is used by mental intent.

3.4 Mental projection of homeopathic remedies

Several people have reported anecdotes to me about transfer of homeopathic effects through mental intent.

One was a world-renowned homeopath who asked that his name not be mentioned in connection with this report. He was phoned in the US by a friend who was visiting in Africa, with a request for help with an infection. The friend was far from any medical facility and the homeopath sent the mental intent to produce the desired homeopathic effects. The friend reported rapid improvements following the phone call.

The other was a spiritual healer who was on holiday and needed a homeopathic remedy for allergies that were triggered. None was available locally and she mentally recalled the benefits she had experienced when previously taking the remedy, finding that the allergic reaction subsided rapidly.

While these anecdotes in no way constitute more than suggestive evidence, they do point in an interesting direction for future research. There is a difficulty here, however, in separating out what might be another form of homeopathic energetic effect from placebo effects and distant healing effects.

Madeline Evans (http://www.madelineevans.com) has an excellent book on homeopathy, including essential, esoteric and chakra relevance [16].

3.5 Theories to explain spiritual aspects of homeopathy

The seeds of grassroots spirituality seem to be springing up everywhere through the cracks in the old order.
- Frances Vaughan

Our body is usually conceived of as our physical corpus that inhabits and interacts with the physical world. Einstein suggested that matter and energy are interconvertible: $E = mc^2$. Conventional physics has amassed sufficient evidence in support of this theory that most people have come to accept. Anyone with even a smattering of knowledge of modern physics will not find it strange if I point out that the chair they are sitting on is more space and energies than matter – from the perspective of Quantum Physics.

This does not mean that we have thrown out classical, Newtonian Physics. Newtonian Physics continues to be essential to sorting out issues at the macroscopic level of our world. We build roads and bridges that provide the required supports for traffic; dental bridges and medical prostheses that support our bodies; and we design buildings to specifications that protect us from forces of nature. All of these require an understanding of Newtonian Physics.

We have come to understand that Newtonian Physics and Quantum Physics simply address the two sides of Einstein's equation. Each side of that equation has its own rules for organizing perceptions, measurements, analyses and interactions with our world. The rules of one side do not apply to the other side.

Newtonian Medicine has been very slow to grasp Einstein's observations. Our body can be addressed as matter or as energies in the same way that a chair can be analyzed. Spiritual healers and intuitives have been saying for generations that they perceive and interact with the energy aspects of people's bodies. Extending this further, they report awarenesses of and abilities to interact with the energetic aspects of people's emotions, minds and spirits.

Homeopaths have proposed that their remedies consist of vibrational patterns of substances that are imprinted in water. This is outside the realms of explanations of Newtonian Physics. However, no other explanation has been proposed for the fact that homeopathic remedies are potent in dilutions where no single molecule of the original substance remains'

This is also paralleled by spiritual healers' imbuing water with healing properties. Research has demonstrated that water which has been given healing will enhance the growth of plants. The most accepted explanation for these effects is that the water carries the healing vibrational pattern. An alternative explanation is that the water becomes a link to the healer, as in radionics the witness creates a link to the healee. The plants might then draw the healing energies/vibrations they need from the healer rather than from the water.

Expanding our focus, Edward Whitmont (1980)[22] proposes that homeopathy creates a link between psyche and substance, in a holographic universe. Accepting that individuals can communicate with each other and with the world at large through parapsychological awarenesses (well validated in research), it follows that there must be a network of individual consciousness that can be termed a collective consciousness – another way of describing a holographic universe. The participation of our individual consciousness in the collective consciousness would appear to be similar to the participation of a single brain cell within the billions of nerve cell interconnections in a physical brain. The collective consciousness includes inanimate as well as animate constituents of the universe.

Homeopathic remedies may link relevant aspects of the collective consciousness in a healing manner. The energetic pattern that constitutes health in a living organism may go awry, creating symptoms or diseases. A remedy may restore the pattern of health through its inherent energetic properties. A remedy may also remind the organism of its normal pattern of health through its metaphoric message to the unconscious mind of the organism. And remedies are now being developed by Peter Chappell that address collective symptoms of chronic diseases rather than just those of the individual (van der Zee, 2009)[20].

3.6 Contributions of wholistic, spiritual awareness in homeopathy

When great forces are on the move in the world, we learn we are spirits - not animals.
- Winston Churchill

Humanity has much to learn from the lessons of homeopathic treatments that include spiritual awareness – defined as the awareness of being part of a world that extends beyond our physical selves.

Mental health in conventional medicine is the ability of a person to conform to the norms of expectations for subjective experiences and behaviours in their society. Deviations from the norm are seen as pathological. Pathology is usually defined in terms of symptoms, which are addressed behaviourally and with medications. Underlying issues often go unaddressed.

Homeopathy addresses each individual in much greater depth, individualizing remedies to the fullest spectrum of issues of a person's being that can be identified, taking into consideration their personalities and other factors in their current life and life history. Remedies are identified to release problematic issues and to harmonize the person to optimal health.

Homeopathy in any form is a major contribution to healthcare today. In addition to the individualization of treatment, there is the major advantage of low risks relative to the serious morbidity and mortality risks with conventional medicine.

Spiritual aspects of a person's health are sometimes overlooked in homeopathy, as they are in conventional medical and mental health interventions. Spiritual aspects represent an area of possible wounding and of potential strengths that can be relevant to homeopathic assessments and prescriptions.

The demonstrated efficacy of imponderable/meditative/metaphoric remedies adds evidence to the theory of consciousness as a healing force in the world. This is an encouragement to activate our consciousness in increasingly healing ways.

The awareness of miasms and of the efficacy of homeopathic remedies that address collective symptoms of chronic diseases adds evidence for a collective consciousness. The practical effects of the Peter Chappell remedies include clearing of emotional traumas.

4   In summary

Personal spirituality, the awareness of our consciousness extending beyond our physical being, is a concept that enables us to begin to appreciate homeopathic remedies in deeper ways. Homeopathic remedies may restore patterns of health that have gone awry through their vibrational patterns or through metaphoric patterns. Within a wholistic framework, mental health is improved through addressing every level of a person's being – spirit, relationships (with others and the environment), mind, emotions and body.

References

This article includes excerpts from Benor, DJ. Healing Research, V. 2 - Professional edition: Consciousness, Bioenergy and Healing, Bellmawr, NJ: Wholistic Healing Publications 2004. www.wholistichealingresearch.com/HealingResearchVolume2-Pro-Ed.html

[1] Asgeirsdottir, Lilja Petra (2009) Waterfall Essences: Energies of a Newborn Land and the Whole Cosmos, *International J Healing and Caring* 2009, 9(1), 1-7

[2] Benor, Daniel J. (2001a) *Healing Research: Volume I*, Spiritual Healing: Scientific Validation of a Healing Revolution, Southfield, MI: Vision Publications

[3] Benor, Daniel J. (2001b) *Healing Research: Volume I*, Professional Supplement, Southfield, MI: Vision Publications

[4] Benor, Daniel J. (2004) *Healing Research, Volume II* (Professional edition), Consciousness, Bioenergy and Healing, Bellmawr, NJ: Wholistic Healing Publications

[5] Benor, Daniel J. (2005) *Healing Research, Volume II* (Popular edition), How Can I Heal What Hurts? Wholistic Healing and Bioenergies, Bellmawr, NJ: Wholistic Healing Publications

[6] Benor, Daniel J. (2006) *WHEE Workbook*, Bellmawr, NJ: Wholistic Healing Publications, http://wholistichealingresearch.com/products.html (Available as immediate eBook download or paperback.)

[7] Benor, Daniel J. (2008a) *Seven Minutes to Natural Pain Release WHEE for Tapping Your Pain Away - the Revolutionary New Self-Healing Method*, Fulton, CA: Energy Psychology Press www.paintap.com

[8] Benor, Daniel J. (2008b) *Using any therapy as an opportunity to heal the collective consciousness and our planet: Lessons from Ho'oponopono and WHEE*, http://www.wholistichealingresearch.com/col_con_hooponopono_whee.html

[9] Benor, Daniel J. http://www.wholistichealingresearch.com/srmeb

[10] Bohm, David. (1980) *Wholeness and the Implicate Order,* London: Routledge and Kegan Paul

[11] Bohm, David and Peat, F David (1987) *Science, Order and Creativity*, New York: Bantam

[12] Brewitt, B et al. (1998) Personality preferences of healthy and HIV+ people attracted to homeopathy, *Alternative Therapies* 1998, 4(2), 99; 102

[13] Cohen, Kenneth (2003) *Honoring the Medicine: The Essential Guide to Native American Healing*, New York: One World/ Ballantine

[14] Cremasco, Karin (2007) Essence of healing: vibrational infusion© of flower essences, *International J Healing and Caring* 2007, 7(1), 1-17

[15] Endler, PC (ed) (1994) *Ultra High Dilution: Physiology and Physics*, Dordrecht, Netherlands: Kluwer Academic Publishers

[16] Evans, Madeline (2000) *Meditative Provings*, Holgate, UK: Rose Press http://www.madelineevans.com

[17] Griffiths, Colin (1995) The Berlin Wall, a remedy proved by group meditation, *Prometheus Unbound* 1995, Spring, 25-30

[18] Mathieson, Andrea (2007) A love affair with nature: Field notes from a flower essence producer, *International J Healing and Caring* 2007, 7(1), Part I: Stepping stones on my path, p. 1-17; Part II: A short primer on the Raven Flower Essences, p. 1-9; Part III: Meditations on destiny, p. 1-10

[19] Radin, Dean (1997) *The Conscious Universe*, New York: HarperCollins

[20] Van der Zee, Harry (2009) Healing humanity with homeopathy: Homeopathy for epidemics, collective trauma and endemic diseases, *International J. Healing and Caring* 2009, 9(2), 1-20

[21] Vargas, Luis A, et al. (1989) Exploring the multidimensional aspects of grief reactions, *American J Psychiatry* 1989, 146(11), 1484-9.

[22] Whitmont, Edward C. (1980) *Psyche and Substance: Essays on Homeopathy in the Light of Jungian Psychology*, Berkeley, CA: Homeopathic Education Services and North Atlantic Books

[23] Whitmont, Edward C. (1993) *The Alchemy of Healing: Psyche and Soma*, Berkeley, CA: Homeopathic Education Services and North Atlantic Books

[24] Whitmont, Edward C. (1996) *The role of mind in health, disease and the practice of homeopathy*, Frontier Perspectives 1996, 5(2), 24-30

[25] Wright, Machaelle Small (1997) *Co-Creative Science: A Revolution In Science Providing Real Solutions For Today's Health & Environment*, Warrenton, VA: Perelandra, Ltd

Chapter 4
Was Hahnemann the Real Pioneer of Psychiatry?

Peter Morrell, BSc MPhil PGCE

Peter Morrell, BSc MPhil PGCE
Stafford College
Earl Street
Stafford
ST16 2QR, United Kingdom
E-mail: petermrrll@yahoo.co.uk

Abstract
This essay explores Hahnemann's treatment of mentally ill patients, his aphorisms in the Organon on the same subject and finally the position 'mental illness' occupies within the conceptual fabric of homeopathy as a whole. The traditional view of the origins of psychiatry has always given the credit to three key figures: Reil, Pinel and Tuke, but Hahnemann seems to have preceded them all.

1   Contemporaries of Hahnemann

As Dudgeon tells us, Hahnemann "*settled for a time in 1792,*" (Dudgeon, p.23) in Georgenthal, and it was while residing there that he "*accepted an offer of the reigning Duke of Saxe-Gotha to take charge of an asylum for the insane.*" (ibid.) In a letter of May 1792, Hahnemann states that the Duke would soon be "*handing over to me his hunting castle in Georgenthal,*" (Haehl, 2, p.32) where he was able to "*pursue his painfully interesting investigations,*" (Dudgeon, p.23) eventually bringing about a dramatic cure of a patient, Herr Klockenbring. The account of this cure was published in 1796 (Lesser Writings, p.243-49) and this proves Hahnemann was "*one of the earliest, if not the very first,*" (Dudgeon, p.23) to advocate a "*treatment of the insane by mildness rather than coercion.*" (ibid.) In fact, it was on 2 September in the year 1793 that "*Pinel made his first experiment of unchaining maniacs in the Bicêtre,*" (ibid.) which was some fifteen months after Hahnemann had commenced treating Herr Klockenbring.

1.1 Johann Christian Reil (1759-1813)

Hahnemann's cure of Klockenbring "*caused a sensation,*" (Haehl, 1, p.41) at the time and certainly reveals him as the originator of "*entirely new methods in the treatment of mental patients, independently of his famous contemporaries Pinel and Reil.*" (Haehl, 1, p.272) "'*We lock up these unhappy beings like criminals in cells,' exclaims Reil in 1803.*" (Haehl, 2, p.31)

The anatomist and psychiatrist Reil (1759-1813), was "*a friend of Goethe and publisher of various medical journals, who was the first to use the term 'psychiatry; he warned against the indiscriminate administration of drugs and instead emphasized the use of psychogogics, occupation, playing music and acting in his therapeutic program, "Rhapsodie" on the application of emotional cures on rain of the mind." The treatment of melancholy included pleasing physical stimuli such as heat, studying aesthetic paintings, strolling, and swinging."* (http://mineralconnection.com/stjohn-3.htm)

1.2 Philippe Pinel (1745-1826)

Philippe Pinel (1745-1826), a French physician, *"M.D. Univ. of Toulouse, 1773. After moving to Paris in 1778, he was appointed (1793) director of the Bicêtre hospital and shortly thereafter of the Salpêtrière. His 'Traité médico-philosophique sur l'aliénation mentale' (2d ed. 1809), based on observations in both these hospitals, advocated humane treatment of mentally ill persons, then called the insane, and a more empirical study of mental disease. He further contributed to the development of psychiatry through his establishment of the practice of keeping well-documented psychiatric case histories for research."* (http://www.slider.com/enc/42000/Pinel_Philippe.htm)

1.3 William Tuke (1732-1822)

William Tuke, *"was head of the Quaker family that founded the York Retreat in 1792...located in a rural setting, provided humane institutional care of people with mental illness. Its reduced use of restraints and confinement, and therapeutic use of occupational tasks, especially farming chores, were duplicated in scores of later institutions."* (Street, 1994) Tuke (1732–1822) was an English merchant and philanthropist, who succeeded at an early age to the family business at York in wholesale tea and coffee. Apart from founding the York Retreat, he spawned a whole family of individuals, all with pioneering links to humane treatment of the poor, the destitute and the mentally ill. The York Retreat was *"an influential early institution for the intelligent and humane care of the insane."* (http://www.infoplease.com/ce6/people/A0849646.html)

2   Treatment of Klockenbring

The chief resource that is alluded to by others in support of Hahnemann's alleged superior and prophetic views on mental illness is his treatment of Klockenbring in Georgenthal in 1792-3. This pivotal event was certainly crucial in moulding his own views on this subject.

Hahnemann's cure of Herr Klockenbring by gentle methods undoubtedly provided him with some pioneering ideas about the nature of mental diseases and how they ought to be treated. Whether it gave him any conception of mental illness, as a separate category of sickness in its own right, seems unlikely, because such an idea clearly flies in the face of the holistic views inherent in homeopathy itself. These events also took place in the decade when Hahnemann was conducting his first provings and just before he published what might be termed his 'first sketch' of Materia Medica in the *'Fragmenta de viribus medicamentorum positivis,'* published in 1805. This incident therefore actually occurred at a very busy and important time when Hahnemann was consumed with his formulation of the homeopathic system for the first time.

At the time in question, Hahnemann declared that he had *"been for several years much occupied with diseases of the most tedious and desperate character in general,"* (Bradford, p.52) including several cases of hypochondria and insanity. Hahnemann then wrote of establishing *"a model asylum for the treatment, by gentle methods, of the insane of the higher classes of society."* (Bradford, p.53) Publicity for the new asylum was given in a local journal, Algemeine Anzeiger, in March 1792, (Haehl, 2, p.20) yet, *"in spite of the clear intention to restrict its use...to persons of...good social standing...the document breaks out compassionately into a plea for a rational treatment of the countless victims of insanity who were kept in confinement in the asylums."* (Hobhouse, p.85-6)

Hahnemann's entry into the psychiatric field *"was four years before William Tuke, the English Quaker had finally established the Retreat in York... and a year before Pinel reformed the Bicêtre Asylum in Paris."* (Hobhouse, p.85) The only drug shown to be capable of producing the precise raft of mental symptoms of Klockenbring was Stramonium, and when given it he was cured. *"One morning during one of his fits, he asked for ink and paper, and wrote a prescription. It was Stramonium. The drug was administered and the patient had no sooner begun to take the medicine when he recovered."* (Hempel, 1859, p.753)

This is how Hahnemann describes the incident: *"One evening, in the midst of the most extravagant paroxysm of folly, he hastily called for pen, ink and paper, and though on other occasions he would not listen to anything about corporeal diseases, he now wrote a prescription[3] which he wished to be made up immediately. The extraordinary ingredients of this were so extremely well arranged and so admirably adapted to the cure of an insanity of this sort, that for the moment I was almost tempted to consider him a very well instructed physician, had not the ridiculous direction he gave as to how it should be used—namely, with a few bottles of burgundy as a vehicle, to be followed up by lard—given another turn to my thoughts. But how was it that in the midst of the very hurricane of its most extravagant passion, his mastless and helmless mind lighted on a remedy so excellent for insanity and unknown to many physicians. 'How came he to prescribe it for himself in the most appropriate form and dose'!"*
(S Hahnemann, Description of Klockenbring during his Insanity, Lesser Writings, p.246)

The background to Hahnemann's use of Stramonium for Klockenbring is interesting in itself. Anton von Stoerck (von Stoerck, 1762) *"asks if Stramonium ought not to be useful in insanity, as it possesses the power to cause derangement of the mind,"* (Dudgeon, p.23) and he had revealed *"the virtues of the mania-producing Stramonium in mental disorders."* (Dudgeon, p.47) Von Stoerck was *"the first who made use of Stramonium in madness...(he) employed it in two cases of mania, and he asserts that he obtained success. According to Engelhart, Smaltz has cured with Stramonium a girl alternately affected with mania and melancholia."* (Guislain, p.156) Hahnemann would certainly have known about *"Von Stoerck with respect to the virtues of the mania-producing Stramonium in mental disorders,"* (Dudgeon, p.47) from his Vienna days (1777) where von Stoerck had been based.

---

3 The commencement was R. Sem, Daturae, gr. ij. &c. [which means a 2-grain dose of tincture of Datura seed; a single grain is approximately 65mg]

At the time of Hahnemann's incursion into this field, the insane were "*treated like wild animals...chained in dungeon-like cells.*" (Cook, p.62) The usual treatment at the time was "*by violence...whipping and dungeons.*" (Bradford, p.54) Haehl states that Hahnemann "*acquired a knowledge of psychiatry...greater than Pinel's...(upholding) the cause of humane treatment,*" (Hobhouse, p.93) and that he additionally laid out "*the foundations of a new medicinal treatment of mental illness.*" (ibid, p.93) Hahnemann also appreciated the importance of the 'law of similars' when he referred to a cure "*by Hippocrates of his friend's mania by the use of Hellebore...(which can) produce the symptoms of mania.*" (Hobhouse, p.92) Apparently, this observation provided one confirmation for his idea of the central importance of similars in medicine.

During the two years following his translation of Cullen's Materia Medica, and the epochal Cinchona bark proving in 1790 that derived from it, Hahnemann "*continued to experiment upon himself and on his family and certain of his friends with different substances,*" (Bradford, p.52) but he had not yet "*tested the truth of this new principle on the sick. The insanity of Klockenbring gave him the opportunity.*" (ibid, p.52) However, for the first few weeks "*Hahnemann simply observed Klockenbring without giving him any medical treatment.*" (Hobhouse, 89)

Klockenbring had been "*Hanoverian Minister of Police and Secretary to the Chancellery... (and) in his fast life, he developed great eccentricity,*" (Bradford, p.53) but he became the subject of a satire claiming he was a close associate of drunken brothel keepers and that he had "*the most dangerous venereal disease and moral vices ranging from drunkenness to fraud.*" (Cook, p.62) As a public figure and family man who could not stand such accusations, he "*became violently insane.*" (Bradford, p.53)

"*In June 1792 he was brought to Georgenthal,*" (Haehl, 2, p.33) being "*so violent that he was escorted by two well-built men to keep him under control.*" (Cook, p.63) His face was "*covered with large spots, was dirty, and imbecile in expression. Day and night he raved. He was afflicted with strange hallucinations...would recite Greek...actual words of Hebrew text...he destroyed his clothing and bedding, took his piano to pieces...and exhibited the most perfect forms of excitable mania.*" (Bradford, p.54) Yet, Hahnemann had succeeded in curing him by "*March 1793.*" (Bradford, p.55) As Cook suggests, it seems likely that his ravings were indeed "*those of the tertiary stages of syphilis,*" (Cook, p.63) as his cruel satirist had suggested in the first place.

3   In the Organon, Hahnemann on so-called 'mental diseases'

There seems little doubt that Hahnemann *"possessed an extraordinary understanding for the nervous and mental activities of his patients...and (possibly) considered psycho-therapy in certain cases to be more important, more applicable than the use of homeopathic medicines."* (Haehl, 1, p.272-3) He also seems to have been *"far in advance of his time in this province,"* (ibid, p.273) by exhibiting a *"fine understanding...for the unfortunate victims of mental derangement,"* (ibid, p.272) and he acquired a reputation for the same, attracting many patients with mental problems. This was in the 1790s before homeopathy was yet established and during the time that he was no longer a regular doctor, having *"retired disgusted with the uncertainty of medical practice."* (Dudgeon, p.21) c.1784.

Several things become apparent to anyone who reads about *"mental and emotional maladies,"* (Aph. 229) and "mental and emotional disease," (Aph. 230) in the Organon. For one, Hahnemann is consistently extremely careful indeed not to fall into the allopathic trap of classing them as a separate category of sickness. He very specifically qualifies his reference to them as diseases, preferring to allude to them as mental symptoms of the whole person. For example, he states that *"what are termed mental diseases...do not, however, constitute a class of disease,"* (Aph. 210) and, employing various phrases, he refers to them as an *"altered state of the disposition and mind,"* (Aph. 212) *"the so-called mental and emotional diseases,"* (Aph. 215) *"the state of the mind and disposition,"* (Aph. 213) *"the symptom of the mental disturbance,"* (Aph. 216) etc.

Hahnemann refers to *"derangement of the mind and disposition,"* (Aph. 215) to *"insanity or mania (caused by fright, vexation, the abuse of spirituous liquors;"* (Aph. 221) *"attack of the insanity;"* (Aph. 223) *"a real moral or mental malady;"* (Aph. 224) *"furious mania...doleful, querulous lamentation...senseless chattering...disgusting and abominable conduct;"* (Aph. 228) *"destruction and injury of surrounding objects;"* (Aph. 228) *"the violent insane maniac and melancholic;"* (Aph. 229) *"an acute mental or emotional disease,"* (Aph. 222) *"periodic or continued mental derangement;"* (Aph. 223) *"mental or emotional disease of long standing,"* (Aph. 222) *"there are incredibly numerous varieties of them."* (Aph. 230) Taken together, these observations clearly demonstrate the degree of careful attention he had personally directed towards such cases.

From the depth and detail of his knowledge of emotional disorders, Hahnemann then reveals a clear familiarity with patients who are *"obstinate, violent, hasty...intolerant and capricious, or impatient...lascivious and shameless;"* (Aph. 210) cases of *"insanity...melancholia...mania;"* (Aph. 216) disease states resulting from *"faults of education, bad practices, corrupt morals, neglect of the mind, superstition or ignorance;"* (Aph. 224) *"the melancholic...the spiteful maniac...the chattering fool."* (Aph. 224) All such references suggest Hahnemann's minute observation of many cases and the thoughtful and compassionate attitude that such experiences must have inspired in him towards *"such unfortunate beings,"* (Aph. 222) who possess a *"clouded spirit,"* (Aph. 229) for he sees in each of them *"the soul that pines or frets in the chains of the diseased body."* (Aph. 229)

He states that even for those he calls *"the accurately observing physician,"* (Aph. 211), such disorders *"can only be detected by the observation of a physician gifted with perseverance and penetration."* (Aph. 216) Being very empathic towards such patients in whom *"the emotional* and mental state ..." constitute "... the principal symptom of such a patient," (Aph. 230) he also offers tentative explanations of mental illness based upon his own extensive observations. He proposes that they "originate and are kept up by emotional causes, such as continued anxiety, worry, vexation, wrongs and the frequent occurrence of great fear and fright;" (Aph. 225) "emotional diseases...first engendered and subsequently kept up by the mind itself;" (Aph. 226) and that they require a "carefully regulated mode of life." (Aph. 228)

Hahnemann also condemns outright the fact that the mentally deranged patient of his day all too "often witnesses the occurrence of ingratitude, cruelty, refined malice and propensities most disgraceful and degrading to humanity, which were precisely the qualities possessed by the patient before he grew ill," (Aph. 210) and which are very clearly uncurative and injurious and only aggravate the condition of the patient. He insists that the physician should adopt an "appropriate psychical behaviour towards the patient," (Aph. 228) employ "an auxiliary mental regimen,", "without reproaching the patient for his acts." (Aph. 228) This should not include "corporeal punishments and tortures," (Aph. 228) or "the employment of coercion." (Aph. 228) He is astonished and appalled at "the hard-heartedness and indiscretion of the medical men," (Aph. 228) for "torturing these most pitiable of all human beings with the most violent blows and other painful torments," (Aph. 228) which he condemns as a "revolting procedure." (Aph. 228)

Such physicians, he says, "debase themselves... (by)...their uselessness." (Aph. 228). He denounces "harshness towards the pitiable, innocent sufferers," (Aph. 228) and proclaims that "they are equally pernicious modes of treating mental and emotional maladies." (Aph. 229). And he advises physicians in general that "I can confidently assert, from great experience, that the vast superiority of the homoeopathic system over all other conceivable methods of the treatment is nowhere displayed in a more triumphant light than in mental and emotional diseases of long standing," (Aph. 230) acknowledging the general point that "the disposition of the patient often chiefly determines the selection of the homoeopathic remedy." (Aph. 211) He then furnishes us with some examples of the key feature of mentals in remedy selection: "Aconite will seldom or never effect a rapid or permanent cure in a patient of a quiet, calm, equable disposition; and just as little will Nux vomica be serviceable where the disposition is mild and phlegmatic, Pulsatilla where it is happy, gay and obstinate, or Ignatia where it is imperturbable and disposed neither to be frightened nor vexed." (Aph. 214)

Always emphasising that "a homoeopathic medicinal pathogenetic force - that is to say, a remedy which in its list of symptoms displays, with the greatest possible similarity, not only the corporeal morbid symptoms present in the case of disease before us, but also especially this mental and emotional state," (Aph. 217) for "a disease of the mind and disposition," (Aph. 218), or a "disorder of the mind," (Aph. 220) Hahnemann then identifies remedies like "Aconite, Belladonna, Stramonium, Hyoscyamus, Mercury," (Aph. 221) as being especially useful for such patients, but though "a lucid interval and a transient alleviation of the psychical disease," (Aph. 219) may thus be obtained, that they can only be truly "cured by antipsorics," (Aph. 223) that "mental and emotional diseases...can only be cured by homoeopathic antipsoric medicine," (Aph. 228) and that one must select "the antipsoric remedies selected for each particular case of mental or emotional disease," (Aph. 230) and administer "a radical, antipsoric treatment," (Aph. 227) as being "the only efficacious mode of curing such disease." (Aph. 228)

Hahnemann has a lot more to say in the Organon on emotional disorders but the above is an accurate précis of his views on the subject.

4   Discussion

Although Hahnemann, in the Organon, and most homeopaths since, do consider the mental symptoms - the *"always predominating state of the mind and disposition."* (Aph. 217) - as being very important and significant in defining a patient's disease and in remedy selection, nowhere in homeopathy is there any coherent theory of mind or mental illness in the same sense as that found in allopathy. Indeed, mind is merely regarded as another part of the whole person: *"the almost spiritual, mental and emotional organs, which the anatomist has never yet and never will reach with his scalpel."* (Aph. 216) In other words, all homeopaths since Hahnemann have predominantly ignored mind as a separate field of disease causation, except insofar as it is merely a field wherein symptoms make themselves manifest either as a product of the drug or of a disease and always when viewed holistically - in the round.

Hahnemann does however acknowledge that such mental disorders do give an impression, an apparition of being a separate class of disease: *"as though it were a local disease in the invisible subtle organ of the mind or disposition,"* (Aph. 215) but because homeopathy fails to take cognisance of mental illness as a separate entity, apart from any other holistic disease entity, it seems to ignore all theories of mental disease in exactly the same way that it ignores all allopathically construed theories of physical disease, as being largely irrelevant to its 'modus operandi' or worldview. It adopts this position because all disease is construed as a *"dynamic aberration of our spirit-like life;"* (Close, p.67) *"a perverted vital action;"* (Close, 70) *"disease is the suffering of the dynamis;"* (Close, p.72) *"disease is primarily a morbid disturbance or disorderly action of the vital force."* (Close, p.74) Close is most emphatic in insisting that disease is *"not a thing, but only the condition of a thing."* (Close, p.70) Since homeopathic drugs correct the vital force, by domino effect (so to say), the entire organism automatically becomes corrected - including mind. We might therefore ask: where is the concept of mental illness in homeopathy? There IS no such concept - there is no concept of mental illness per se in homeopathy.

Clearly, the Organon's conception of 'mental illness' is not congruent with the conventional definition or with the way it is applied by modern practitioners. In this sense, homeopathy clearly has no separate category of 'mental illness'. Even though the symptom of the one-sided illness may involve mental illness (in the conventional sense) an obsession, illusion, delusion, hallucination, fear (phobia?), suicidal impulses, depression, etc., to homeopathy it is only an illness of a deeply deranged vital force, deranged at the most fundamental level, never of the mind itself in isolation from the whole person.

The essence of this view is peppered throughout the Organon and in Kent and Close and Boger - it states simply that mind and body comprise one holistic unit (whereas conventionally regarded as two arenas) in which symptoms manifest themselves. It depicts a *"functional unity of the psychic state...and somatic state."* (Verspoor, p.103) Boenninghausen also repeats this dual unity of Aphorisms 224-226 (ibid, p.118). However, Hahnemann is clear that the ultimate source of all symptoms is derangements in the *"life force"* - a view incidentally he shared with Paracelsus,

Stahl, and van Helmont. Remedies remove these derangements and so the flow of symptoms - to whichever arena - is slowed and then ceases. These views are stated repeatedly by Close and Kent, for example, and are echoed constantly by all the 'greats'.

4.1 Vitalist predecessors

Hahnemann leaves no doubt about the fundamentally holistic nature of homeopathy and rails repeatedly against materialistic and allopathic constructs, which seek to slice the person up into organs or systems and condemns any 'treatment of parts' that always flows from such a re-ductionist perspective. Kent likewise condemns this approach in his own emotional manner. The only option therefore is to regard all so-called 'disease' as an expression of an internal disorder resident in the life force, which remedies reach and eliminate, and then the flow of symptoms ceases. Clearly, the remedies must be chosen on the basis of their totality and similarity to the entire person, rather than upon the disease as an entity. This was originally an idea of Paracelsus which inspired contrasting interpretations: the material school leading to allopathy, and the vitalist schools represented by van Helmont (Paracelsus' chief interpreter) and Stahl. This stream leads directly to Hahnemann - even though he never states this overtly.

'Disease as entity' was a spiritual concept of invasion of the life force - this concept was created by Paracelsus, but poorly described by him, and articulated much more clearly by Van Helmont. The same point was also amplified extensively by Kent in his idea that the cause of disease invades the vital force first, as a spiritual entity, and then outflows its bad effects into the entire organism 'from within outwards'. This view comes close to that of some modern homeopaths who believe in *"the all-encompassing state of mind."* (Verspoor, p.125)

Whether this is truly *"Hahnemann's conception of the 'highest disease'...those that are 'spun and maintained by the soul' but ultimately rooted in the arch beliefs of the human spirit (Aph. 224),"* (Verspoor, p.130) is very hard to say. It almost suggests *"the idea of disease as a delusion,"* (ibid, 268) which again sounds like Hahnemann as a disease *"first spun and maintained by the soul."* (ibid, 299) However, it is hard to see to what extent such modern ideas about the significance of mind or mental symptoms in homeopathy truly derive from the words of Hahnemann. One suspects that his own words have been hammered on an anvil of modern psychology into very distorted word shapes, belonging to a lexicon of concepts that would have been entirely alien to Hahnemann himself. This clearly remains a matter of opinion and debate.

5   Summary

As we have seen, Hahnemann appears to have been the first to recommend gentle and humane methods for the treatment of the mentally ill, a year or more before Pinel, Tuke or Reil, thus making him the true pioneer of psychiatry. In his work with Klockenbring — coinciding as it did with his first provings — Hahnemann realised that only by careful matching of the symptom picture of the patient with a drug shown to be capable of creating the same symptom pattern can a true cure for mental suffering be achieved. Fortuitously, it was Klockenbring's insistence on *Stramonium* for his own condition that enabled Hahnemann to appreciate the unerring similarity between a drug's proving symptoms and the sufferings of the patient. This case superbly exemplifies Hahnemann's absolute break with the ideas and methods of his contemporaries in his early focus on the single drug, his use of medical simile, his long interest in studies of poisonings and hence of proving symptoms. In this sense, the Klockenbring case arrived exactly at a time when Hahnemann was able to seize the conceptual and practical realities of the case, which coincided with the evolution of his own medical ideas at a crucially embryonic stage in homeopathy's development.

We have also seen how homeopathy takes a very different view of 'mental illness' compared to that in the predominating allopathic medical system. By viewing 'mental illness' within the wider holistic concept of patient symptom totality, homeopathic conceptuality dismisses as an artificial construct any separate categorisation of mental sickness as adopted by allopaths. Always extolling a profoundly holistic viewpoint, Hahnemann's Organon repeatedly emphasises that mental symptoms, though often very important in remedy selection, form only one facet of the symptom totality of an individual patient. Finally, we have also seen that homeopathy, with its emphasis on the vital force, on mentality and potency energy, shares some common conceptual ground and stands in a direct line with such previous vitalist medical systems as those of Paracelsus and Van Helmont.

References

[1] Bradford, Thomas L. (1895) *Life and Letters of Hahnemann*, New Delhi: B Jain Publishers

[2] Close, Stuart (1924) *The Genius of Homeopathy, Lectures and Essays on Homeopathic Philosophy*, New York: Reprint New Delhi: B Jain Publishers

[3] Cook, Trevor M. (1981) *Samuel Hahnemann, the Founder of Homeopathic Medicine*, Wellingborough: Thorsons Publishers

[4] Dudgeon, Robert E (1853) *Lectures on the Theory & Practice of Homeopathy*, London: Henry Turner

[5] Guislain, Joseph (1826) *Traité sur L'Alienation Mentale*, Paris: Joseph Gulslatn, Médecin à Gand

[6] Haehl, Richard (1922) *Samuel Hahnemann His Life and Works*, 2 volumes, Reprint, New Delhi: B Jain Publishers

[7] Hahnemann, S. (1893) *The Organon of Medicine*, combined 5th/6th Edition, Translated by R.E. Dudgeon, and edited by William Boericke, New Delhi: B Jain Publishers

[8] Hahnemann, S. (1895) *Lesser Writings* edited by R.E. Dudgeon, London: Henry Turner & Co

[9] Charles Julius Hempel (1859) *A Comprehensive System of Materia Medica and Therapeutics*, Philadelphia: William Radde & Boston: Otis Clapp

[10] http://books.google.co.uk/books?id=d4ZNAAAAMAAJ&pg=PA753&dq=klockenbring+stramonium

[11] Hobhouse, Rosa W. (1933) *Life of Christian Samuel Hahnemann*, Harjeet, India, Reprint New Delhi: B Jain Publishers

[12] Street, W. R. (1994) *A Chronology of Noteworthy Events in American Psychology*, Washington, D.C.: American sychological Association, Addenda, http://www.cwu.edu/~warren/addenda.html

[13] Verspoor, Rudi & Steven Decker (1999) *Homeopathy Re-Examined*, Ottawa: Heilkunst

[14] Von Stoerck, Anton (1762) *An essay on the internal use of thorn-apple, henbane, and monkshood: which are shown to be safe and efficacious remedies, in the cure of many obstinate diseases.* Translated from the original Latin: "Libellus quo demonstrator: Stramonium, Hyoscyamus, Aconitum non Solum tuto posse Exhiberi usu Interno Hominibus," Vienna. Electronic reproduction, Farmington Hills, Mich.: Thomson Gale, 2003

Section 2: Integration, Case Applications, and Therapeutic Process

Chapter 5
Homeopathic Treatment of Children with Behavioural and Learning Problems

Judyth Reichenberg-Ullman, ND DHANP LCSW
& Robert Ullman, ND DHANP

Judyth Reichenberg-Ullman, ND DHANP LCSW
Robert Ullman, ND DHANP
The Northwest Center for Homeopathic Medicine
131 Third Avenue, N.
Edmonds, WA 98020
USA
drreichenberg@gmail.com
www.healthyhomeopathy.com

Abstract
This chapter is a practical, case-oriented discussion of homeopathic treatment of behavioural and learning problems in children. Included are an overview of the problem, conventional diagnoses, case taking, case analysis, prescribing, case management, potency selection, case studies, and what to expect from homeopathic care of this group.

1   Overview of clinical experience

We are licensed naturopathic physicians board certified in homeopathic medicine, and have been in practice for twenty-six (Judyth) and twenty-eight years (Robert). In addition, Judyth received a Master's in Psychiatric Social Work in 1970 and worked in both in-patient and outpatient psychiatric settings. Robert pursued graduate work in psychology and gained inpatient experience with developmentally-disabled children. Although our practice was initially focused primarily on adults, Judyth began, in the late eighties, treating foster children whose problems ran the gamut of behavioural and learning problems. This led to presentations at case conferences, articles in homeopathic professional journals and in mainstream publications such as *Mothering* and *Natural Health*.

By the time our book, *Ritalin-Free Kids*, was published, we had treated over a thousand children; now it has been well over five thousand. We have heard from many of our colleagues that our book brought many parents and their children to their practices as well. The epidemic of ADHD (Attention Deficit Hyperactivity Disorder) began in the United States, but spread internationally over time, first to the United Kingdom, then beyond. As we taught seminars to professional homeopaths and the public throughout the U.S., Canada, New Zealand, Australia, Scotland, and even Pune, India, we found the same constellation of symptoms and the same challenges facing children and adults. In fact, one of the largest crowds was in one of the most out-of-the way locations, Perth, Australia, which has documented an unusually high incidence of ADHD.

The diagnosis of ADHD was the primary one when we entered this field. Since that time, numerous other co-morbid diagnoses have evolved, and most children that we see who have received formal psychological testing and medication carry more than one diagnosis. Since that time many other so-called "co-morbid" diagnoses have been added. Many of the youngsters in our practice suffer from behavioural, attitudinal, and developmental issues in addition to learning challenges, which led us to document additional paediatric cases in two other books: *Rage-Free Kids* and *A Drug-Free Approach to Asperger Syndrome and Autism*, as well as including a few cases of childhood Obsessive Compulsive Disorder in *Prozac-Free*. There are so many special considerations in treating children on the autism spectrum that we will focus primarily on behavioural and learning problems, although one of our cases is that of a child with Asperger Syndrome, which a decade ago was easily confused with Obsessive Compulsive Disorder.

A decade ago, the children who arrived at our practice, if medicated, were taking a single stimulant medication, initially Ritalin[4], later Adderall[5], and the new amphetamine drug, Vyvanse, also known as Concerta[6]. Now the population that we see is broader and the diagnoses and medications multiple. Children brought to us may be on a stimulant medication, even two, as well as an atypical antipsychotic, anticonvulsant, and/or antidepressant. Whereas the side effects were initially the classical ones resulting from stimulant use - sleeplessness, lack of appetite, weight loss, and stimulant rebound - there are many more as a result of the additional medications, including significant weight gain, thyroid inhibition, diabetes, and, rarely, tardive dyskinesia (involuntary, repetitive movements of the face, tongue, or limbs).

Some of the more common labels attributed to the children in our practice include the following:
- ODD (Oppositional Defiant Disorder)
- OCD (Obsessive Compulsive Disorder)
- SID (Sensory Integration Disorder)
- BPD (Bi-Polar Disorder) also known as MDD (Manic Depressive Disorder)
- RAD (Reactive Attachment Disorder)
- AS (Asperger Syndrome)
- AD (Anxiety Disorder)
- DD (Depressive Disorder)
- TS (Tourette Syndrome)
- LD (Learning Disability)
- CD (Conduct Disorder)
- PTSD (Post-Traumatic Stress Disorder)

Homeopathy treats patients, not diagnoses. Therefore, regardless of nomenclature or abbreviation, we endeavour to understand the child as a whole, from inside to out. Although the diagnosis may at times help provide a prognosis, ultimately we, as homeopaths, do not base our prescriptions upon that child's so-called label, but rather upon the uniqueness of that individual.

---

4 Generic name: methylphenidate

5 Generic name: amphetamine and dextroamphetamine

6 Generic name: Lisdexamphetamine (L-Lysine-d-amphetamine)

2 Why homeopathic treatment?

Let us clarify from the outset that although homeopathic self-care can be quite effective for first-aid and acute conditions, parents should not even think about treating their children with attention, behavioural, and learning problems themselves. We are talking about two thousand-plus potential remedies, expertise in case taking, and subtleties in differential diagnosis. It's absurd to think of a parent doing a surgical procedure on his/her child. Parents should find skilled and experienced homeopaths to assure the best possible outcome for their children.

There are numerous compelling reasons to seek out homeopathic care for these children:

1. Homeopathy is safe, gentle, and natural. There is no need for a *Physicians's Desk Reference* listing all of the side effects, as with conventional medicine.
2. Homeopathic treatment is highly individualized. There are basically a dozen or fewer conventional medications used for most children with behavioural and learning problems. The prescription is based on the common symptoms shared by children with the same diagnosis. Homeopathic treatment is based on what is unique about each child, and how that child is different from every other child with the same or similar diagnosis. S/he may need one remedy from a choice of over two thousand.
3. The effects of a single dose of a homeopathic medicine can last for weeks, months, or, occasionally, years. This is in stark contrast to stimulant medications which, unless of the time-release kind, may last only a few hours, then produce an unpleasant rebound effect. The homeopathic pills taste like sugar, go down easily, and are palatable even for infants.
4. Homeopathy treats not only the mental and emotional symptoms of the child, but also any physical symptoms and strengthens the child's immunity as well. Suppose, for example, that a child has migraines, asthma, or eczema, along with the behavioural and learning challenges. These too will resolve or improve significantly with the correct homeopathic remedy.
5. Homeopathy treats the root of the underlying imbalance rather than merely putting a Band-Aid on symptoms. Parents find all-around, global changes in their children, even in behaviours or tendencies which they considered to be simply a party of the child's personality or makeup.
6. Homeopathic remedies will not dull or blunt a child's affect, but will rather allow the child to become more vibrant, relaxed, and to optimize abilities, creativity, awareness, and natural gifts. Homeopathy does not remove any of the positive aspects of a child's expression or personality; it just frees the child to be more of who s/he can be. This includes greater confidence, ability to interact with peers and adults, and greater overall happiness and well-being.
7. Homeopathic remedies often eliminate the need for conventional medications, depending on the individual and the condition. It is also possible to take them in conjunction with pharmaceutical drugs.
8. Treatment with homeopathy often enhances the effectiveness of other therapies and interventions so that they can occur less frequently and sometimes eliminates the need for them entirely.
9. Homeopathic medicines are very inexpensive and appointments with homeopathic practitioners occur much less often than with other health care providers.
10. Homeopathy is easy to administer, does not require dietary or lifestyle changes, and is much less restrictive than many other approaches.

3   Homeopathic treatment

3.1 Case taking

Since this chapter is our contribution to an international homeopathic publication, we will not assume that all homeopaths take cases in a similar fashion, and will outline clearly our approach. In cases of children up to fifteen years old we schedule an hour and a half for the initial visit. The first half of the appointment, whether in person, by telephone, or by video consultation, is with the parent(s). This allows us to get the lie of the land, so to speak, before interviewing the child.

We are aware that some homeopaths choose to do the entire interview with parents and child together, but this is not our style. The parents may have attention issues themselves, they may have other siblings present as well, and we endeavour as much as possible to give the parents and the children privacy so they are free to speak their minds. Parents may not always have a sense of what is therapeutic for the child to hear and what may be damaging. We prefer to run the risk of the child feeling left out during the first part of the interview rather than find ourselves in an awkward situation of wishing the child were not in the room to hear certain revealing information. This private time with the parent(s) allows us to tease out marital problems, confidential family history, circumstances of birth, adoption, parental frustrations with the child, etc.

Similarly we offer the child whenever possible the opportunity to speak with us alone. S/he is likely to be more candid and less influenced by the responses of the parent(s).

There are of course exceptions. Some children are so shy that they are unwilling to speak with us unless their parents are present. Others are simply too developmentally disabled, ill, or nonverbal. Although the interview itself yields the most compelling and revealing information, we do find periodic feedback from teachers, counsellors, and other caregivers to be helpful.

We have found the most essential aspects of the case taking to be:

- *Observation*: Child's and parents' actions, body language, movements, countenance, activities, gestures, habits, play.
- *The exact words used*: Even when we interview parents about their children, we attempt to elicit the precise words used, rather than the parents' translation or interpretation of the child's responses.
- *Engage the child*: We invite the child to speak candidly about his/her favourite topics, hobbies, movies, books, video games, likes and dislikes, school. We are simply interested in finding an inroad to get the child to open up so that we can enter into her mind, reality, point of view.
- *Follow the energy*: We first heard this term from one of our colleagues and teachers in India, Sunil Anand, who also specializes in homeopathic paediatrics. It is the best term we have heard to sum up the intention of case taking. We are simply trying to immerse ourselves in the flow of the child and to follow that energy where it leads us. You may have heard the expression, "If you give him enough rope, he will hang himself". We use that approach in a positive sense. If we allow someone, child or adult, to talk more and more about himself, it will generally lead us, if not to the correct remedy, at least in the ball park.
- *Flexibility*: This approach to case taking is the complete opposite of that of a homeopath who may be limited to prescribing polychrest remedies[7], who will not stray from a particular potency or style of prescribing, and who may even have a list of questions that s/he asks each

---

7 Polychrest is the term used in homeopathy for a remedy that has many uses.

and every patient during the initial interview. We make every effort to be open to what the individual brings, so that it is a fresh, new, and never-before experienced interaction. This flexibility of perception, prescribing, and ongoing case management means that we continue to be open, even years into the case, to new information, symptoms, and remedies emerging.

- *Listen for what has never before been heard*: The homeopath can make the mistake of thinking, "He is so much like that *Lycopodium* child that I saw in my office last week". Or, "he is fearful and aggressive, so he must be a *Stramonium*, like the boy in that article". What is most exciting and what will most reveal the correct remedy is that each and every child is unique. If we delve deeply enough into the case, there will usually be something that we have never before heard. It is that aspect of the child that makes her different from every other child with the same diagnosis - that strange, rare, and peculiar symptom that will lead us to perceive why she needs a different remedy from our last ten patients, or perhaps a remedy that we have never before prescribed, or possibly, never even heard of in our studies. Or, to step even further afield, a remedy that has not even yet been proven or is even not yet available in a homeopathic preparation.

3.2 Case analysis

Homeopaths are often independently-minded individuals, so it is no surprise that there is controversy surrounding the treatment approaches of different practitioners. We have studied closely with Dr. Rajan Sankaran of Mumbai, India since 1993. Our methodology has evolved along with his. In our experience, his technique is best applied to adults, and it is often challenging to find the same degree of sophistication and vocabulary with children, though there are certainly exceptions. This brings us back to the importance of flexibility and following the energy of each case.

Whenever possible, we do apply Dr. Sankaran's schema of classification to our prescribing, identifying first the kingdom (mineral, plant, animal, nosode[8]), then the family (according to his homeopathic periodic table of minerals, plant classification system) (Sankaran 2005) and his characteristics of those needing mammal, insect, arachnid, reptile, bird, or mollusc remedies. We also identify wherever possible the appropriate miasm[9], or hereditary layer of predisposition in the case. This is very important in order to choose the exact remedy according to Dr. Sankaran's schema. In some cases we rely on information from the internet in order to learn about substances that have not yet been prepared as homeopathic remedies. In summary:

- *Children needing mineral remedies*: Tend to have issues of performance, relationship, identity, roles, structure, security, and attack and defence. They are organized, literal, logical, numbers-oriented, by-the-book, and systematic. A few of the most common remedies for this population that fit into this group are *Calcarea carbonica* (calcium carbonate), *Baryta carbonica* (barium carbonate), *Sulphur* (sulfur), and *Natrum muriaticum* (sodium chloride). Any mineral or mineral salt, however, could be needed for a particular child.
- *Plant remedies*: Sensitive, emotional children whose physical symptoms have a number of

---

8 A nosode is a homeopathic remedy prepared from a pathological specimen.

9 Hahnemann's view of a miasm is one where a contagious infection has been medically mismanaged and in consequence becomes a systemic illness that permeates the entire physical body to such an extent that the disease imprint can now be genetically transferred from one generation to the next.

modalities and sensations. These children are adaptable and changeable, compared to the fixed nature of minerals. They exhibit sensitivity to emotions, pain, the environment, interactions with others. There are thousands, eventually millions, of potential plant remedies, but a few of the most common that everyone familiar with homeopathy will recognize are *Veratrum album* (white hellebore), *Stramonium* (thorn apple), *China* (Peruvian bark), and *Hyoscyamus* (henbane).

- *Animal remedies*: Primary issues are of survival, competition, dominating and dominated, victim/aggressor, predator and prey, sexuality, animation, attention. You will find a number of animal cases in this article because they tend to be fascinating and the children are charismatic. Common animal remedies for this population are *Tarentula* (tarentula), *Lyssinum* (Hydrophobinum or rabies nosode), and *Lachesis* (bushmaster snake).

When we do not have sufficient information to use the schema mentioned above, we do the best we can to prescribe a remedy in another way, relying on information from homeopathic *Materia Medica* and our previous experience.

3.3 Homeopathic prescribing and case management

We are often asked about potency selection. In our early years of homeopathic practice, we used exclusively high-potency remedies in dry doses, ranging from 200C to 10M, with occasional 30C and 50M prescriptions. Then for several years we experimented with using repeated 6C and 12C dry doses, but we basically found them cumbersome and to yield less satisfying results than what we were doing previously. Over the past ten years or so we have added liquid LM potencies and, more recently, plussed[10] liquid remedies, both given up to once a day or in some cases once a week or month. We are not wedded to one particular type of remedy administration, in line with our theme of flexibility. Contrary to practitioners who claim that LM potencies are the safest, we have seen at least as many reactions to LMs as to high potencies, resulting in our using multiple-glass

---

10 Dr. Ramakrishnan's "Plussing Method" involves agitating the remedy before each dose, according to the classical method. These are the instructions we give to our patients:

1. Shake bottle 10 times against the heel of your hand or a book.
2. Take 5 drops under tongue according to the schedule indicated on the bottle. If it burns your tongue, you can place the drops in a small amount of water (about 1 oz.) and hold the water in your mouth before swallowing.
3. If your symptoms worsen, stop taking the medicine. Resume when the symptoms subside. If you become worse after beginning to take it again, stop and contact your doctor.
4. If you continue to feel well, you can keep on taking the medicine at the prescribed frequency OR take it less often. If after that you begin to relapse, start taking it again or increase the frequency.

11 LM Multiple Glass Method to reduce initial aggravation. Instructions for patients:

1. If you are very sensitive or your symptoms are extremely aggravated after taking your LM medicine, we may suggest using 2, 3, or more glasses to prepare your LM medicine. Check with your doctor.
2. Follow the instructions above for LM Medicine. Then, instead of taking the ? teaspoon, put it in a second glass with 4 oz. water and stir. If you have been instructed to use the two-glass method, take 1/2 tsp. from this glass as your dose.
3. For the three-glass method, put the 1/2 tsp. from the second glass into a third glass containing 4 oz. of water, stir, and take 1/2 tsp. as a dose.
4. For four or more glasses, repeat the same procedure the prescribed number of times, taking 1 tsp. from the last glass as your dose.

methods[11] with many of our patients who take LM remedies. The kinds of reactions we have seen with patients using LM remedies include agitation and nervousness, a general sense of discomfort, an exacerbation of previous symptoms or new symptoms. This seems to result from proving the remedy as a result of taking it too often, and can often be corrected by reducing the frequency of administration or increasing the number of dilution glasses.[12]

Here is a brief summary of our considerations in potency selection:

- Children not on other medications: We often use single-dose, high-potency remedies administered infrequently. These doses can be effective for months at a time.
- Children on other medications: LM or plussed, repeated remedies, though single-dose remedies can still act in many cases.
- Children exposed repeatedly to substances or medications that we feel may interfere with treatment (aromatics, corticosteroids, antibiotics): LM or plussed remedies.
- Highly sensitive children or children with severe suppressed eczema: Single dose of 30C or lower potency or LM remedies.

3.4 Course of treatment
Many of the parents who contact us have never even heard of, much less tried, homeopathic medicine. They have come to us via other patients or health care practitioners, our books, the internet, and, occasionally, school counsellors or psychiatrists. They share the desire to improve their children's concentration, attitude, behaviour, health, and happiness. These parents often feel desperate. They know there must be an answer for their beloved children and, in the case of those who contact us, hope for an alternative to conventional medications. Frequently these parents have just received report cards, evaluations, or other types of feedback about their children, and are in hurry to set up an appointment with us. More often than not, following the initial appointment, they ask that we have a remedy ready for the following day. This speaks highly of the initial motivation of the parents.

Following the initial appointment we send out the remedy as soon as possible. If the parents are open to it, we collect a seven-day diet diary and after two weeks do a naturopathic appointment in which we discuss diet, nutritional supplementation, exercise, and lifestyle. Our first homeopathic follow-up visit occurs after one month. Subsequently, as the child improves, the appointments decrease in frequency, first to six-week intervals, then two or three months or longer. There are adolescents and young adults whom we have been treating for many years that may have appointments twice, or even once, a year. Many of our patients are treated by telephone or video consultation, since there are few homeopaths who specialize in this area and parents, often having already tried a number of therapeutic approaches, seek out the "experts".

Compliance varies with the attention and staying power of the parents and with the cooperation of the child. Parents may also suffer from ADHD, may try a number of approaches simultaneously, and have little patience to stick with homeopathy. In some cases either we find the correct remedy the first time or the parents do not return to give us another opportunity to help their children. It

---

12 We use the plussing method according to the handout of the Hahnemann pharmacy, which is very similar to Dr. Ramakrishnan's method (footnote 8).

may also be that parents have less of a commitment to a practitioner they do not meet in person. In addition, they are likely to have little encouragement and support to pursue homeopathy, either from other family members, psychiatrists and psychologists, or teachers. The prevailing wisdom continues to be that overactive children should be managed with stimulant medication.

When parents do continue with homeopathy long enough for the simillimum to be found, which may happen at the first visit, or months, or, occasionally years, later, they are usually very satisfied with the outcome and eagerly refer other parents. When we say it may, in rare cases, take years, it is not that positive results will not occur sooner, but rather that the most dramatic and profound results occur after the one best remedy is found. Our expectations, with the right remedy, are at least a seventy percent improvement in all or most symptoms in at least seventy percent of the children we see.

4   Illustrative cases

4.1 A thirteen-year-old-boy with Oppositional Defiant Disorder

The word that best described Daniel was "intense". The first sound that he made as a newborn, upon exiting from the birth canal, was a roar. "Like a lion or an airplane," his mother explained. "Not like you would imagine a baby sounding. We were waiting at a restaurant when he was about six months old. He let out a loud cry. Like the call of the wild! Daniel had such an anger thing from the time he was so little. He can be the sweetest, kindest kid one moment, then tell you to 'shut the hell up' or that he's 'not gonna eat that dog crap'. Daniel demands to be served first. He shouts, 'Don't eat that!' because he wants a second helping before the rest of us have even had our first servings. Or he puts his face up in front of yours and yells, 'What???' "

"One of Daniel's most common complaints is, 'I haven't eaten all day. I'm hungry. I'm starving!' He plays his dad against me and makes both of us squirm. Daniel is always telling us that we like the cat better than him. He's quite an amazing rapper and loves to rap at the top of his voice. We call him a prima donna. He wants to be the greatest.... to get the most attention." Daniel's mother reported, over time, a number of his expressions verbatim. They were uncanny, as you will see, given the homeopathic medicine that he received and the fact that he was never aware of its name. "I have to be at the top of the food chain … I'm nursing my wounds … I'm the king of my domain … king of the food chain."

Much of Daniel's oppositional, aggressive behaviour centred on food. Quoting his mother again, "He goes ballistic over food. He is a meat eater". He is dominant and dictatorial. "He thinks he rules the roost." Other comments provided wonderful insight into the animal kingdom. "Mom, you're not predatory enough on the road … All you want to do is prowl into people's lives." Daniel was quite lazy. He much preferred to sit around and have others wait on him. There were of course many interviews with Daniel himself. But it was his mother who had the most insight into him and that is why we focus here on her comments.

The homeopathic medicine that Daniel needed was *Lac leoninum* (lion's milk). Rest assured that the animal was not harmed in the extraction of the substance. Some of the main symptoms that emerged in the homeopathic proving of lion's milk that fit this case are: vehement assertiveness, a delusion of being king, intolerance of domination, abruptness, abusiveness, snappish answers, delusion of being a great person, egotism, intolerance, irritability at trifles, quarrelsomeness, love of power, rage, blunt speech, disregard for the feelings of others, and outrageous or uncivilized behaviour. Other themes of the proving of this substance were: an underlying feeling of timidity, the perception of any dared insult as a challenge to one's position and authority, a need to fight or leave the pride/group, the importance of being a successful predator, the necessity of maintaining strength, and dreams of hurt pride.

Daniel needed six doses of Lac leoninum MK in seven years, then five doses of a 10MK. His parents describe a dramatic attitude shift each time he took the remedy. "His siblings can't believe how nice he is!" His insolence and defiance diminished markedly after every dose and lasted until he relapsed after a number of months. We last saw Daniel nearly a year ago. He had graduated from high school, was 6' 3 $^1/_2$" tall, weighed 270 pounds, and was working at a 24-hour fitness centre with the goal of becoming a personal trainer. At this time his obsession was with eating a high-protein, muscle-building diet, with the goal of "pumping more blood into the muscles to increase strength". He described a recent car accident as being "T-boned." It was the first time we had ever heard that phrase in over twenty-five years of practice ... quite appropriate for a carnivore needing Lac leoninum!

4.2 An interesting teaching case: finding the simillimum

"Caroline is a little terror" is how our telephone interview with her mother began. The family lived in New York City. She was born five weeks early with an induced delivery. She was furiously angry from the moment she was born.

The child's mother expressed concern about Caroline's phobias to her paediatrician from the time her daughter first demonstrated compulsive tendencies. She could never take baths. Whenever she drank water, she complained of choking. Caroline was petrified of swimming. She felt annoyed by the textures of clothes and food. Doctors were another source of terror and she wouldn't even allow them to weigh or measure her. Another fear was cockroaches, although she loved parrots and lizards. Caroline also had an aversion to dirtying her hands.

When Caroline made up her mind, there was no changing it. Caroline sometimes cried all day long and often woke up crying in the middle of the night. She loved birthday parties, but insisted she was a little girl who never wanted to grow up. Another peculiar characteristic was her attraction to anything white. Chocolate, clothing, and everything else had to be white. It is not surprising that she loved marshmallows.

Caroline could be very aggressive. She struck out, threw objects, and her moods changed like the weather. Her parents never knew what to expect. One moment she would fawn over her older brother, call him her prince charming, and affectionately blow him a kiss. The next she'd spit in his face. Caroline frequently behaved like a dog. Barking, crawling, growling, scratching, licking her parents or the floor, walking on all fours. She had bitten when younger. Caroline carried around her stuffed animals wherever she went, especially her all-white teddy bear and rabbit.

She had frequent belching and had a particular fondness for chocolate and fish. We first prescribed her *Lyssinum* (rabies nosode), which is indicated for children who spit, growl, scratch, bark, crawl on all fours, act like dogs, and are full of rage, then remorseful.

We spoke with Caroline's mother seven weeks later. After four days of diarrhoea, a previous symptom, an aggravation of behaviour lasted for two weeks. After that she was able to play for long periods, she calmed down considerably, and began to act "like a normal kid." The growling and other dog-like behaviours stopped. She was better able to play with other children, was quickly potty trained, and her teacher reported excellent behaviour.

Four months later her father reported that she was still much calmer and softer, anger was no longer a problem, but she had become much more clingy and fearful of strangers, witches, monsters, ghosts, the dark, and animals with sharp teeth. In addition, she began to insist that she was a baby and didn't want to grow up.

We now prescribed homeopathic *Chocolate*. It can be a very beneficial for people who want to remain a child and never grow up. They love cuddly animals, whether stuffed or real. Children and adults needing Chocolate often demonstrate animal-like behaviour, which is particularly interesting given that Caroline had previously benefited from Lyssinum. They love and often hoard chocolate. And like Caroline they often have fears or disgust of cockroaches (interesting to note that a certain percentage of cockroach content is allowed in cacao) and either an aversion to or liking for lizards.

Three months later, Caroline's mother exclaimed that she had seen a ninety-seven percent improvement across the board:

> "She's a miracle child. Like night and day. Everything changed ten days after she took the medicine. It's so incredible. She went from naughty to nice. Now she's always saying 'Good'. Water no longer bothers her. She never wakes up crying. I was worried about her starting a new school, but she's fine. Quite easy to handle. Her father is amazed. I was hoping for at least a seventy percent improvement when we began. I never even dreamed of this much of a change. Her teachers and occupational therapist say she's doing great. She would never sit through church before but now we've started going again. And you know what? She seems to have lost her taste for chocolate."

Caroline needed four doses of the *Lyssinum* 200C, then MK potencies and three of the *Chocolate* MK over two years.

4.3 Case: a fascination with blood and core

Jeffrey, Caroline's brother, was according to our perceptions a child who was misunderstood by mental health professionals. Not only were they unable to agree on a diagnosis or help him to any significant degree they had widely varying interpretations of Jeffrey's inner world.

Aged seven, he was likeable, friendly, and charming. This little boy was extremely sensitive to the least slight. He would nearly collapse whenever his parents suggested that he hadn't done something just right. Taunting by his friends left him devastated. But what was the most out of proportion about Jeffrey was his obsession with blood, practically his only topic of conversation. "Mommy, I imagined cutting the monster's throat. The blood is coming out!"

It all began when Jeffrey was three and a half and the kids at school bullied him for the entire year. They beat him up almost daily, which rendered him psychologically traumatized. Around the same time the child became very accident-prone. One kid kicked him in the mouth and he lost two front teeth, both of which were already loose. The only tactic that this gentle boy could come up with to defend himself was to make up scary stories. And at this he was a master. His tales were so convincing that the school complained because kids were having sleep problems after hearing them.

This child also had an incredible ability to memorize poetry, but he was only interested in scary poems. At first his parents thought this habit was humorous and entertaining. Then it got out of control. Blood, monsters, and vampires were all that Jeffrey would think and talk about. For instance: "It was dark. A boy was walking through the forest. He found an alien's house. The alien had lots of arms. Suddenly out came a big hand. Then the alien spit poison and the boy died." Jeffrey's stories always seemed to end with someone dying or the conclusion was left unfinished.

Jeffrey exhibited obsessive tendencies. He picked his arms until they bled and even fantasized about drinking blood and blood oozing from someone's throat. He loved Dracula and any kind of story in which there was cutting or stabbing. As he shopped with his mom at the supermarket, Jeffrey would playfully grab at her neck. At two, he picked out a vampire costume for Halloween then delighted in wearing it for months after. While driving in the car with his mother, he would launch into one of his tales, oblivious to the fact that she had got out to fill the gas tank. When she eased herself back into the car, he was still talking as if she had never left.

In addition to his obsession with blood, Jeffrey was also preoccupied with germs. If someone coughed, he'd leave the room. He was a frequent hand-washer and wouldn't let anyone touch his food. He brushed his teeth excessively to avoid any possibility of cavities. The word "germs" came out numerous times each day. Jeffrey was quite attached to rituals and needed his mother to repeat over and over that she loved him.

Jeffrey experienced lots of fears. He was scared of the dark, of ants, sharks and dogs, of being grabbed by something frightening, and of being buried alive. Quite fearful of losing his mother, he ran out to protect her whenever she went outside. Whenever he left the house he was afraid another child would hit him. Jeffrey was even afraid of his own scary stories. Jeffrey awakened every night between 2 and 4 AM and fled to his parents' bed for protection. Reassurance came in the form of his imaginary friends in a pretend attic who came down and rescued him from danger.

Jeffrey suffered from frequent headaches, sometimes brought on from having to make even the simplest decision. He had a history of asthma and had taken antibiotics off and on from age two to four for recurrent bronchitis and ear infections.

Although a seven-year-old at a tenth grade level, Jeffrey was placed in a school for learning-disabled children. His teacher described his writing as disorganized and dyslexic. When he drew pictures of people or creatures, all of the limbs came out of the head. Diagnosis of Jeffrey's condition ranged, according to who was assessing him, from Obsessive Compulsive Disorder and Bi-Polar Disorder to Asperger Syndrome.

The medicine for Jeffrey was *China officinalis* (Peruvian bark). China is an important remedy for imaginative, dreamy children who feel weak within but fantasize about being superheroes. Interes-

---

13 Dr Seuss is a whimsical, wacky collection of illustrated children's stories, mostly about animals

tingly, it is a remedy for weakness after blood loss and also for excitement after hearing (or imagining) horrible things, which was the central feature of Jeffrey's case.

Immediately after taking China, Jeffrey became more active for four days. Then, "as if by magic", he started exhibiting greater awareness of his surroundings. Six days later, he spontaneously illustrated three pages of karate techniques. His interest in television diminished and he began to read avidly. When his teacher asked him to read one book, he read ten. The talk about monsters stopped and upon his sister's request to read to him he now selected Dr Seuss[13]. Jeffrey's father was amazed at his transformation. His progress continued and within nine months he was moved to a programme for gifted children in a mainstream classroom where he was considered one of the best students. He was selected as the most promising student in his entire school. For the first time in his life, Jeffrey now had several friends. Jeffrey's mother now mentioned that a prominent psychologist in her area had previously evaluated Jeffrey as having the profile of a serial killer.

One year after beginning homeopathic treatment, Jeffrey's conversational abilities were vastly improved. He mentioned monsters now and then, but was more occupied with baseball and basketball. In fact his ambition was to be a great basketball star or an actor. Jeffrey did so well in school that the other children asked him regularly for help with their assignments. He needed five doses of the *China* (200C then MK) over three years, one following a setback after moving to a new school and feeling rejected by the other children. Jeffrey blossomed beyond his parents' wildest dreams.

4.4 Case of a perfectionistic child with Attention Deficit Disorder

Charlie, a bright, loveable, carrot-topped seven-year-old with artistic talent came for treatment of his ADD, food sensitivities, and perfectionism. Charlie daydreamed in school and had difficulty focusing and staying on task. His teachers said they had never seen another child like him in all their years of teaching. His verbal IQ tested at 122, despite feedback from the psychologist that he was barely paying attention. As a result, Charlie's performance IQ tested at only 91.

If Charlie made a mistake he would say, "I'm a failure", or "I didn't do it." Quite self-critical, he did not want to disappoint anyone, and felt his mistakes deeply disappointed his parents. When he received all outstanding grades but one, he was very upset. Highly anxious, Charlie worried about numerous things, especially about trying new things. His fears included burglars, water, bees and wasps, and spiders, especially poisonous spiders.

His mother described him as an extremely creative boy and a talented artist who loved to draw. Charlie tended to fixate on certain things, so he drew various themes at different times, like police cars, dinosaurs or wild cats. He created detailed three- dimensional images of dinosaurs and big cats, complete with teeth and claws. Charlie produced up to fifty drawings a day, and his aspiration was to be a famous artist. Despite his obvious artistic talent, however, he refused to draw at school until he used a Magna-doodle, which allowed him to erase his mistakes easily. Charlie seemed wise beyond his years, with encyclopaedic knowledge.

Charlie's social skills were limited, as was his ability to recognize social cues. He had only had one good friend, who had also been diagnosed with ADD. Despite his lack of friends, Charlie was very affectionate and loved to hug people. The child had the nervous habit of biting his nails down to the quick, often to the point of bleeding. His body was covered with numerous moles and the child had a *café-au-lait* birthmark on his chest. There was also a strong history of cancer of various types on both sides of Charlie's family, including cancers of the breast, lung, colon, stomach and throat.

When Charlie was interviewed on his own, he expressed how much he enjoyed drawing, reading and writing. He was fascinated by large, wild cats, and by dinosaurs, as his mother had described. "I think of all the dinosaurs I can imagine. When I find a plastic dinosaur, I think of how it could fight. The Stegosaurus swings his tail at the Allosaurus, but the Allosaurus eats the Stegosaurus. The Allosaurus goes 'R-a-a-a-h!'" Charlie elaborated: "Sometimes I draw evil things, like evil men and women, or I draw snakes as big as two men or lizards as small as ants. If I make a mistake, I feel bad. Anger comes to my mind and I get upset or go g-r-r-r. If I get in trouble, I worry that I could get suspended from school."

Charlie was given *Carcinosinum* 1M, one dose, and has received this remedy only during his two years of treatment. Carcinosinum is a nosode whose main feature is a strong need to perform exceedingly well, with the feeling that one's survival depends on it. Carcinosinum types feel that they must go far beyond their limits in order to maintain control over their lives.

Children needing this remedy may have a history of strong parental expectations. The Carcinosinum child is sensitive to any situation that might suggest he is less than perfect. This makes Carcinosinum patients fastidious and sensitive to reprimands. In Charlie's case he was highly sensitive to doing anything less than perfectly. The mere suggestion that he had made a mistake affected him deeply and made him feel as if he were a failure. They are typically quite sympathetic, like Charlie. Children needing Carcinosinum often have moles and birthmarks, especially *café-au-lait* spots or *latte*-coloured skin.

After Carcinosinum, Charlie's mother reported that his bedwetting stopped and that he became better able to deal with things. The child became even more loving, more relaxed, and his nail biting diminished considerably. He developed a transient red rash under his arms, one in the vicinity of the *café-au-lait* birthmark.

At his third visit, Charlie's mother told of her surprise that the holes in his eardrum left by a previous myringotomy (tubes in ears for chronic ear infections) had repaired themselves, resulting in slightly better hearing. He was better able to handle disappointments, to reason more when things were not going his way. Moods improved and he brought into our office several freehand drawings of dinosaurs and big cats, which were of a quality well beyond his years in detail and artistic ability, and with which he seemed quite satisfied. Concentration was improved as well. His mother was quite happy with the response.

Charlie needed several doses of Carcinosinum 1M, then he progressed even further with a 10M potency. His food sensitivities to additives, preservatives and salicylates decreased significantly. His bedwetting and nail-biting disappeared. His academic work was progressing well, his grades were very good, and he was reading at a seventh grade level at the end of the fourth grade. At his last visit Charlie reported, "I'm calmer. I feel more relaxed and peaceful. I'm happier with where I am. I'm not bothered by anything now."

5   What to expect from homeopathic care

In conclusion, homeopathy can be excellent in treating children with behavioural and learning problems, either as a sole therapy, or in conjunction with diet, nutritional supplementation or pharmaceutical treatment. We expect the following symptoms to improve considerably with the appropriate homeopathic care, especially if the simillimum is found:

- concentration, attention, memory
- academic performance
- social interactions with peers
- self-confidence
- moods
- aggressive, defiant, angry behaviour
- improved relations with parents and siblings
- increased resistance to acute illness
- improvement in chronic health complaints
- reduced overall sensitivity
- often less need for prescription medications
- more appropriate affect

In our experience, parents are frequently averse to medicating their children for behavioural and learning problems, far more averse than to using pharmaceuticals themselves. These families present an excellent opportunity for homeopathic intervention. We hope that the information in this chapter educates and informs parents, physicians and other health care professionals, educators, and anyone else who makes decisions regarding treatment of children with behavioural and learning problems. There is potentially much to be gained from homeopathic treatment of this population.

[Cases 4.1 and 4.4 are reprinted from *The Townsend Letter for Doctors and Patients*; Cases 4.2 and 4.3 are excerpted from Reichenberg-Ullman, Judyth and Ullman, Robert: *Rage-Free Kids*. Edmonds: Picnic; Rage-Free Kids; 2003: 174-8 and 248-253.]

References

[1] Reichenberg-Ullman, Judyth and Ullman, Robert (2005) *A Drug-Free Approach to Asperger Syndrome and Autism*. Edmonds, WA: Picnic Poit Press

[2] Reichenberg-Ullman, Judyth and Ullman, Robert (2003) *Rage-Free Kids*. Edmonds, WA: Picnic Point Press

[3] Reichenberg-Ullman, Judyth and Ullman, Robert (2000) *Ritlain-Free Kids* (2nd ed). Rocklin, CA: Prima Publishing

[4] Reichenberg-Ullman, J and Ullman, R. (2008) *The Townsend Letter; A Family of Animals: Two Mammals and a Mollusk. Homeopathic Treatment of Oppositional-Defiant Disorder, Eczema, and Depression*; Fall, 2008

[5] Reichenberg-Ullman, J and Ullman, R. (2003) *The Townsend Letter; A Perfectionist Child with ADD: A Picture of Carcinosin*; Fall, 2003

[6] Sankaran, Rajan (2005) *Sankaran's Schema*. Mumbai, India: Homoeopathic Medical Publishers

[7] Sankaran, Rajan (2008) *The Other Song: Discovering Your Parallel Self*. Mumbai, India: Homoeopathic Medical Publishers

Chapter 6
Homeopathic Treatment of Multiple Personality Disorder

Dr Philip M. Bailey MbBs MFHom DipHyp

Dr Philip M. Bailey MbBs MFHom DipHyp
89 George St, East Fremantle
West Australia 6158
baileypm@iinet.net.au

Abstract
Multiple Personality Disorder is a serious psychiatric condition usually associated with childhood sexual abuse, and generally difficult to treat. In this article three cases are presented that illustrate quite clearly the usefulness of homeopathy in the treatment of Multiple Personality Disorder.

1 Introduction

This chapter presents my experience in treating five cases of Multiple Personality Disorder homeopathically. It includes three case histories. The names of the patients have been changed for privacy reasons.

I have had a homeopathic general practice for the past eighteen years, where I have offered both homeopathy and psychotherapy. I have found that the two modalities go very well together. Very often treatment with a constitutional homeopathic medicine can give the patient enough clarity and emotional security to cope far better with psychotherapy than they would otherwise. The remedy can both strengthen them and help them to get in contact with suppressed feelings. Consequently, psychotherapy can proceed at a quicker pace and achieve more if homeopathy is used as well.

2 Multiple Personality Disorder

In my own practice, I have seen a lot of patients who had been victims of childhood sexual abuse. As a result, I have seen more cases of Multiple Personality Disorder than most general practitioners, since this condition occurs almost exclusively in people who have experienced serious childhood sexual abuse. A study by Boon and Draijer in 1993 found that 94 per cent of patients with Multiple Personality Disorder had a past history of childhood sexual abuse [1].

Multiple Personality Disorder is not common, but neither is it rare. A study by Bliss and Jeppen in 1985 found that ten per cent of psychiatric patients in an American hospital met the criteria for Multiple Personality Disorder [2]. A study by Kluft in 1987 found that the disorder is underdiagnosed, and 'is not rare' [3]. Amongst psychiatrists it is very controversial. Many assert that the syndrome does not exist, and that patients said to have it are actually just hysterical and manipulative. However, I have found that those therapists who work a lot with victims of childhood sexual abuse tend to believe in the reality of Multiple Personality Disorder, because they actually come across it.

In my own practice I saw five cases of MPD over a period of twelve years. All of them responded significantly to homeopathic treatment, though none could be said to have been cured by it.

When small children are exposed to extreme trauma, there are several ways they can protect their conscious minds from an overload of impressions so disrupting that it would otherwise cause insanity. One is to enter a kind of catatonic state, where they withdraw, become mute and seem to be in a dream. This can resemble infantile autism. Another is to split the psyche into separate compartments, each of which carries part of the traumatic impressions. Typically these sub-personalities are age-determined, with later traumas creating new sub-personalities to carry the new load of painful impressions. There are usually many child sub-personalities, since the early traumas are the most devastating, and are shared amongst several identities. As long as these sub-personalities remain separate and by and large unaware of each other, the individual is only conscious of one at a time, and is therefore not bombarded with the full weight of traumatic impressions. However, people with MPD instead experience periods of missing time, periods when they cannot remember what they said, did or experienced, since the dominant or often the more adult sub-personality was not the one who experienced the period which they cannot recall.

The popular image of MPD is of a bizarre individual who shifts between different voices and facial expressions, different beliefs and different personalities. In most cases the truth is a lot more subtle. There are usually one or two dominant sub-personalities which interact with the outside world. When they are 'overtaken' by another sub-personality, the person may talk in a different manner, usually more immaturely or impulsively, but seldom with a totally different voice. And, although the younger identities are often very anxious and emotional, it is not usually obvious that the person is suffering from MPD, but rather that they are unstable and unpredictable. In my own practice I found that it would sometimes take a year or more of therapy before I discovered that the client had many distinct sub-personalities. We all have sub-personalities, but they are not cut off from each other in the way they are in MPD. Because our sub-personalities are more integrated, they cannot take over and affect us as distinctly as they can in a person with Multiple Personality Disorder.

Many patients with MPD do not realize that they are 'multiple', since the different personalities are not aware of each other. It can be a shock to discover in therapy that they have numerous sub-personalities with lives of their own, and sometimes it is better not to tell the patient the diagnosis.

Two of my patients with MPD have responded to the remedy *Mandragora*, one to *Stramonium*, one to *Mercurius vivus*, and one to *Boron metallicum*. In selecting the simillimum I have found that the process is much the same as in any other case. In other words, the fact that the patient has Multiple Personality Disorder is of little help, when compared to the consideration of individual symptoms and themes running through the case. In homeopathy we treat the person rather than the diagnosis.

I have found that both psychotherapy and homeopathy can make a big difference to patients with Multiple Personality Disorder.

I have referred some of my patients to a psychiatrist who specialized in this condition, and she was able to help them a great deal. (The therapy which made all the difference involved speaking with each sub-personality separately, then helping them to get to know each other, and then getting some of them to agree to merge. This took a long time, but it enabled patients who were very fragmented and poorly functioning to begin living more normal lives, including returning to work).

I shall now present three cases of Multiple Personality Disorder which responded well to constitutional homeopathic treatment.

3   Cases examples

3.1 Wendy

My first case that responded to the remedy *Mandragora* was a thirty-year-old psychiatrist whom I will call Wendy. She was thin, with medium length dark hair, and a very intense manner. The more I saw her, the more I noticed how her sharp analytical mind hid a person who felt very young inside.

She first came to see me about infertility. She was trying to get pregnant, having had a very difficult history of two miscarriages, one abortion, and one successful pregnancy where the child had died at the age of two from a 'cot death'. She had woken to find her daughter dead beside her in bed. Not surprisingly, this had generated a lot of fear in her about her ability to take care of children. However, as I came to know her better, I realized that she had had a lot of fears throughout her life.

It gradually became clear that this woman kept very much to herself. She had a couple of close friends, and a partner, and otherwise was very much a recluse. She said that she had a tendency to cancel appointments with people, because she could not face seeing them.

"I don't know how to manage other people. I feel intruded upon by the instability of others. I feel their emotional undercurrents. It comes into me, like a demand. It is as if they can get into me, under my skin. My only defence is to avoid people. Otherwise I lose myself, and then I get anxious. My man gives me space, which I need. I am unpredictable. I don't know how to control my feelings.
I want to maintain my buffer with other people. I need to escape their demands."

"As a child I felt separate, in my own world. I was the eldest. I was very maternal towards my siblings. I wasn't bonded enough with Mum. She was busy. There wasn't enough of her left. I was permanently confused and scared. I felt really powerless as a child. Maybe that's why I stole things. I stole a candlestick, an antique ring, money and clothes."

"Later when I had my daughter I was a very uncertain mother. I felt I didn't know how to look after her. I used to dream she was someone else's baby. When she died I felt as if I had killed her.
I have a recurring dream of tidal waves coming down on me."

"I feel too young, as if I am missing the facts. And I feel like I am an outsider, separate from other people. For a while I practised Wicca (a form of witchcraft), which helped to give me a feeling of connection and empowerment."

"In the past I have been used by men. I had lesbian relationships, and strong desires to revenge myself against men. My father sexually abused me as a child, though he has never admitted it. I feel powerless around him. I have chosen a very gentle partner, very unlike my father. During sex sometimes I feel like I want to kill him (my partner)."

Initially I found it difficult to find a remedy that covered the case. There seemed to be a great deal of fear, a lack of trust in her own boundaries, as if people almost literally got under her skin, and great distrust about her ability to care for children.

I gave her several remedies over a period of a year, including *Beryllium muriaticum*, with its keynote of an *uncertain mother* [4]. However, there was little effect either physically or mentally. Then she volunteered some important information.

"I have been seeing a therapist, who says I am schizoid, that I have cut off from part of myself. It is a kind of dissociation. I am very good at compartmentalizing my mind, so I don't always know what is going on in another part."

I asked how she experienced it and she told me about her 'delusions'.

"I have delusions that there are dead children who I am responsible for. They might be my forebears. I pay attention to them, which helps them. It makes me unavailable to the outside world. They are not at rest. Some can appear to be demonic. They have little wings. I sense them rather than see them. They fly around. I call them 'owl children'. When they are around I feel grief, or terror. They fly around my head like birds. I have a fear of birds. I can't watch movies about possessed children. They terrify me. There have been a lot of children who died in my family tree.
Sometimes I dream of graveyards. It is scary. I get a sense of someone behind me, anytime, but especially at night. It can startle me. When I am scared I get a crawling sensation on my skin and face."

"I was attacked recently by three small dogs. I don't like noise or bright light. I don't eat much. I get migraines before my period, with a lot of nausea."

At this point, it was clear that this was a highly unusual woman who needed a highly unusual remedy. Her description of her mind as compartmentalized, along with her inner 'family' of small children, immediately reminded me of accounts I had read of Multiple Personality Disorder. In this disorder, early childhood trauma is so intense that it threatens to destroy the young mind. As a defence against annihilation, the mind splits into many separate compartments. Each compartment carries its own sub-personality, and each sub-personality carries its own traumatic experiences. If these sub-personalities were to merge before the person was ready, the combined traumatic impressions would result in insanity. Multiple Personality occurs pretty much only in cases where there has been severe early childhood sexual abuse.

Wendy was a keen painter, so I asked her to bring in one of her paintings. The painting she brought in showed a family sitting in the sun on a grass area. The other half of the painting was in shade. It had dark high buildings with red windows. Some of them were churches. In front of them a little girl was standing. A black and white dog stood at the border of the shade and the light area.

The painting was very striking, particularly the division into two equal halves, one dark and one light. I was immediately put in mind of the *solanaciae* (the nightshade family), particularly *Stramonium*, with its fear of the dark, and of dogs, and its need for bright light, and aggravation from shimmering light. Stramonium also includes the theme of possession, which runs through this case, and the powerful theme of death and graveyards. However, I was reluctant to give Stramonium because I had never seen a case of Stramonium where the functional capacity was so high. Although she avoided people, she was able to maintain a busy psychotherapy practice. Also, her anger seemed more suppressed than that seen in Stramonium cases.

In my search for a remedy for Wendy, I decided to concentrate on the solanaceae family, since her paintings of dogs and of black and white schisms seemed so reminiscent of these remedies. Using MacRepertory ReferenceWorks [5], I repertorised using the search words 'possessed', 'kleptomania' and 'solanaceae'. There were four remedies which came up in all three searches, *Belladonna*, *Stramonium*, *Mandragora* and *Hyoscyamus*. I decided to research Mandragora, since I knew the other three remedies quite well, and knew they did not fit the case well enough. There were two sources of information which helped me select Mandragora as Wendy's remedy. Besides information from the homeopathic Materia Medica there was a wealth of lore on the mandrake root available on the internet.

3.1.1 *Mandragora (Mandrake root)*

The latter was invaluable in gaining a deeper insight into the remedy, since there was so little homeopathic information available. The name *Mandrake* reminds us that the root of the mandrake plant resembles a human figure, and this coincidence, coupled with the hallucinogenic properties of the plant, gave rise to its use in magic and witchcraft, and contributed to the rich folklore surrounding the plant.

The belief arose in the Middle Ages that the root was itself a magical being, known as a mandragora, which could confer special powers on its owner, but also attract the Devil. It was believed that the mandragora gave out a terrible scream when dug up, which could kill those hearing it or drive them to madness. Hence dogs were trained to dig up the root, and elaborate rituals were used to protect the master of the dog, who had to sound a trumpet as the root surfaced, so as to drown the deadly scream. The dog had then to be slaughtered and buried at the site of the excavation, presumably to propitiate the dark powers.

Theocritus describes how the root was associated with the goddess Kirke, who turned men into animals, and with Hecate, who chased whining dogs whilst walking over the graves of the dead through streams of blood. (Whitmont, Psyche and Substance [6]). Interestingly, mandrake has been used for over two millennia as a treatment to draw demons out of the possessed. Many used to believe that if you possessed a mandragora you could make the spirit of the little man do your bid-

ding, but that if you died whilst in possession of the root, the Devil would take your soul.
The belief in ages past that the mandrake root was a manikin, a little man with special powers, is pertinent when we consider the remedy Mandragora and its relationship to Multiple Personality Disorder. Basically, the root was seen as a manifestation, an embodiment, of a little demon or spirit. In Multiple Personality Disorder, many 'little spirits' inhabit a single body. If we were to look for a remedy that covers the phenomenology of Multiple Personality, it would have to include the tendency for the mind to split. This is basically a tendency of the syphilitic miasm[14], and there are many syphilitic remedies that cover mental schisms. However, I have found few of them useful in the treatment of Multiple Personality Disorder.

There is another element to the phenomenology of the disorder that is covered by fewer remedies. That is the personification of psychic contents. Not only does the mind split into numerous compartments, but also each compartment has its own personality, complete with appearance (inner self-image), name and personal history. It is this personification of mental compartments which lends itself to a comparison with the idea of possession, and which must be contained in the picture of a remedy chosen to alleviate the syndrome. With this stipulation in mind, most of the remedies which seem to fit belong to the solanaceae family, which includes *Belladonna*, *Hyoscyamus*, *Mandragora* and *Dulcamara*. The whole family is associated with the dark side of the unconscious, with madness, violence, possession and uncontrolled sexuality. An association with both violence and sexuality is likely to be found in any remedy which resonates with Multiple Personality Disorder, since the syndrome is almost exclusively a sequela[15] to extreme sexual abuse.

The other source of information I found helpful was Krista Heron's case history in *The American Homeopath* in 2001, entitled 'Mandragora - The darker side of Belladonna' [7]. In it she describes the case of Emily, a young girl with Attention Deficit Disorder, who responded well to the remedy. There are several features in Emily's case that resemble Wendy's. First of all, like Wendy, Emily was attracted to magic and rituals (Wendy used to practice Wicca, a form of witchcraft). Secondly, she had a history of stealing things. (Mandragora is listed in the Millennium Repertory [8] under the rubric 'Kleptomania'). Heron describes how Emily was unusually detached for a girl of her age, and this dissociated quality also characterized Wendy's relationship with the world. Both patients were also highly private, allowing nobody into their inner world. And both were highly functioning individuals when compared to most Stramonium or Hyoscyamus cases I have treated. Emily was fascinated by graveyards, and dreamt of owls. Wendy dreamt of graveyards, and called her inner children 'owl-children'. Clearly owls and graveyards belong to those parts of the collective unconscious which we associate with magic and witchcraft. Extraordinarily, Emily wrote a book for her school project about a boy with Multiple Personality Disorder.

Wendy's use of language often betrayed a sense of feeling possessed. Speaking of feeling invaded by other people, she said, 'It is as if they can get into me, under my skin'. Furthermore, she could not

---

14 Hahnemann categorized chronic diseases into three miasms and postulated that chronic diseases originated from one or a combination of them: Psora, Sycosis, Syphilis. See other chapters for a more detailed and updated description.

15 A disease or disorder that is caused by a preceding disease or injury in the same individual.

bear to watch films about possessed children. Her sense of dead 'demonic' children flying around her head with wings is an extraordinary example of feeling possessed. And her description of these children as 'Owl-children' connects her story more closely to mandragora, with its characteristic fascination with the hidden side of life.

The similarities between descriptions of possession and of Multiple Personality Disorder are not hard to see. It was my assumption that the children Wendy perceived were in fact cut-off parts of her own psyche, which carried the worst traumatic experiences from her own sexual abuse. Most cases of Multiple Personality Disorder include several child sub-personalities, and often infant sub-personalities. Of course, Wendy's experience of losing her small child to sudden infant death syndrome could also have produced hallucinations of dead children. In either case, the content of the 'delusion' fits particularly closely with the content of Mandragora provings and mandrake mythology.

It is interesting that the dog is closely associated with the mandrake root, and dogs appear in Wendy's paintings. To the Ancient Egyptians the dog was associated with the realm of the dead, and dog-headed guardians guarded this realm. Furthermore, Wendy was attacked by three dogs shortly before she told me of her owl-children. These kinds of synchronicities are seen all the time when one works at the level of essence, or the patient's central delusions. It is as though the energetic field of the patient manifests in her external reality.

One of the principal symptoms of Mandragora is that the patient feels that they are in their own world - hence its association with magic. Wendy felt separate, and literally said that she was in a world of her own as a child. This accounts for her feeling like an outsider, and being diagnosed as schizoid by her therapist. *Schizoid* refers to being cut off from part of oneself, and is thus a precursor of Multiple Personality Disorder, where there are many schisms in the psyche. Given the strong associations between mandrake and witchcraft, it is fascinating that Wendy was drawn to witchcraft in the form of Wicca, and that this gave her a sense of belonging.

Being a member of the solanaceae family, the remedy Mandragora includes violent elements. In my experience these elements are usually a part of the patient's inner landscape, and are not visible to outsiders. Wendy felt sometimes when having sex that she wanted to kill her partner. It is the internalized, hidden quality of violent symptoms that separates Mandragora from other well-known remedies in the solanaceae family like Stramonium and Belladonna.

Although there are not many mental symptoms in the provings we have of Mandragora, and the classical literature gives a very sketchy picture of the mental constellation, one rubric listed in the Millennium Repertory under Mandragora is highly pertinent to Multiple Personality Disorder, namely 'Ailments from mortification'. Extreme sexual abuse is almost always found in the history of cases of Multiple Personality Disorder, and this kind of horrifying trauma is what is meant by the rubric 'Mortification' (literally, something that has shocked you to death).

Once I realized the strong resonance between Wendy's case and Mandragora, I commenced treatment with Mandragora 200C weekly (the only potency I had at the time).

3.1.2 Follow-up

Follow-up after five weeks

"I don't feel so paranoid. I am not withdrawing so much from other people. And I have more sense of my own personal power. On the other hand, I started showing my anger more, and feeling less in control. I had a blowout with my father, and told him he was full of shit. And that I had had enough of his crap. I walked out. It's the first time I have had a confrontation with my father without breaking down, without becoming afraid, and without feeling guilty afterwards.
I have less mental confusion, and since the confrontation with my father I feel I can control my anger again."

"I am struggling with the fear that babies in my care will die. We offered to care for a three-month- old baby for a weekend, and I couldn't do it. I was afraid something terrible would happen. (Cries). I would have to watch her constantly whilst she slept."

"I have a fear of getting pregnant too. The owl-children are still around me. I have a heavy sense of being haunted. I get nausea a lot, worse when I leave the house."

Comment: Clearly the remedy was having an effect. Her ability to stand up to her father, who had abused her as a child, seemed particularly encouraging, as did her comments that her paranoia and her confusion were less. I have subsequently found that Mandragora cases often report a feeling of being haunted, and nausea is a prominent symptom of Mandragora Materia Medica.

Treatment: Mandragora 1M, single dose.

Follow up at eleven weeks

"I got gastroenteritis shortly after taking the remedy. It was a huge purge. I felt a lot of anger toward my sister. My paranoia increased for a while after the 1M dose. I have told a lot of people a lot of things I had suppressed for years, about wanting respect, especially from my parents and my sister. And my own sense of self-respect has increased."

"I haven't felt the owl-children around so much.
I feel less hidden from other people. It is very uncomfortable. Sometimes I am hidden from myself - com partmentalised. I used to not feel very much. Now I feel a lot more. And I hate it."

Comment: It is common after taking a high dose of a constitutional remedy for suppressed feelings to surface, and for unsaid things to be said. Wendy's reduced awareness of the owl-children was the first sign I had that the remedy could help Multiple Personality Disorder. Wendy had not mentioned Multiple Personality Disorder, and neither had I. So it was interesting when she commented upon how compartmentalized her mind could be. She was an experienced psychiatrist, and I got the impression that she knew she had Multiple Personality Disorder, but chose not to face the diagnosis directly.

At this follow-up I noticed that Wendy appeared more present, and it felt like I could make better contact with her. Thus I was not unduly perturbed by her increased sense of vulnerability. When the mental compartmentalization that maintains Multiple Personality Disorder begins to break down, the patient is flooded with emotions which had previously been hidden from her. This appears to be an unavoidable part of the reintegration of split-off psychic contents. I reassured Wendy that she was moving in the direction of wholeness, and gave no remedy, since the 1M dosage was still acting.

Follow up at seventeen weeks

"I feel more comfortable in my body. I am coping better generally, and especially with my feelings. I feel less disconnected, and more aware of my feelings. My anxiety is much better. There have been no owl-children now for several weeks."

Comment: Wendy seemed like a different person from the woman I first met. Then she had appeared very intense, and very secretive. Now she appeared relaxed, and so much more open. Her use of language tends to confirm the diagnosis of Multiple Personality Disorder. At the previous visit she had commented on the compartmentalization of her mind, and now she comments on how her feeling of disconnectedness has improved. The disappearance of the owl-children speaks for itself. (Wendy's case illustrates well one of the main differences between Multiple Personality Disorder and Psychosis. In psychotic patients there is a breakdown in the connection between the patient and reality. In Multiple Personality Disorder this connection is maintained, thanks to, rather than in spite of, the splitting of the psyche into many compartments.)

Treatment: Mandragora LM6 once a day.
This was given to help maintain the improvement brought about by the 1M potency.

Follow-up at 27 weeks

"I feel more powerful, less like a doormat. And I feel more in control. Suddenly our application to adopt a child is moving forward, after years of delays. I am trusting my feelings a lot more. It gives me a sense of being a whole person. I am not so paranoid, so I am able to be around people more. I am persevering with my new supervision group, which is unusual for me. Usually I find some excuse to back out of groups. I have noticed that I am taking on my partner's feelings a lot less. His sadness. Now I can feel my own feelings. I no longer have the fear of the owl-children. They are a split-off part of me, and of my siblings, all the dead kids in my family. I don't feel them very often now."

Comment: Once Wendy had been able to integrate the dead children sub-personalities, her adoption application began to move forward. And she finally acknowledged that the children were a split-off part of herself.
Wendy's case is a clear example of how the homeopathic remedy Mandragora can help a person with Multiple Personality Disorder

3.2 Sabine
20-year-old woman, thin, wearing a man's black hat.

"I have come about trouble I have with myself and my mind. For as long as I can remember I have had conflict within myself, not knowing who I am. It seems like I don't have a single identity, but several. There are people inside of me that tell me different things at different times. Whether it is about a big decision that needs to be made, or a little thing, there are people arguing inside. It can be the stereotypes that I have created inside myself."

Question: For example?

"Well, there is a wise old woman who gives her opinion on certain subjects. And a conservative nerdy person, and a criminal type who is quite rebellious and a bit bad. They all give different views, so there is this bantering in my mind. Sometimes it seems to me that they are all versions of a single me. Sometimes it seems like they are completely different people, and I have no idea who they are or where they come from. Sometimes they will agree with each other, and sometimes they are completely absent, and then I will feel lost. Lately they have been absent, and sometimes I have been feeling lost without them. I am used to hearing them, and if I want some specific input on a subject and they're not there, I can feel lost."

Question: Can you think for yourself if they're not there?

"I don't know. For my whole school life I have had this noise in my head. Sometimes it is specific and I can understand it, and sometimes it's just like background noise. Sometimes if there are no voices I suddenly feel that my world has changed and I don't know who I am or where I am or what I am doing. Then I have to walk out. I have walked out of school several times when that happens. If I lie down for half an hour and close my eyes, then usually its better when I get up."

Question: Do the voices express any crazy thoughts?

"I would say yes. I will be talking to someone, and I will say something, but it feels like it doesn't come out of my mouth, but that it has been blurted out from I don't know where. I might say something that I don't really believe."

Question: Do the voices say anything bizarre?

"Yes. Really strange things, like wondering whether or not Charles Manson was a good person. Or whether Hitler did a lot of good things. For some reason I confide in people like that, because they stand up for what they believe in, which is something I always do. I listen to a lot of music that is very dark and black and 'out there'. I will listen to the lyrics and think 'they're beautiful' or nice. Other people will read them and think 'That's really fucked up. What is wrong with you?' I don't think it is a problem. I just think that is how I am. It is just a bit dark. There is nothing really wrong with that."

Remark: Sometimes it can be a problem if people act out their dark sides.

"Yes I know. But I also have a very light side as well."

Question: Do you ever feel you want to express your dark side?

"Yes. I usually act it out by wearing certain clothes or badges. That is enough expression for me. Or I will wear a hat, do something different. I am very conscious of these kinds of things. I have been reading about it for the longest time. I have kind of diagnosed myself."

Question: Which diagnosis have you settled upon?

"Dad doesn't believe in it, but I think I have a personality disorder. At one extreme there is schizophrenia,

and at the other manic-depressive illness. And there are a whole load of personality disorders in between."

Question: Have you considered Multiple Personality Disorder?

"Yes, but I have read things about it that I don't fit. For example, people with that don't realize there is anything wrong with them."

Remark: There are actually some with MPD who are not so extreme, and who have insight into their condition.

"I have read that people with MPD are either geniuses or very twisted and don't know what is going on around them, because they are stuck in their own world. Charles Manson had Multiple Personality Disorder and he got so lost in his own world that he was convinced his own beliefs were right and true. Lately I have felt that I have been comfortably numb. I have felt that I have grown a lot in myself. The people that are supposedly inside me have been absent for a couple of weeks. But I still get those times when I feel lost and I have to leave school.

I can talk openly with you today about this, and tomorrow I could come in and say 'No, the problem is something completely different'. I change so fast. I will know what I am saying, but I am not sure that I believe it. Like the way I am talking to you now is very broad, and I am not sure if that is a certain identity in me that is talking, or me as a whole. If you took them all away, I don't know that I would have a single identity. I have only told two friends about this, and they ask me, 'But which one is you?', and I don't know if there is a 'me'.

Everyone can sit down and have a thought, and next minute think something different about the same topic, but with me it's a thousand times per second."

Question: Do the voices have specific sounds?

"Yes. They are quite specific. I can see a woman, about 45 years old, in a tweed suit. I can see her. Maybe not a detailed face, but the body is clear, and her voice. I can also see the criminal in a leather jacket, holding a knife, wearing a checkered shirt and glasses.

Sometimes I act out these people. I put on fingerless gloves and I act out the bad side. I have nice long white dresses and a cape, which I wear when I act out the wise old woman. I have always acted them out, but I didn't used to be aware of it.

Because I am so conscious of the dark side, I inflict it on myself, not on others. I have punched walls many times. And I banged my head against the wall in the shower, just to get my head to be quiet."

Question: What are you studying at university?

"Forensic science. I have always been into forensics. I would like to study criminology. I don't know if my mind would be stable enough right now. I couldn't work full-time right now. But if I was to get a grip on what is going on, then I could.

Also, I don't want to exclude 'mediumship'. This could be something completely separate from what we have been talking about. I hear the voice of an entity, which I believe is my father's dead father. Even though I never met him, and know nothing about him. That voice always says the same thing: 'We are going to get it right this time'."

Question: What do you think he means?

"He means 'don't kill yourself'. He took his own life, and that is why he is with me. I don't know why I believe it so strongly."

Question: Do you get a desire to take your own life?

"No. I have never thought that closely about it. But it kills me to think that people commit suicide. Sometimes I think about it. It is one of the biggest questions in philosophy – whether it can be right to commit suicide. At that point a person is at a point of no return, in oblivion to themselves. If they are going in that direction, is it even possible to turn them back? I also think that if I get so down about things, if I have so much trouble in this life, how will I be able to enjoy the next life? I don't know what I believe in, but I do believe in guardian angels. Sometimes I feel my guardian angel is my father's father. At other times it is so completely oblivious to me. So I don't know. That is why I think it is not always just one person. It could be a whole bunch of people that are your guardian angels. But something tells me that far away someone is watching me. I have never been one to pray much. Once recently I asked this person, this guardian, to do something for me, and whether or not it was by chance, it happened. We were driving in the bush towards a campsite. It was dark and we couldn't find where to meet up with our friends. So I stopped and asked for a sign, and the next minute we drove right up to them. That is the only time I have prayed.
Do you think this mind chatter is an issue?"

Answer: That's for you to decide.

"It is definitely there."

Sabine is a most extraordinary young woman. She describes her inner world so clearly, and has insight that these people inside her head are probably parts of herself. Like many people with Multiple Personality Disorder, she has the sense that she doesn't know who she is, and that she is in conflict with herself. And it is typical of people with Multiple Personality Disorder to feel surprised when they say something, because it was another sub-personality that said it. The diagnosis of Multiple Personality Disorder was clear to me immediately, even though Sabine did not report any childhood trauma. The next question was: which remedy could help her.

The aspect of Sabine's case which stood out above the rest, once I began to look beyond the fact that she had multiple personalities, is her preoccupation with the darker side of life. She listens to songs with very dark lyrics, and is fascinated with the darkest examples of human beings, like Charles Manson and Hitler. She is also preoccupied with suicide, without being suicidal. And when she thinks of other people committing suicide, she says 'It kills me'.
At this point, it is essential to stress that my contact with Sabine felt very easy and very good. There was good eye contact, and her facial expressions were natural and congruent. Also, I had no sense of being with a dangerous or warped person. This is important, because many remedies which resonate with the dark side of life (or death) tend to fit people who feel dangerous to you as a therapist, or mad. Sabine not only seemed perfectly rational, but also pleasant and calm, and able to make contact with me. Her interest in forensics seemed like a relatively healthy way to pursue her fascination with the dark side.

At this point *Mandragora* had already come to mind, since it covers cases of mental splitting where the dark side is prominent, but the patient is not overwhelmed by it. There is a detachment that protects the Mandragora patient from her own demons, as it were. Mandragora, like *Anacardium* and *Stramonium*, may see angels and demons, but as this case illustrates, Mandragora's angels are not hallucinations which take her totally out of the present physical reality. Sabine's angel was one of her sub-personalities, none of which totally dominated her and deprived her of her sanity. Similarly, her dark side manifested as an interest in dark people and things, not possession by the Devil. This 'possession-lite', or once-removed, is highly characteristic of the Mandragora cases I have treated. They appear sane and rational, because they are. Julian [11] describes Mandragora as a 'cool, attenuated *Belladonna*', reflecting this contradictory combination of control and wild dangerous psychic contents. Sabine's interest in suicide is interesting in that Mandragora is found under the rubric 'suicidal' in the Millennium Repertory. Thus the theme of suicide is part of the remedy picture.

The next aspect of Sabine's case which must be included in the remedy picture is her sense of being a medium. She feels that some of the characters inside of her are spirits rather than sub-personalities. I have come across this phenomenon in other cases of Multiple Personality Disorder, and they responded to either Stramonium or Mandragora homeopathically. All of the solanaceae family seem to cover states where spirits are perceived, or at least are believed to be perceived. Those cases of Multiple Personality Disorder I have treated successfully which did not have this experience of being a medium did not respond to solanaceae remedies, but to others such as *Boron metallicum* and *Mercury*.

Treatment: Mandragora 1M

3.2.1 *Follow-up*

Follow up after six weeks

"I felt the sense of being lost was really bad the day after I took the pills. And it lasted longer than usual, about two hours. But since then I have only had it once, which is much less than usual. And the second time it was only for about half an hour. Generally I have been feeling better. More confident, and less different from other people. The people inside my head have been less apparent, like they are really far in the background, and I have to look hard to find them."

No treatment.

Follow up at twelve weeks

"I have been well. I haven't had that sense of being lost since last time I was here. Occasionally I see one of the people inside, but it's like other thoughts, if I give them no attention they just go. I feel a lot more together than I used to. I find I am getting a lot more work done for my degree."

Follow-up at six months

"Things have been going well for me. I feel a lot clearer about who I am, and it feels like the people inside of me are just aspects of myself. I can choose whether to visit them or not, and they don't argue with each other any more. I have only had one episode of feeling lost since last visit, and it was only for about 15 minutes. I still feel attracted to dark subjects, but I don't think that it's a problem."

Comment: Sabine's case was unusual for Multiple Personality Disorder in that she had always known about all of her sub-personalities, and there was no known history of early trauma. Perhaps because there was no early trauma, she did not have numerous child sub-personalities. In cases of Multiple Personality Disorder, it is usually the child sub-personalities that carry the worst of the person's traumatic feelings and memories. The question naturally arises, if there was no early trauma, why did she have Multiple Personality Disorder? I do not know the answer. It seems possible that MPD can also arise out of a miasmatic background. In other words, that someone can be born with a strong tendency for their mind to split and compartmentalize. This case illustrates the potential for the homeopathic remedy Mandragora, when correctly chosen, to bring about a profound integration in a more or less 'full-blown' case of Multiple Personality Disorder.

3.3 Diedre

Diedre first came to see me about depression. She was thirty-eight years old, though she looked younger. She had a manner that was very innocent and open, and she laughed easily during our first consultation. She worked as a masseuse, and had not been getting enough work. She said she had begun to feel depressed and anxious, with a sense of hopelessness about the future. Strangely, she appeared very animated and in good humour during the consultation. She came from Ireland, where she had been put in a Catholic children's home at the age of one, when her mother fell ill. At the age of four her mother had taken her home, and she had been a bit of a wild child, skipping school to play with the horses in a nearby field, or paying visits to the zoo instead of going to school. She laughed as she described her childhood antics, and I could see that she enjoyed adding a bit of drama to her stories. During our first interview she would sometimes make sweeping statements which suggested that she did not always think logically or in an adult way. For example, she complained that her sex drive had diminished, and then said, "It is a fact that a woman's sexual desire disappears at the age of 38".

I would later come to recognize that she had a concrete way of thinking and understanding the world which was very immature. She would gather statements she had heard or read, misinterpret them, and then repeat her incorrect interpretation very dogmatically, as if she were the best judge of the truth of things. This was in fact a comical manner of speaking, but she had no insight into the effect she was having.

During the first interview she described how she felt "bad" inside, but could not be more specific. Her vivaciousness, combined with her sense of being somehow "bad", led me to give her *Thuja* initially. (Thuja is a constitutional remedy which suits states where there is a sense of self-loathing or disgust, usually in people who are very passionate. They tend to be escapist, and to use bravado to hide their vulnerability [9].) Thuja appeared to help her mood for a while, but then stopped acting. She became more anxious, particularly when out in public, and her mood generally became more unstable. She appeared to be isolating herself more and more, and so I offered her psychotherapy.

From the start of our psychotherapy sessions Diedre began to talk about her suspicion that she had been sexually abused whilst in the orphanage in Ireland. Whenever she talked about the priests who visited the orphanage, she would become agitated and anxious. Over a period of several weeks I encouraged her during sessions to stay with the feelings in her body, and during this process she began to remember incidents of sexual abuse in the orphanage. When the memories arose she would experience terror, and required a very slow and gradual pace in therapy to allow her to integrate the suppressed feelings associated with her traumas.

One day during a therapy session Diedre was remembering some detail from her life in the orphanage when she referred to herself as "Dotty". She said that had been a nickname her mother had given her. It seemed strange to me at the time, that she would refer to herself in the third person, and using a different name. As the therapy progressed she began to use other names for her previous selves. When she talked about herself as a young teenager she called herself Nickie. Instead of saying "I was a bit of a rebel" she said "Nickie was a bit of a rebel". I asked her more about Nickie, and she talked at length in the third person about her teenage self. Then she said, "I think Nickie is still a rebel. It is her that wants to smoke dope and get drunk". At this point it was becoming clear to me that Diedre could be suffering from Multiple Personality Disorder. She went on to talk about four more aspects of herself, giving them all names, three of which she had used in her own mind all her life. Thus the very young child of 1-2 years old was called Susie, Dotty was 2-4 years old, Dierdie was 4-10 years old, Nickie was the rebellious teenager, Dierdre was the adult with problems, and Diana was the spiritual adult who was wise and always calm. In addition to these female sub-personalities there was also a male teenager named Mike, who was tough and never felt fear.

Once the diagnosis of Multiple Personality Disorder was considered, I was able to understand why Diedre had always appeared so unstable, flighty and unpredictable in therapy. One moment she was serious and sensible, talking about her illness, the next she was teasing me in a little girl's voice, and pulling funny faces. She was extraordinarily escapist, changing the subject whenever she didn't want to face a painful subject, smoking marijuana in binges, and downplaying the seriousness of her symptoms.

Although Diedre had two adult sub-personalities, she seldom talked in a truly adult manner. Generally she either talked like a child, or like a child trying to appear adult, using long words inappropriately, and jumping to conclusions because she did not understand the complexity of the adult world. She was, for example, extremely impressionable. Any statement expressed to her with confidence would be taken on board as fact. She could then defend these 'facts' enthusiastically, despite having no real knowledge about them.

One other very important characteristic of Diedre was her all-or-nothing extremes. Either she was the most talented person in the world, or she was useless. She was especially liable to idealize people on first meeting them, and later demonize them. Anyone she idealized would become the focus of her hopes for friendship, support and even employment. She joined various spiritual groups, and was always initially absolutely thrilled with them and their teachings, but before long she would reject both the teacher and the adherents in a most vehement manner.

She seldom succeeded in realizing that it was her own positive and negative projections which lent these people such strong shades of good and bad. When on occasion she did have such insights, she was both shocked and depressed by them for a brief time, before forgetting them.

In the course of treating Dierdre I gave her many homeopathic remedies. With time I came to realize how fragmented, immature and unstable she was, and this led me initially to the prescription of *Lithium bromatum*. Lithium is found in the first stage of the Periodic Table. This means that it has one spare electron, and is thus rather unstable and reactive as an element. Scholten [10] has shown that remedies made from elements in the first stage of the Periodic Table suit cases where the patient is very young emotionally, naïve and innocent. Furthermore, Lithium belongs to the Carbon series. Scholten has shown how remedies made from elements in the Carbon series help patients who are developing a sense of self, and who tend to see the world in terms of good and bad [10]. I used the Bromide salt of Lithium because it covered Diedre's strong feelings of guilt, as well as her passionate, intuitive nature. *Lithium bromatum* had little effect, and so I focused on other remedies for immaturity and fragmentation.

3.3.1 *Boron*

Jan Scholten's description of *Boron* [10] immediately caught my attention. He says that Boron cases are 'jumpy', and this fitted Diedre's case very well. She had the kind of anxiety that made her jump or startle easily. Regarding their childishness, according to Scholten Boron cases cannot grasp how things work. This was exactly the impression I had of Diedre. It was as if she was a three-year-old trying to negotiate the complexities of the adult world alone. Scholten says that Boron cases dare not say no. Diedre was often angry with me during the course of therapy, but she was terrified of telling me. She would often begin a session by saying she was afraid I would not see her again, because she had said something terrible to me in the previous session. It always turned out that she had said something very mild, but was afraid I would be offended by it. This was a very young way of reacting, like a small child who thinks that if Daddy gets angry her world could collapse.

Under causes of Boron's pathology, Scholten lists abuse, incest, and loss of parents. Diedre's pathology was intimately linked to her experience of sexual abuse in an orphanage. Finally, perhaps the most interesting part of Scholten's description of Boron as a remedy is his observation that it is a remedy for cases of Multiple Personality Disorder.

To try to confirm the prescription, I asked Diedre whether she would go on a roller-coaster. She screwed up her face and said she couldn't bear them. I have confirmed in my Boron cases what Scholten has written, that Boron is aggravated not only by downward motion, but also by round-abouts and roller-coasters.

Treatment: Boron 1M

3.3.2 *Follow-up*

Follow up at four weeks

Diedre looks different. More composed, more together, more 'presentable'.

> *"That remedy was amazing. After I took it I had all these realizations. It was a bit shocking. I realized that I have been taking dope not just to escape, but because I wanted to fit in, to feel a part of a group. And I realized that I am so dishonest with myself. I can make up any excuse to avoid something difficult or painful, and I believe it myself."*

126

This had been one of Diedre's chief defence mechanisms -- to excuse herself from any situation which could be stressful, and in practice this meant most situations. It seems that the only time in her life when she had felt secure around other people was when she lived in a spiritual community, had set routines, and was in a sense looked after by the community. Living on her own she had coped mainly by isolating herself.

> "After those realizations I felt this enormous sense of love and gratitude for being looked after by Existence. It is still there. I haven't been tempted to take dope, and suddenly I have lots of energy, and I am getting all the things done around the house that had been piling up for months. I am talking more with my neighbours, and it's like I am seeing them for the first time."

She really was shining, and positive in a centred way, not manic like she had sometimes been before. After taking Boron she seemed a lot more settled, and she was able to look at feelings that had been too threatening previously. We therefore made a lot more progress in therapy, and she never again fell into the serious depressive episodes that she had been prone to before Boron.

As for her Multiple Personality Disorder, it took a back seat in our therapeutic focus. She did not wish to focus on herself as divided, and indeed she appeared a lot less divided after taking Boron. This showed itself in her being more stable generally, more present during therapy sessions, and more able to stick to plans she made for herself. I doubt that the schisms in her psyche healed completely, but they ceased to be dominating features in her life. After taking Boron she remained more positive and better able to look after herself.

I have since treated several patients successfully with Boron, though no others with Multiple Personality Disorder. However, they all had certain features in common. All appeared very young emotionally, and also very friendly, in an innocent kind of way, as young children are before they learn to be circumspect. All were terrified of making commitments, and used a variety of excuses to get out of commitments. In this sense, they were all very 'slippery'; one could not hold onto them. And all were prone to extreme idealization and demonization of other people.
I believe that Boron is particularly likely to be indicated in cases of Multiple Personality Disorder where parents were absent, and hence the child grew up without even the most basic sense of identity, security or mirroring.

4 Conclusion

The above cases illustrate quite clearly the usefulness of homeopathy in the treatment of Multiple Personality Disorder. Since MPD is one of the most serious psychiatric disorders, it is not surprising that homeopathy can also help many other psychological problems. In my own practice I have had a lot of success using constitutional remedies for the treatment of anxiety, depression, anger problems and emotional immaturity. Correctly chosen homeopathic remedies not only help alleviate symptoms of psychological disorders, they can also resolve the underlying mental patterns which perpetuate mental disorders.

References

[1] Boon and Draijer (1993) Multiple Personality Disorder in the Netherlands, *American Journal of Psychiatry*. 1993:50: 489-494

[2] Bliss and Jeppen (1985) Prevalence of Multiple Personality Disorder among inpatients and outpatients, *American Journal of Psychiatry*. 1985:142 p250

[3] Kluft (1987) An update on Multiple Personality Disorder, *Hospital Community Psychiatry*. 1987:38:363-376

[4] Scholten J. (1996) *Homeopathy and the Elements*. Utrecht, Netherlands: Alonnissos, p151

[5] MacRepertory ReferenceWorks (2005) (Homeopathic software) San Rafael CA: Kent Homeopathic Associates

[6] Whitmont E. (1991) *Psyche and Substance*. Oakland CA: North Atlantic Books, p167

[7] Heron K. (2001) Mandragora - The darker side of Belladonna, *The American Homeopath* 2001:18

[8] van Zandvoort R. (2005) *The Complete Millennium Repertory* 2005, MacRepertory, San Rafael CA: Kent Homeopathic Associates,

[9] Bailey Ph. (1995) *Homeopathic Psychology*. Oakland CA: North Atlantic Books

[10] Scholten J. (1996) *Homeopathy and the Elements*. Utrecht, Netherlands: Alonnissos

[11] Julian O.A. (1979) *Materia Medica of New Homeopathic Remedies*, Translated by Virginia Munday, M.A., Beaconsfield, UK: Beaconsfield Publishers Ltd.

Chapter 7
Homeopathic Treatment for Post-Traumatic Stress Disorder

Edward Shalts, MD DHt ABPN ABHT ABHM*
(*ABPN = American Board of Psychiatry and Neurology; ABHT = American Board of Homoeotherapeutics; ABHM = American Board of Holistic Medicine)

Edward Shalts, MD DHt
Museum West Medical
123 West, 79th Street, Suite PH4
New York, NY 10024
USA
E-mail: dr.shalts@gmail.com
Website: www.HomeopathyNewYork.com

Abstract
Homeopathy has powerful tools for treatment of Post-Traumatic Stress Disorder (PTSD). Conventional psychopharmacology does not have medications specific for PTSD and fails to provide cure or even significant relief for this fairly prevalent illness. Experience of treatment of patients in the post-9/11 era is presented in clinical vignettes. The strategy of homeopathic treatment of PTSD in adults and children is discussed and illustrated with clinical cases.

1   Introduction

Post-Traumatic Stress Disorder, or PTSD, is a major adverse sequela that occurs following the experience or witnessing of life-threatening natural and man-made disasters such as earthquakes, hurricanes, military combat, terrorist incidents, serious accidents, or violent personal assaults like rape [1-7]. People who suffer from PTSD often relive the experience through nightmares and flashbacks, have difficulty sleeping, and feel detached or estranged, and these symptoms can be severe enough and last long enough to significantly impair the person's daily life.

PTSD is classified as a variant of a broader category of Anxiety Disorders.
Data from a number of studies indicates that up to 30% of individuals of various age groups, including children and adolescents, exposed to life-threatening events present with a clinical picture of PTSD [8-11].
Unfortunately, only about a quarter of victims discuss their problems. For example, in the USA, despite universal health coverage and the benefits of an employee assistance programme for all employees, only 28.5% of those with PTSD symptoms have talked to a health professional about the events of Hurricane Katrina or issues encountered since the storm [11].
The easiest way to identify PTSD is to remember the PTSD mnemonic presented on the next page.

PTSD Mnemonic
  E - Event/experience (threatening to life or physical integrity of self or others)
  R - Re-experiencing (flashbacks, nightmares etc)
  A - Arousal (anxiety, startle, hypervigilance, irritability)
  A - Avoidance (of things, places, images reminiscent of event)
  D - Duration of more than one month

It is also helpful to know that:

- PTSD is generally more severe or long-lasting when the trauma is of human design (e.g., torture, terrorist attack) vs. a natural disaster (e.g., earthquake).
- The chance of developing PTSD increases as the severity, duration, and physical proximity to the trauma increases. Other factors that increase the risk of developing PTSD include history of previous trauma and negative reactions from friends and family.
- Although symptoms of PTSD usually begin within the first three months after the trauma, there may be a delay of months or even years before symptoms appear. Delayed onset of PTSD is said to have occurred when the symptoms begin at least six months after the trauma.
- Research on individuals at risk of developing PTSD shows that the highest rates of onset (30% to 50%) are in survivors of rape, military combat and captivity, and ethnically or politically motivated internment and genocide.
- PTSD can occur at any age, including childhood.
- Individuals with PTSD often report painful feelings of guilt about surviving when others did not or about things they had to do to survive.

2   History of PTSD

Anyone who watched "300" or "Braveheart" can easily imagine that PTSD has always been present as a prominent illness throughout human history.
Below are some highlights of the development of public and medical awareness of this disease.

- 1900 B.C. Egyptian physicians report hysterical reaction.
- 8th Century B.C. Homer in *The Odyssey* describes flashbacks and survivors' guilt.
- 490 B.C. Herodotus writes of a soldier going blind after witnessing the death of a comrade next to him.
- 1597 Shakespeare vividly describes war sequelae in King Henry IV
- 1600 Samuel Pepys describes symptoms in survivors of the Great Fire of London.
- 1879 Rigler coins term *compensation neurosis*
- 1880s Pierre Janet studies and treats traumatic stress. Describes "hysterical and dissociative symptoms, inability to integrate memories, byphasic nature" of suppression and intrusion.
- 1899. Helmut Oppenheim coins the term *traumatic neurosis*
- WW I: "Shell-shock"
- WW II: Battle fatigue, Combat exhaustion, Traumatic Neurosis
- 1980: PTSD becomes a diagnostic category in DSM III[16]

---

16 Diagnostic and Statistical manual of Mental disorders

Careful research into and documentation of PTSD began in earnest after the Vietnam War.

Although PTSD has been noted in many patient populations, the largest potential population of people manifesting PTSD symptomatology are those who would be directly or indirectly affected by nuclear war. Lifton (1967) has described the course of PTSD in respect to hibakusha, the survivors of the atomic bombs dropped on Hiroshima and Nagasaki, Japan during World War II [12].

3   Official criteria for PTSD

Comprehensive knowledge of symptoms of PTSD is one of the key components to successful homeopathic prescribing. As you can see from the official criteria represented below, patients may be experiencing a wide variety of symptoms. But, as stated above, an overwhelming majority of victims do not volunteer information about their psychological state. An experienced clinician might be able to elicit at least initial information of the current state of the patient following the guidelines. As the patient starts revealing information in response to direct questions, a homeopath might be able to assess individual characteristics of the patient and arrive at the remedy this particular individual needs.

For example, shortly after the terrorist attack on 9/11/2001, one of the doctors at the Center for Health and Healing of the Beth Israel Medical Center in New York was conducting a routine physical examination of a young female. This doctor had gone through homeopathic training with the author of this chapter as a part of the Fellowship programme. At the end of the exam the patient asked the doctor: "is it normal that sometimes I see airplanes flying into the building out of the corner of my eye?"

The doctor was alarmed and proceded with detailed questioning following the diagnostic criteria for PTSD. After just a few direct questions, it became apparent that the patient was re-living the events of 9/11 she had witnessed just a few months earlier. In less than 30 minutes the patient was evaluated by me and prescribed a homeopathic remedy for what turned out to be a severe case of PTSD. Luckily the remedy was effective and the patient was cured in the course of a few weeks.

Clinical criteria characteristic of the majority of patients is best described in the Fourth Edition of the *Diagnostic and Statistical Manual of Mental Disorders* [13]:

- Exposure to a Trauma – The person has been exposed to a trauma, in which he or she has experienced or witnessed an event involving the threat of death, serious injury, or a threat to the physical well-being of him/herself or others. Note that only physical threats count in the definition of a trauma in PTSD. Situations that represent a psychological threat (e.g., a divorce, being criticized by a loved one, being teased) are not considered traumas in the definition of PTSD, even though they may lead to difficulties for the individual.

- A Response of Fear, Helplessness, or Horror – The immediate response to the trauma is one of fear, helplessness or horror (in children, it may be a response involving disorganized behaviour or agitation). So, if an individual's response to the trauma is one primarily of sadness or loss rather than fear (this is often the case following the death of a loved one who was ill), PTSD would likely not be diagnosed.

- Symptoms of Re-Experiencing the Trauma – The individual persistently re-experiences the event in at least one of the following ways:
  - o Recurrent and disturbing memories, images, and thoughts about the trauma.
  - o Recurrent and disturbing dreams or nightmares about the trauma.
  - o Acting or feeling as if the trauma were occurring again (these experiences are often called flashbacks). This may include hallucinations (e.g., seeing things or hearing voices that were present during the trauma, even though they are not really there currently), misinterpreting things that are heard or seen (e.g., being convinced that the sound of fireworks in the distance is actually the sound of gunfire).
  - o Becoming emotionally upset upon being exposed to reminders of the trauma, including physical sensations that were present during the trauma or situational reminders (e.g., the street where the trauma occurred, the anniversary of the trauma).
  - o Becoming physically aroused (e.g., breathless, heart racing) upon being exposed to reminders of the trauma, including physical sensations that were present during the trauma or situational reminders (e.g., the street where the trauma occurred, the anniversary of the trauma).

- Symptoms of Avoidance and Emotional Numbing – The individual avoids triggers and reminders of the trauma, or experiences a sense of emotional numbing, as indicated by at least three of the following features:
  - o Avoiding thoughts, feelings, or conversations that remind the individual of the trauma.
  - o Avoiding activities, places or people that remind the individual of the trauma.
  - o An inability to remember important aspects of the trauma.
  - o A lack of interest or participation in significant activities, such as socializing, work, and hobbies.
  - o Feeling detached or different from others.
  - o An inability to enjoy things or to experience positive emotions (feeling "flat").
  - o A sense that one's future will be shortened. For example, it may be difficult to imagine having a career, getting married, having children, or having a normal life span.

- Symptoms of Increased Arousal and Vigilance – The individual has symptoms of arousal and vigilance that were not present before the trauma, as indicated by at least two of the following features:
  - o Difficulty falling or staying asleep - sleeplessness.
  - o Feeling irritable and grumpy, or experiencing outbursts of anger and temper tantrums.
  - o Difficulty concentrating.
  - o Hypervigilance (e.g., always being on guard, looking over one's shoulder while walking down the street, etc.)
  - o Becoming startled very easily (e.g., jumping when the telephone rings).
  - o The problem must last at least one month for a diagnosis of PTSD to be assigned.
  - o The individual's fear, anxiety, avoidance, or other PTSD symptoms cause significant distress (i.e., it bothers the person that he or she has the symptoms) or significant interference in the person's day-to-day life. For example, the symptoms may make it difficult for the person to perform important tasks at work, meet new friends, attend classes, or interact with others.

4   Types of PTSD

There are four main types of Post-Traumatic Stress Disorder. All involve the same symptoms and are only differentiated by the length of time the symptoms have been manifested.

Acute Stress Disorder: Acute Stress Disorder is diagnosed when symptoms occur within four weeks of the traumatic event and last for more than two days but less than four weeks.

Acute Post-Traumatic Stress Disorder: Acute post-traumatic stress disorder is diagnosed when symptoms last for more than four weeks.

Delayed Onset Post-Traumatic Stress Disorder: This form of the disorder may not appear until years after the initial traumatic experience.

Chronic Post-Traumatic Stress Disorder: This form of PTSD is diagnosed when symptoms last for more than 90 days. The patient will likely experience lapses in symptoms for a number of days or weeks in a row, but the symptoms will always return.

5   Examples of traumas that can lead to PTSD or Acute Stress Disorder

- military combat
- violent personal assault (e.g., physical attack, mugging, robbery)
- being kidnapped or taken hostage
- torture
- incarceration as a prisoner of war or in a concentration camp
- natural disaster (earthquake, fire, tornado, hurricane)
- terrorist attack
- serious automobile accident
- serious accident at work or in the home
- sexual abuse during childhood
- sexual assault or abuse
- being diagnosed with a life-threatening illness
- unexpectedly observing the serious injury or unnatural death of another person

It has also been my experience that young children may develop PTSD as a result of parents having loud and/or violent arguments in front of their children. Unfortunately, I have seen many cases of this. As a matter of fact, while I am writing this chapter, one of my young patients is recovering from such a terrifying experience. In these cases family therapy is essential. In some cases, individual homeopathic prescribing for one or both parents might also be indicated as there may be some significant psychological pathology, including PTSD, undiagnosed in one of the parents.

6   Conventional treatments for PTSD and Acute Stress Disorder

Most of the treatment guidelines suggest psychotropic medications (psychopharmacology) and /or various types of psychotherapy [14-16]. While certain types of psychotherapy have been consistently shown to be effective in treatment of PTSD [15,17], evidence for the effectiveness of psychotropic medications has been at best inconclusive [16,17]. Remarkably, one of the most frequently used prophylactic psychological tools, a brief psychological intervention (debriefing), which is conducted immediately after exposure to a stressful event, has also been reported as ineffective in preventing the development of PTSD [18]. A large proportion of female PTSD victims opt for psychotherapy over medication [19]. The reasons most frequently cited are the effectiveness (or lack thereof) of a treatment, including potential masking of symptoms with the medication and, more logical, long-lasting effects with the psychotherapy.

There is also evidence suggesting that, in depressed patients with a history of early childhood trauma (loss of parents at an early age, physical or sexual abuse, or neglect), psychotherapy alone was superior to antidepressant monotherapy [20].

Various ethical issues [21] that exist around the research, production, and marketing of antidepressants and other psychotropic medications also make the efficacy and safety of psychopharmacology highly questionable.

Amazingly, some allopathic physicians have suggested that there is no evidence that conventional medication, including psychotropic medications, "are likely to do more good than harm in the long term" and that "although several drug classes (and possibly some antidepressants) are known to induce psychic indifference, the utility and desirability of this effect is doubtful" [22].

As a matter of fact, the authors cited above represent a group of physicians who question the so-called "drug-centered approach;" at the core of their objections is the fact that conventional drugs, instead of treating the target problem, create a different state in the brain or the body (i.e. sedation) that simply suppresses symptoms of the illness rather that treating them.

Dr. Hahnemann would be very happy to read such a statement coming from the "old school!"

7   Homeopathic approach to PTSD

While there is ample evidence characterizing the risks and benefits of conventional treatment of PTSD, there are no controlled studies that I was able to identify on the efficacy (or lack of thereof) of homeopathy for this fairly prevalent disease.

This comes as no surprise to anyone involved with homeopathy. The need for well-funded, well-designed studies of homeopathy has been acknowledged on numerous occasions by the homeopathic community. The problem is that no one with significant funds wants to finance such studies. The only attempt to conduct such a study was undertaken in 2006 by Dr. Iris Bell [23], who received funding from the Samueli Institute for a pilot study on PTSD. The writer of this chapter was one of the homeopaths contracted to conduct the study. Unfortunately, this very well designed study had an early termination owing to one of the most common phenomena of PTSD described above [11]: most of the subjects refused or were unable to participate in the study [24]. This issue could have been easily resolved if the study had had significantly more funding in order to pay subjects for participation and completion of the study, and/or if military personnel, rather than civilians, had been the targeted population.

There are also very few peer-reviewed papers on homeopathic treatment of anxiety disorder available as of this writing [25-27]. Those that do exist offer only very general guidelines on the homeopathic treatment of this pathological state.

However, homeopathic literature has an almost 200-year history of clinical reports on successful application of homeopathy starting with the original proving of *Aconitum* described by Hahnemann [28].

While the helpful presence of homeopaths during World War I is a strong possibility, the writer was not able to gain access to any records of their success. Unfortunately, with all the man-made catastrophic events beginning with World War II and up to September 11, 2001 probably there was a lack of trained homeopaths owing to limited access to patients and an obvious decline in the number of homeopathic practitioners per capita. India's vast number of trained homeopathic practitioners is an exception to the rule, but, again, the author has no access to reports from this part of the World.

The terrorist attack on 9/11 produced numbers of patients suffering from PTSD comparable to the Vietnam War or a nuclear disaster in Japan during WWII [29,30]. Researchers at the nonprofit RAND group used random digit dialling three to five days after the September 11th attacks to interview a national representative sample of 560 U.S. adults about their reactions to the terrorist attacks and their perceptions of their children's reactions. According to their report[29], 44% of adults reported one or more "substantial" symptoms of stress, 90% of adults had at least one stress-related symptom to some degree, 35% of children had one or more stress symptoms, and 47% of children were worried about their own or their loved ones' safety.

This time a number of homeopaths (although not as large as one would wish) were able to participate in the treatment of victims of this catastrophic event. Some of them, including the writer, have published case reports [31-37]. Despite differences in training and theoretical approaches to assessment and treatment of homeopathic patients, the results reported were uniformly impressive. Those treated with homeopathy were able to recover completely and go on with their lives. Later Roger Morrison and Nancy Herrick participated in the treatment of victims of a terrorist act in Bali and reported amazing results using only very basic homeopathic remedies [38]. Some of the homeopaths also participated in the homeopathic treatment of victims of natural disasters and reported overwhelming success using just a few basic homeopathic remedies [39,40].
As a result, the homeopathic community has gained an insight into the practical aspects of treating PTSD.

7.1 Main principles of homeopathic approach to treatment of PTSD

7.1.1 Acute Stress Disorder
If you hear hoof beats, think Horse, not Zebra. One should clearly understand the difference between an acute and a chronic illness, especially in the case of a massive terrorizing disaster. The latter produces a Genus Epidemicus-type [41] response. A few remedies will most likely

be very frequently required for the majority of the population. In the case of a natural disaster, such as an earthquake or a hurricane, the majority of relatively healthy people are going to respond with the picture of a limited number of remedies. For example, victims of earthquakes in Honduras responded very well to *Aconitum* [39], while victims of hurricane Katrina frequently presented with a clinical picture of *Ignatia amara* [40]. Roger Morrison and Nancy Herrick reported an amazingly good response by victims of the Bali terrorist attack to *Aconitum* and *Arnica* [38]. One should know the Materia Medica of these frequently prescribed remedies very well. In the first few hours/days after the disaster the clinical presentation of victims will be very clear. The response to the remedy is going to be very dramatic and satisfying to both the patient and the practitioner.

Sometimes you have to think of Zebra. There are going to be individuals who are constitutionally predisposed to being sensitive to stressors characteristic to terror-inducing events. To illustrate, a patient whose constitutional remedy is *Natrum muriaticum* will most likely respond with a clinical picture that indicates this remedy. For example, shortly after 9/11 I saw a young cardiologist, whom I'll call Dr. Michael. His main complaint was large painful aphtae deep in the mouth that did not allow him to eat any solid food. Visual: Very quiet, reserved. Neat. Laughs while talking about serious problems. Complaints: 1). Wakes very anxious from scary dreams; 2). Large aphthae in the mouth – unable to eat; 3). These problems – since 9/11 – made him feel "very disappointed", "abandoned". Some History: Responsible, serious since young age. Does not tolerate abandonment too well. When upset, needs to stay alone. Recently started craving salt "like crazy". His girlfriend says, "he would eat it in tablespoonfuls if he could".

I selected the following rubrics:
1. Mind – Reserved
2. Mind - Laughing, serious matters over
3. Mind – Anxiety, dreams, on waking from, frightful
4. Generals – Aphthae
5. Mouth – Aphthae
6. Mind – Ailments from disappointment
7. Mind – Consolation aggravates
8. Generals – Food and Drinks – Salt, desires

This resulted in a pretty straightforward repertorisation that put *Natrum muriaticum* at the top of the list of suggested remedies (See Fig. 1).

Fig. 1: Repertorisation (using RADAR 7.3)

	1 nat-m.	2 merc.	3 lyc.	4 calc.	5 arg-n.	6 sil.	7 chin.	8 sulph.	9 staph.	10 sep.	11 nit-ac.
	19/58	15/25	15/20	14/23	14/22	14/20	14/18	14/18	13/31	13/22	12/21
1.	3	1	1	2	1	1	1	1	2	1	1
2.	2	-	1	-	1	-	-	1	-	-	-
3.	2	-	1	1	-	1	1	-	3	-	-
4.	2	1	-	-	-	-	1	-	-	-	-
5.	2	3	2	2	1	1	1	3	2	-	2
6.	3	3	2	-	-	-	-	-	4	1	-
7.	4	1	1	1	1	3	1	1	1	4	2
8.	4	1	-	2	3	1	2	1	-	1	2

Here are Dr. Michael's e-mails after I gave him one dose of Natrum muriaticum 200C:

2 days later: "Ed, I CAN EAT NOW. I think I'm 50% better. Had my first normal meal today. First time in almost three weeks. Thank you very much. This small pill really worked".

5 days later: "I'm 90% better. Going to a steakhouse tonight."

6 months follow-up: Remains well. No anxiety. No aphthae. Now realizes that he was "quite depressed too". That is better too. "The depression is gone."

Even where Genus Epidemicus has been clearly identified, one must remain alert and conduct thorough evaluations as different people will still react differently to the same stressor. Mitch Fleisher [33] reported a case of Acute Stress Disorder when two people both exposed to the events of 9/11 developed two different clinical pictures. One required *Aconitum* (in my observation, a leading remedy after 9/11); another *Gelsemium*. I described a similar situation that happened with two experienced homeopaths during our trip to the International Academy of Homeopathy (Alonnisos, Greece) [41]. They were riding on the same motorbike and fell rather suddenly. Both were shaken up. They were evaluated and treated by Paul Herscu. One presented with a clear picture of *Pulsatilla*, another with *Arsenicum album*. A "typical" fall with psychological sequelae. Actually the homeopath who needed *Arsenicum album* stated he was fine. But *Arnica* still was not indicated (to deny any need for help is typical of an Arnica state).

Automatic "protocol" prescribing should never be a part of homeopathic practice. This principle does not exclude consideration of remedies that are most likely to be effective in a particular situation. But there always has to be differentiation of presenting symptoms. In another paper [32] I presented a case of two people who were sleeping in the same house when a part of the fuselage of the airplane that crashed in Bell Harbor on November 12, 2001 landed in the garage of their house. One required *Stramonium*, another *Opium*. Both were morbidly scared and both went into a state belonging to their constitutional remedy, bypassing the Aconitum state.

There is a continued argument between firm believers in one, and only one, constitutional remedy that "works" on each and every occasion for a particular person and homeopaths who believe in prescribing different remedies to the same person depending on a particular acute situation. It has been my experience that even in cases when long-term follow-up reveals that the initially prescribed remedy was not constitutional, one still can see significant improvement after accurate acute prescribing.

For example, one of the first patients I saw after 9/11 was in both Twin Tower bombings (1993 and 2001). On the morning of 9/11 Richard (not his real name) was in a subway station under the WTC when the first aeroplane hit the building. After being evacuated with everyone else, he realized that his attaché case had been left at the subway station. He went back, and crawling in the dark, retrieved the case and went to his office in the building right across from the WTC. He stayed glued to the window and watched the bodies flying through the air. These pictures have stayed with him day and night ever since. He became progressively more withdrawn. He was morbidly afraid of the dark, and had terrible nightmares and flash-backs. Usually a mild-mannered man, he became extremely argumentative. At one point two young men attempted to mug him at the parking lot. He bit them viciously until the police came. Even then he had to be pulled away from the criminals. He was literally unable to sleep because of constant nightmares. He also felt very guilty that he is alive while his colleagues and friends from the WTC are dead. He lost all powers of concentration. A very prominent computer analyst, he was paid a high salary, but was unable to perform. Richard had all the symptoms of PTSD.

I selected the following rubrics (Repertorisation – see Fig. 2):
1. Mind – Ailments from mortification
2. Mind – Anguish
3. Mind – Concentration, difficult
4. Mind – Fear, dark, of
5. Sleep – Sleeplessness, room, in, dark
6. Mind – Delusion, danger, impression of
7. Mind – Company, desire for, night

Fig. 2: Repertorisation (using RADAR 7.3)

	1 stram.	2 camph.	3 lyc.	4 acon.	5 caust.	6 puls.	7 calc.	8 carb-v.	9 phos.	10 ars.	11 arg-n.
	16/40	16/23	11/29	11/26	11/23	11/22	11/21	11/21	11/21	11/17	11/16
1.	1	1	3	2	1	2	1	1	1	1	2
2.	2	1	3	4	3	2	3	2	2	4	2
3.	2	1	3	2	3	2	2	3	3	1	1
4.	4	2	2	2	2	2	2	2	2	1	1
5.	3	·	·	·	·	3	1	·	·	·	·
6.	2	1	·	·	·	·	·	·	·	·	·
7.	3	2	·	·	·	·	·	·	·	·	·

Follow-up after two weeks: after one dose of Stramonium 200C. No nightmares for the last five days.

Follow-up after six weeks: Only two nightmares since the remedy; mood is much better, significantly less irritable.

An apparent success? Actually Richard continued to complain of feelings of guilt and poor concentration. Although significantly improved, he was still suffering from some consequences of PTSD. It needed two re-takes using the Sensation method (Sankaran) for me to arrive at his constitutional remedy. It has been over 1.5 years since he presented with no complaints after a few doses of *Aurum bromatum*. A rare remedy, a long process of finding it. But even the first relatively superficial prescription already changed Richard's life rather dramatically.

I am sure that Roger Morrison and Nancy Herrick would probably have used more than two remedies in Bali. But even such a narrow selection of powerful polychrests frequently required for psychological trauma brought about profound healing changes in their patients.

7.1.2 Acute and delayed onset PTSD
All basic principles of constitutional homeopathic prescribing apply in this situation. As has been seen in the last example, so-called "small" or "rare" remedies may be required depending on the individual characteristics of the patient. However, it has been my experience that an overwhelming

majority of patients who suffer from PTSD require just a few usually easily identifiable remedies. All of these remedies are thoroughly described in numerous reputable sources [42-47]. I find it nonetheless appropriate to present key features of these remedies as applied to treatment of PTSD. Remedies are presented in order of importance (based in my experience) in prescribing for patients with PTSD.

Aconitum napellus. Brilliantly described by George Vithoulkas [43]. In my experience this remedy remains one of the most frequently indicated for PTSD. To those familiar with the Sensation method, the importance of Aconitum in treatment of PTSD should be obvious. It belongs to the acute miasm and is a member of *Ranunculaceae* family which is characterized by being very easily excited, having "raw nerves". In a way, Aconitum is the "Mr Supersensitive" of homeopathic Materia Medica.

The main characteristic of this remedy is a feeling of TERROR that drives the person to move, to run. Such a patient is visibly scared and restless. For example, the majority of people who run away from a disaster zone in a state of panic will most likely respond very well to a dose of Aconitum.

I have seen numerous cases of people with chronic panic disorders who responded very well to Aconitum, which turned out to be their constitutional remedy. As I am writing this chapter, I am following a 55-year-old successful artist who presented with severe symptoms of chronic PTSD. He is constantly scared, claustrophobic, feels a need to move. He also gets angry very easily at the slightest provocation and has terrible, horrifying nightmares. It all started many years ago after he was awakened by an armed burglar. The patient presented with numerous other symptoms. The initial evaluation was very difficult. But a few things were very clear. The patient is extremely sensitive. He even said that he is like a "bunch of raw nerves". He feels in constant, endless danger, making him to want to run away. After a single dose of Aconitum 1M he gradually improved to the point of being able to function normally. He is not anxious any more, does not have panic attacks and nightmares. He is not as easily offended as before.

Stramonium. Inspired by Vithoulkas, Paul Herscu wrote a great book on Stramonium [44]. This remedy is another member of the Acute miasm. But it represents "the dark side" of terror. Death, night terrors of extreme intensity, violent behaviour. Extremes of panic and rage. I have seen many cases of Stramonium. All of them without exception presented with elements of violence and violent nightmares.

Opium. The patient is paralyzed by terror. One of the best examples I know is a dog brought to Paul Herscu's class. The dog developed severe constipation after a scary encounter with a car. Placed on the desk this little dog looked frozen. But it was also trembling in fear. It was frozen in shock. After a dose of Opium the dog jumped on the floor and defecated, producing a very impressive specimen of what had been stuck in its body for a few days. The next thing everybody knew was a happy, personable dog. As if nothing had happened.

Arsenicum album. A frequently required remedy. The person becomes very organized, fruitlessly busy, anxious. In my experience, "Arsenicum anxiety" has a critical, slightly paranoid streak. Patients are very needy (attention seeking) and hypochondriac.

7.1.3 Homeopathic approach to PTSD in children

Children are (indirectly) more and more frequently exposed to physical and sexual abuse. They also silently watch their parents argue, get divorced, behave violently towards each other.

It has also been my experience that violent, terrifying events that occur in a mother's life during pregnancy may affect the foetus quite dramatically. On more than one occasion I found a correct remedy based on the history of the pregnancy.

Children who suffer from PTSD experience the event over and over again through strong memories, flashbacks, and nightmares. They also often worry about dying at a young age.

The main psychological mechanism that young children and teenagers use is acting out. Naturally, children cannot express clearly their feelings. Observing their behaviour in the office is key to successful prescribing. Oppositional, at times violent behaviour in a child should alarm health providers to the possibility of PTSD.

In my experience, the most frequently prescribed remedies for PTSD in children are *Ignatia amara*, *Aconitum* and *Stramonium*. Ignatia is a very important remedy in this age group. I have successfully treated numerous children of unstable argumentative parents with this remedy. Frequently, but not always, children who need Ignatia, have a hysterical component to their behaviour.

Another very important remedy, especially during adolescence, is *Mancinella*.
Children who need this remedy present with a unique feeling of being controlled by some outside entity. The remedy is derived from Hippomane mancinella (Manzanillo), a euphorbiaceaous tree that grows on a territory spreading from Mexico and the West Indies through Colombia. Provers of this plant reported feelings of "being taken by the devil" (possessed) [48]. The remedy state frequently first appears in adolescence. The following case illustrates how one of the adolescent boys I met benefited greatly from Mancinella.

7.1.3.1 Case of Mancinella

Jordan came to my office by accident. I had met his father at a mutual friend's party. After learning that I was a board-certified psychiatrist, he asked me whether I could do anything to help his thirteen-year-old son, and he gave me the following details.

Jordan seemed to be constantly preoccupied and worried. When asked what was going on, he would answer that he had the same thought going through his head. He also had to repeat certain activities every day. Before leaving for school, for example, he had to touch the door exactly five times in the exact same spot, and then he had to walk five steps forward and five steps backward. He also had to repeat certain words many times in a row before he felt he could sit down at the dinner table. Pretty disorganized before the problem arose, Jordan absolutely had to have certain things on his desk in a certain order now. He was also very anxious and couldn't concentrate at school. All these problems had started cropping up about a month after the attack on 9/11. Jordan had seen the footage on TV and got very upset.

I explained to Jordan's father that I practise homeopathy and I'd be glad to help, but he needed to understand clearly what I do. I recommended a book to read. Soon after our conversation, he set up an appointment.

When Jordan and his parents came to my office, I could tell that Jordan was a quiet, timid young man. He told me that something weird was sitting inside of him and "this thing" controlled what he was doing. He couldn't stop thinking about this problem. He was tormented by it, preoccupied with these thoughts day and night. He felt depressed and had developed vertigo that was much worse in the morning. He also felt dull. Often he caught himself forgetting why he'd gone to the kitchen or what he was looking for in a drawer. His concentration was terrible. Formerly happy, easygoing, and sharp, now he was constantly afraid that something bad was going to happen to him or to his family. He wanted to stay around people all the time.

The family was seriously considering heavy-duty psychiatric medications. The conventional diagnosis of this condition would be PTSD with strong elements of OCD (Obsessive Compulsive Disorder). Preoccupation with this "thing" that was telling Jordan what to do could have been also classified as a delusion - maybe he was hallucinating. The selection of conventional medications could have been daunting, and likely would have included an antipsychotic.

The Mancinella worked beautifully for him. Jordan's symptoms gradually went away.

8   Conclusion

Numerous case reports and my own clinical experience suggest very strongly that homeopathy is effective in the treatment of PTSD.

In my opinion, not only professional homeopaths but also other health professionals, emergency response personnel and military personnel in particular, should be trained in basic homeopathy for Acute Stress Disorder and acute PTSD.

I also hope that one day soon funding will become available to conduct a full-scale well designed study on the treatment of PTSD with homeopathy.

Until then, we have to continue sharpening our prescribing skills and try to help as many patients as we can.

References

[1] Zatzick D. (2003) Posttraumatic stress, functional impairment, and service utilization after injury: a public health approach. *Seminars in Clinical Neuropsychiatry* 2003; 8(3): 149-57

[2] Frueh BC, Hamner MB, Cahill SP, Gold PB, Hamlin KL. (2000) Apparent symptom over-reporting in combat veterans evaluated for PTSD. *Clinical Psychology Review*. 2000; 20(7): 853-85

[3] McCarroll JE, Fagan JG, Hermsen JM, Ursano RJ. (1997) Post-traumatic stress disorder in U.S. Army Vietnam veterans who served in the Persian Gulf War. *Journal of Nervous & Mental Disease*. 1997; 185(11): 682-5

[4] Veenema TG, Schroeder-Bruce K. (2002) The aftermath of violence: children, disaster, and post-traumatic stress disorder. *Journal of Pediatric Health Care*. 2002; 16(5): 235-44

[5] Orcutt HK, Erickson DJ, Wolfe J. (2002) A prospective analysis of trauma exposure: the mediating role of PTSD symptomatology. *Journal of Traumatic Stress*. 2002; 15(3): 259-66

[6] Barrett DH, Doebbeling CC, Schwartz DA, Voelker MD, Falter KH, Woolson RF, et al. [2002] Post-traumatic stress disorder and self-reported physical health status among U.S. Military personnel serving during the Gulf War period: a population-based study. *Psychosomatics*. 2002; 43(3): 195-205

[7] Bremner JD, Southwick SM, Johnson DR, Yehuda R, Charney DS. (1993) Childhood physical abuse and combat-related post-traumatic stress disorder in Vietnam veterans. *American Journal of Psychiatry*. 1993; 150(2): 235-9

[8] Howgego IM, Owen C, Meldrum L, Yellowlees P, Dark F, Parslow R. (2005) Post-traumatic stress disorder: An exploratory study examining rates of trauma and PTSD and its effect on client outcomes in community mental health. *BMC Psychiatry*. 2005; 5: 21

[9] Jane Liebschutz, Richard Saitz, Victoria Brower, Terence M. Keane, Christine Lloyd-Travaglini, Tali Averbuch, and Jeffrey H. Samet. (2007) PTSD in Urban Primary Care: High Prevalence and Low Physician Recognition. *J Gen Intern Med*. 2007 June; 22(6): 719–726

[10] Nilamadhab Kar, Prasanta K Mohapatra, Kailash C Nayak, Pratiti Pattanaik, Sarada P Swain, and Harish C Kar. (2007) Post-traumatic stress disorder in children and adolescents one year after a super-cyclone in Orissa, India: exploring cross-cultural validity and vulnerability factors. *BMC Psychiatry*. 2007; 7: 8

[11] Karen B. DeSalvo, Amanda D. Hyre, Danielle C. Ompad, Andy Menke, L. Lee Tynes, and Paul Muntner. (2007) Symptoms of Post-traumatic Stress Disorder in a New Orleans Workforce Following Hurricane Katrina. *J Urban Health*. 2007 March; 84(2): 142–152

[12] Paterson KC, Prout MF, Schwartz RA. (1991) *Post-traumatic Stress Disorder. A clinician's Guide*. New York: Plenum, Edition 2. p. 58.

[13] DSM-IV-TR; American Psychiatric Association, 2000

[14] Edna B. Foa, Terence M. Keane and Matthew J. (2000) Friedman Guidelines for Treatment of PTSD. *Journal of Traumatic Stress* 2000 Volume 13, Number 4: 539- 588

[15] VA/DoD clinical practice guideline for the management of post-traumatic stress. Version 1.0. (2004) Washington (DC): Veterans Health Administration, Department of Defense. National Guideline Clearing House: http://www.guideline.gov/summary/summary.aspx?ss=15&doc_id=5187

[16] Kozarić-Kovačić D. (2008) Psychopharmacotherapy of Post-traumatic Stress Disorder. *Croat Med J*. 2008 August; 49(4): 459–475

[17] Treatment of PTSD: An Assessment of the Evidence. Report from the Institute of Medicine, released on October 18, 2007: http://www.iom.edu/CMS/3793/39330.aspx

[18] Wessely S, Rose S, Bisson J. (1998) Review: a brief psychological intervention (debriefing) is ineffective in preventing post-traumatic stress disorder. *Evidence-Based Mental Health* 1998; 1: 118

[19] Bryan N. Cochran, Larry Pruitt, Seiya Fukuda, Lori A. Zoellner, and Norah C Feeny. (2008) Reasons Underlying Treatment Preference: An Exploratory Study. *J Interpers Violence*. 2008 February; 23(2): 276–291

[20] Charles B. Nemeroff, Christine M. Heim, Michael E. Thase, Daniel N. Klein, A. John Rush, Alan F. Schatzberg, Philip T. Ninan, James P. McCullough, Jr., Paul M. Weiss, David L. Dunner, Barbara O. Rothbaum, Susan Kornstein, Gabor Keitner, and Martin B. Keller. (2003) Differential responses to psychotherapy versus pharmacotherapy in patients with chronic forms of major depression and childhood trauma. *Proc Natl Acad Sci USA*. 2003 November 25; 100(24): 14293–14296

[21] L McHenry. (2006) Ethical issues in psychopharmacology. *J Med Ethics*. 2006 July; 32(7): 405–410

[22] Joanna Moncrieff and David Cohen (2006). Do Antidepressants Cure or Create Abnormal Brain States? *PLoS Med*. 2006 July; 3(7): e240

[23] Southwest College to conduct PTSD research (2006). Homeopathy in the News. *Homeopathy Today*. July/August 2006

[24] Personal communication with the study coordinator

[25] Martin P. (2006) Sexual abuse and pregnancy - a homeopath's perspective. *Midwifery Today Int Midwife*. 2006; (77): 22-3, 68-9

[26] Coll L. (2002) Homeopathy in survivors of childhood sexual abuse. *Homeopathy*. 2002 Jan; 91(1): 3-9

[27] Davidson JR, Morrison RM, Shore J, Davidson RT, Bedayn G. (1997) Homeopathic treatment of depression and anxiety. *Altern Ther Health Med*. 1997 Jan; 3(1): 46-49

[28] Hahnemann S. (1996 – originally 1811) *Materia Medica Pura*. New Delhi: B. Jain Publishers (P) Ltd., Vol I. pp.25-46

[29] AU Schuster, MA; Stein, BD; Jaycox, LH; Collins, RL; Marshall, N; Elliott, MN; Zhou, AJ; Kanouse, DE; Morrison, JL; Berry, SH. (2001) A national survey of stress reactions after the September 11, 2001, terrorist attacks. *New England Journal of Medicine*. 345(20):1507-1512

[30] Schlenger WE, Caddell JM, Ebert L, Jordan BK, Rourke KM, Wilson D, et al. (2002) Psychological reactions to terrorist attacks: Findings from the national study of Americans' reactions to September 11. *Journal of the American Medical Association*. 2002; 288: 581–588

[31] Shalts E. (2002) A Story of Survival. *Homeopathy Today* 22(8):8-10

[32] Shalts E. (2002) Two Different "Faces" of Terror. *Homeopathy Today*. 22(8): 24-25

[33] Fleisher M. (2002) Post-Traumatic Stress. Two Different Reactions to 9/11. *Homeopathy Today* 22(8):10

[34] Gahles N. (2002) A NYC firefighter finds relief with homeopathy. *Homeopathy Today*. 22(8):12-13

[35] Gahles N. (2002) Firefighters in the wake of 9/11. Guilt, anger, denial, suppression… hope. *Homeopathy Today* 22(8):14-15

[36] Sonz S. (2002) In the shadow of the Twin Towers. A personal story of 9/11. *Homeopathy Today* 22(8):16-19

[37] Fassler K. (2002) Anxiety since 9/11. *Homeopathy Today*. 22(8): 26-27

[38] Morrison R, Herrick N. (2002) The Bali tragedy - Homeopaths on hand to help. *Homeopathy Today*. 22(11): 4-5

[39] Shalts E. (2005) *Easy Homeopathy*. New York: McGraw-Hill, p66

[40] Sebastian I. (2006) Hurricane Katrina and the Many Faces of Ignatia. *Homeopathy Today*. 26(4):10-12

[41] Shalts E. (2005) Our Children Were Attacked on 9/11, too. *Homeopathy Today*. 25(5): 20-23

[42] Hahnemann S. (1996 – originally 1811) *Materia Medica Pura*. New Delhi: B. Jain Publishers (P) Ltd.

[43] Vithoulkas G. (1995) *Materia Medica Viva*. London: Homeopathic Book Publishers. Volume I. pp. 45-96

[44] Herscu P. (1996). *Stramonium*. Amherst, MA: New England School of Homeopathy Press

[45] Sankaran R. (1997) *The Soul of Remedies*. Mumbai: Homoeopathic Medical Publishers

[46] Vermeulen F. (2002) *Prisma*. Haarlem, Netherlands: Emryss

[47] Morrison R. (1993) *Desktop Guide to Keynotes and Confirmatory Symptoms*. Berkeley, CA: Hahnemann Clinic Pub.

[48] Hering C. (1997) *The Guiding Symptoms of our Materia Medica*. New Delhi: B. Jain publishers (p) Ltd. Vol VII, page 263

[49] Shalts E. (2005) *The American Institute of Homeopathy Handbook for Parents*. San Francisco, CA: Jossey-Bass A Whiley Imprint, pp. 270-272

Chapter 8
Healing Collective Trauma with Homeopathy
Applying the Genus Epidemicus Approach to Trauma

Harry van der Zee, MD Hom

Harry van der Zee, MD Hom
P.O. Box 68
9750 AB Haren
Netherlands
E-mail: harry@homeolinks.nl
www.homeolinks.nl
www.ARHF.nl

Abstract

Homeopathy has proved to be a potent and effective system for healing individuals because individualising each case is the essence of its methodology. Homeopathy's possibly greatest asset, however, appears to be in individualising treatments for larger totalities, such as epidemic diseases (the Genus Epidemicus approach). There are impressive historical examples of such broader applications of homeopathy in the 19th and 20th centuries and recent experience in treating epidemic diseases like AIDS and malaria shows similar consistent results. This article presents a new development in which the Genus Epidemicus approach is applied to collective trauma (Genus Traumaticus). Case histories from early explorations of these possibilities in today's world are presented as examples. This approach would allow homeopathy to realise its full potentials and would allow use of the Law of Similars on which it is based to bring healing to collective psychological trauma.

1   Introduction

Homeopathy is a holistic form of medicine. This means that it is impossible to look only at the physical or psychological dimension without including the other, or, in an integrated approach to both, to exclude the spiritual dimension of meaning and purpose. This realization has as a consequence that despite the focus on mental health care, a proper discussion of it cannot be given without including physical diseases and their expression. Also the border between individual diseases and collective diseases is an arbitrary one, which is another important realization that has consequences for the discussion of either.

The basic thrust of this article is that it is possible to treat collective trauma with homeopathy in the same way as collective infectious diseases (epidemics) can be treated. A proper discussion of how epidemics are most effectively treated therefore logically has to precede the introduction of a proposed theory and practice of treating collective trauma.

A definition of *collective trauma* is needed here. The meaning used in this chapter is any kind of trauma that can be clearly defined as a situation, and in its signs and symptoms, that either occurs to a large group of people at the same time and place (e.g. tsunami, earthquake, war or genocide), or that has a high incidence and is of an archetypal nature (e.g. burns, rape, incest), meaning that the experience is never many generations away from an individual and therefore exists in the subconscious memory of practically every human being.

The line of thought that I hope to convey in this article includes the following steps:

1. The basic modus operandi in homeopathy is to individualise every case (individual approach).
2. An exception to this rule involves epidemic diseases, where a homeopathic prescription is based on individualising for the disease (collective approach). The analysis of this so-called *Genus Epidemicus* usually results in a limited number of remedies from which a homeopath can choose the one that best fits an individual patient. There are examples from history to show how long before the introduction of antibiotics and other drugs homeopaths successfully treated epidemic diseases.
3. It is postulated that this as-if-one-person approach can also be used for trauma (*Genus Traumaticus*) as the experience of trauma is of an archetypal nature and often takes place on a collective scale.
4. A new technology is introduced making it possible to design a remedy for a specific disease or state that fully covers the totality of all relevant signs and symptoms, and examples are presented of its efficacy in practice.
5. The consequence of this development is that one single remedy that is cheap, safe and effective can be used for one type of trauma.
6. This in turn makes it possible for non-homeopaths to use homeopathic resonances for trauma effectively. Considering the millions of traumatised people on the planet and the limited number of available skilled homeopaths, this is obviously a huge advantage. Homeopaths can then focus on those indications that require the classical approach of individualised treatment.

2   The principles of homeopathy

The general principles of homeopathy are discussed in different chapters of this book. Here only a short mention of those relevant to the subject of this chapter.

Law of Similars: This law is the bedrock of homeopathy and is also known as *"like cures like"* or *Resonance*.

Provings: In order to discover the curative properties of a broader range of substances, Dr Hahnemann introduced a method of testing called '*proving.*' In a proving, healthy individuals (the provers), take a small dose of a substance and by very carefully observing themselves document any symptoms which are at odds with their normal state. By this method symptoms connected to the substance are discovered.
It is important in the context of this article to mention that, for disease-specific remedies, either for epidemic diseases or for trauma, the current situation is that practically no single substances are known in the Materia Medica that cover the totality for one disease/condition (more on this later).

The smallest possible dose: Owing to the potentisation process a homeopathic remedy can induce a healing response in the diseased individual without causing side-effects. Thus homeopathic remedies, applied in the correct way, can be safely used for everyone, including small babies and pregnant women.

Individualising remedies for each person: No two people are the same and so to apply the Law of Similars most effectively a homeopath needs to find a remedy which best matches the totality of the symptoms in a patient. Those symptoms which stand out because they are strange, rare or peculiar are the most important. In these the individuality of the patient is most visible, that which makes him or her different from other people. Those symptoms which are very general, in that most people have them, are considered to be among the least important.

3   As if one person

The one exception Hahnemann made to the rule of individualising for each person was in the case of epidemic diseases. In epidemic diseases the personal history and traits are not important because they have little or nothing to do with the disease, as opposed to chronic diseases that emerge, as it were, from the history of the patient. In the case of these collective diseases we now do not need to individualise on the level of each patient but on that of the disease as expressed in the whole group – as if one person.

I will go into the subject of epidemic diseases in more detail because understanding the principle and realising the potential of the 'as-if-one-person' approach in infectious diseases, and projecting that as a possible approach to treat collective trauma, can have huge implications for global mental health care.

The role and purpose of an epidemic disease is on the level of the collective, even though it is expressed through individuals who belong to that collective. So here we need to collect all the symptoms that are typical of the disease and make it different from other diseases. This totality of a disease complex of symptoms Hahnemann called *Genus Epidemicus*. Again in this application of homeopathy, anything strange, rare or peculiar for a specific disease is of the utmost importance in defining a remedy which matches the totality of the symptoms of the disease. To find this remedy, homeopaths bring the symptoms of a group of patients suffering from the same disease together as if they were one person. All symptoms typical of individual persons are excluded, and all symptoms typical of the disease are included. So if, for instance, a person always worries about money matters and during the epidemic illness does this even more so because now he cannot work, this is not typical of the disease and can be ignored. But, if a person is always very thirsty and during the illness refuses to drink at all, this symptom, thirstlessness, is typical of the disease and is to be included in the analysis. Once all the symptoms of the disease have been gathered in this way, a remedy can be selected that best matches the totality of the disease, and this remedy can be given to all those who suffer from the same condition. In practice this often means a group of remedies, as usually no single remedy fully covers the totality of the epidemic disease, so, on the basis of the individual expression of the disease in a patient, a remedy is selected from the Genus Epidemicus group.

It is interesting to go back in time to the nineteenth century and early twentieth century, the peak era of Western acceptance of homeopathy, and read the results homeopaths reported in applying the Genus Epidemicus principle to infectious diseases. A century ago homeopathy was at its zenith, in terms of public acknowledgement and scientific recognition, and also in terms of clear and significant therapeutic results. The reason for this is that homeopaths were using homeopathy's best asset – the treatment of epidemics.

In *The American Homeopath* – 'As If One Patient' - *Greg Bedayn* (1998) describes Hahnemann's discovery of how to treat epidemic diseases:

"In 1799 Hahnemann first applied the Genus Epidemicus: the single homeopathic remedy to treat a similarly affected population, during a scarlet fever epidemic he treated in Königslutter, Germany. The story of how he accidentally discovered the Genus Epidemicus is interesting: There was a large family that had members with scarlet fever.

Hahnemann noticed that one of the children who had been taking Belladonna for another reason did not have symptoms of scarlet fever. He discovered that by giving the other members of the family Belladonna as a prophylactic, they did not get scarlet fever. Hahnemann concluded that a remedy that rapidly cures at the onset of an illness would be the best preventative.

This serendipitous discovery led Hahnemann into developing the principle of Genus Epidemicus - where if one takes the symptom-totality from each person in an epidemic population and then puts those features together into one case, as if one person, and gives the indicated simillimum (a remedy selected that in its signs and symptoms is similar to the disease) to the entire affected population - that it will cure."

This approach, as Hahnemann found out, worked well. Bedayn continues:

"The curative results of the Genus Epidemicus were so positive during the epidemics in the ensuing decades that they not only cured the majority of those affected where nothing else had worked, but they also drew international acclaim towards homeopathy, the new, the rational, medicine. There is something intrinsically powerful about the success of homeopathy in curing large populations that is undeniably attractive to anyone gifted with the power of observation, and it was through these early cures with epidemics that Hahnemann was able to quickly and widely spread the word: Homeopathy. It was from his discovery of the Genus Epidemicus that Hahnemann later developed his theory of miasms; the taints that color and shape all family trees, as representing the basis of chronic disease."

Hahnemann later writes about the Genus Epidemicus principle in his 'Organon' §101:

"It is possible that a physician meeting with the first case of a certain epidemic should fail to perceive at once its perfect image, because every collective disease of this kind will not manifest the totality of its symptoms and character until several cases have been carefully observed. But after having observed one or two cases of this kind a physician may approach the true condition of the epidemic and is thus enabled to construe a true characteristic image of the same and to discover the true homoeopathic remedy."

Hahnemann broadens this general principle in §102, when he says that complete knowledge is only to be obtained in a perfect manner by observations of the symptoms of several patients of different bodily constitutions.

Using this as-if-one-person approach, homeopaths impressed the medical establishment with their results. Here are a few quotes to illustrate this:

> "In epidemics the mortality per 100 patients is 1/2 to 1/8 in homeopathic hospitals (a century ago there were more than 100 homeopathic hospitals in the US) compared to allopathic hospitals." (Bradford, 1900)

> "Homeopathy had become very popular in North America during its early years due to its amazing successes obtained by the 'old guard' during the epidemics - epidemics of diphtheria, scarlet fever, cholera, malaria, yellow fever." (From its Roots Upwards, Interview with André Saine, N.D., D.H.A.N.P., Vienna January 1994.)

> "Ever since Samuel Hahnemann homeopathy has time and again been able to successfully treat epidemics/pandemics with a small number of remedies." (Stahl, Hadulla, Richter, 2006)

Different authors from Europe and the US reported impressive results with diseases like Cholera (Gebhardt 1929, Humphreys 1849), Yellow Fever (Saine 1994) and Spanish Influenza (Winston 2006, Dearborn 1923, Dewey 1921, Hoover 2006) and the data concerns many thousands of patients.

The great advantage of the homeopathic treatment of epidemics is that the individuality of the patient is not an issue, and as a result, nor are the skills of individual homeopaths. Once a successful group of remedies is identified, any homeopath will be successful. The collective case is a lot simpler and the skills of the homeopath have less influence on the results. This means that in situations of a rapidly evolving killer pandemic any person who can make the diagnosis can effectively use the homeopathic Genus Epidemicus remedy, or, where a group of remedies are involved, only needs brief instruction to choose from them. Given that developing countries in particular suffer from epidemic diseases and that homeopaths are often scarce in these countries, this approach is also ideal there.

Currently homeopaths have followed in the footsteps of the old masters by offering sustainable treatment for the epidemics of our time. The (medical) world is gradually realising that the principle of waging war on micro-organisms (antibiotics, antivirals), on diseases (like cancer) or on terror, has a counter-productive effect in the long run. As can be read in other chapters of this book, the same applies to mental health care. An attitude of fighting a mental condition alienates the patient from the doctor, but more importantly also from himself, and although medication may seem to cure because symptoms have been reduced, the true state of the patient instead gets worse.

It has become very clear that 'Big Pharma' does not and will not have all the answers and actually creates many of the problems we are facing today. The use of conventional medicine is the third leading cause of death in the modern world, ahead of automobile accidents and all other causes other than cancer and heart disease (Lazarou, Pomeranz and Corey, 1998; Null, Dean, Feldman et al., 2005). Hahnemann concluded in his day that the suppression of infections is also a causative factor in the emergence of chronic diseases, meaning that conventional medicine is co-responsible for the increase in conditions like cancer and heart disease (which are Numbers One and Two respectively on the list of leading causes of death today) (Hahnemann 1828). The simultaneous rise in the use of antibiotics and the prevalence of chronic diseases suggest he may be right.

Moreover, increasing numbers of deadly strains of bacteria and viruses are created as a result of the war against them. The term used for this is therapy resistance, meaning that the bacteria or viruses are no longer killed by the medication used. For the major epidemics in Africa, malaria, TB and HIV-AIDS, this is a serious problem. The problems surrounding resistance are being increasingly acknowledged within the healthcare community.

"The threat of large-scale drug resistance is 'real and scary.' " (Marani 2007).

"Resistance develops naturally, in response to the selective pressure from drugs or from the body's own immune system." (World Bank 2003)

The World Health Organization (WHO) is aware of these issues and so should any doctor be, but an alternative has not been developed because the alienation of the diseasing agent as an enemy that should be eradicated is deeply seated within mainstream medical philosophy. Fighting bacteria with antibiotics simply leads to ever more resistant strains. Hospitals have now become dangerous places to be in because of 'super-infections' with dangerous, antibiotic-resistant bacteria.

4   Miasms

4.1 Infectious diseases and miasms

The concept of miasms is an essential aspect of homeopathic philosophy and important to consider here.

In §78 of his 'Organon' Hahnemann declares that true natural chronic diseases are those that arise from a chronic miasm. He defines a miasm as the result on an organism of the suppression of an infectious disease that can cause signs and symptoms later in life and can also be passed on to the next generation. Hahnemann postulates that these miasms are the very basis of chronic diseases. (Hahnemann 1810)

In his analysis Hahnemann defines three miasms: Psora, Sycosis and Syphilis. In modern terms, Psora could be seen as 'the mother of all chronic diseases', as Hahnemann in his analysis concludes that ultimately all other miasms must have grown out of this one.

Hahnemann's observation is that an episode of an infectious disease can have a lasting influence on an individual and is even passed on to later generations. In modern terminology, he supposed that an infection can cause hereditary genetic changes. These changes can be recognised as an individual or collective diathesis (predisposition, tendency) that initially may only be expressed as general signs (e.g. sensitivities) but at a later stage can be triggered into full-blown pathology.

Homeopaths recognise acute and chronic miasms. An *acute miasm* is defined as a disease-producing power which causes acute, specific, infectious disease having almost fixed manifestations. An acute miasm according to Dr J.T. Kent (1900) is "the one that comes upon the economy, passes through its regular prodromal period, longer or shorter, has its period of progress and period of decline and in which there is a tendency to recovery." Acute miasms, as with other true acute diseases, have a relatively sudden onset, climax and resolution, and thus are self-limiting.

Chronic miasms, in contrast, have a slower onset, seldom grow to any climax (although there are periodic flare-ups) and continue until one's death. Their course cannot be altered but only slowed by favourable circumstances.

According to Hahnemann, uncured miasms cannot be eradicated by the life force; (§79) he thought only homeopathy can do this. This may be too bold a statement, as I believe the 'like cures like' principle is broader than homeopathy and a general law underlying all creation.

Further miasms have been recognized since the time of Hahnemann, although not all homeopaths accept them. I have no doubt that somewhere in the future these will be broadly accepted and it will be recognized that many influences besides the three infectious diseases Hahnemann identified determine states of health and can cause a miasmatic disturbance.

I suggest that our understanding of miasms needs to be updated to be able to bring homeopathic treatment of collective issues to a higher level in today's world. A broader definition of the term *miasm* would allow us to also use it for trauma. A miasm would then be defined as a lasting effect on an organism owing to any outside influence including infections, but also trauma. Or, stated differently, an infection can be seen as a traumatic event with possible lasting (miasmatic) impact. The concept of miasms also forms a bridge between (collective) infectious diseases and (collective psychological) trauma. The impact of (collective) trauma lowers the immune system, making the individual/collective more vulnerable to infectious (epidemic) diseases.

4.2 Miasms and process

My own theoretical understanding of the miasms underwent a revolutionary change as a result of an accidental observation that I made. I was fascinated to discover the work of Stanislav Grof (a Czech psychiatrist who later moved to the US) on the birth experience (Grof, 1995).

All the miasms homeopaths have come to recognize (e.g. Psora, Sycosis, Syphilis, tubercular, cancer, leprous, etc.) can be clearly traced back to a certain phase in the birth process, and the main remedies representing them can be understood using the symbolic language of that aspect of the birth experience. Since birth is a process, it became clear that miasms are related to development, and each of them to a specific phase or theme in development, both on an individual and a collective level (van der Zee, 2000).

The birth process shows us life in a nutshell. All phases of human development and of the individuation process are represented. Analysis of an individual birth shows amazing similarity to the states of physical and psychological health and illness observed later in life, so the birth experience already displays the central theme of an individual's life. Birth seems at first to be causing a trauma but after having analysed many cases I have come to think of it differently. Birth is not causing that state but expressing it, since in cases where there is information from pregnancy, conception or previous life experiences, the same patterns can be observed. Stated differently, there is a high level of synchronicity between the birth experience and the circumstances surrounding it and a pre-existing state in the incarnating soul. So no *tabula rasa* but an already existing pattern that 'creates' / 'encounters' circumstances optimal for its expression.

Case example:

A person with anxiety disorder when in narrow places that seemingly started after a history of drowning may show an earlier history of severe whooping cough, a birth history of near-suffocation, an anxious situation the mother experienced during pregnancy that points to the same remedy indicated for the child, and images of a tsunami coming up in regression therapy or recurrent dreams.

Phases of birth and miasms:

- The onset of birth is related to Psora (departure from Paradise, learning to take care of oneself, formation of the Persona);
- The dilatation phase irreversibly entered related to the Tubercular miasm (longing to return to Paradise and resenting being 'fixed' on any level; fighting socialization);
- The dilatation phase itself by Sycosis (fixed, victim, powerless, no exit, identification with the Shadow);
- The transition from dilatation to the propulsion phase by the Cancer miasm (taking on responsibility for others but insufficient care of and space for oneself) and the Malaria miasm (wanting to express individuality and trying to break loose from tribal rules and customs that restrict);
- The propulsion phase itself by the Syphilitic miasm (death-rebirth struggle; Anima and Animus issues; egotism versus altruism); and
- The actual moment of birth by the Acute miasm (sudden change, seeing the light, death-rebirth experience).

A fuller discussion of the marked analogy between Hahnemann's miasms and the stages of birth can be found in 'Miasms in Labour' (van der Zee, 2000) and 'Homeopathy for Birth Trauma' (van der Zee, 2007).

From my work on the miasms the following conclusions can be drawn:

- Miasms have a role and serve a purpose. In homeopathy we have only highlighted their pathological side, the results of something going wrong during development. From analyzing each miasm and its corresponding phase, it becomes clear that each cultivates qualities in humanity and plays a role in the individuation process. For example, if one suffers from a situation that one perceives as incapable of being changed, a quality like endurance is nurtured, along with love in the form of friendship and loyalty with others who are in the same position. Dissociation can be a pathological expression of an inner escape from a painful situation but becoming free from identification with the ego is a positive side of the same miasm.

- Disease induces change within an individual, and miasmatic diseases that we could also call collective diseases induce change within society, the group, tribe, nation or mankind as a whole.

- Diseases and miasms induce the development of qualities within an individual and within humanity. Miasms are subconscious archetypes that pervade not only the psyche but also the physical form. If the normal process of development and growth is blocked, diseases can manifest themselves in order to bring this to awareness and to induce the changes needed to restore a healthy, balanced state of being.

- Diseases and miasms are both the problem and the solution, they seem to stunt development but are actually the path to further growth. Diseases and miasms are the teachers of mankind, and, in infectious diseases, microorganisms carry the message.

- About 95% of our DNA originated in the dawn of our evolution from viruses and bacteria. This means that these germs today bring pieces of information to us and integrating these pieces is a significant part of what drives evolution. This also makes very clear why killing the bug, as allopathy proposes, can never support the role and purpose of the disease, and forces the organism to acquire the same lesson/information following a different route, one that may involve even more suffering. This is the deeper meaning of suppression of individual and collective diseases and miasms and the cause of chronic diseases.

4.3 The logic of miasms

1. According to Hahnemann *symptoms* are a sign of the dynamis (Life Force) restoring balance in the organism (Hahnemann 1810).
2. A *disease* is a combination of symptoms.
3. A *disease* is a sign of the dynamis restoring balance in an individual by bringing it to a higher level of functioning. The fact that balance is restored does not mean that the individual is brought back to a previous state, but rather moved on to a new one that includes the qualities induced by the disease.
4. An *epidemic disease* is a sign of the collective dynamis restoring balance and inducing growth and awareness in a group.
5. *Miasms* are a sign of the dynamis restoring balance and inducing growth in the collective, and the expression of collective diseases can be part of that process.
6. Epidemic outbreaks are acute collective manifestations of this process involving a large group, whereas miasmatic diseases are more of a chronic expression of the same energy afflicting those individuals that apparently are working on the same issues in their individual development.
7. Epidemics that are endemic for long periods of time, like malaria (the conflict between the individual and the tribe), are concerned with major shifts in humanity that take many generations.

The idea that an epidemic disease has a role and purpose is a concept whose elaboration would need much more space than this chapter can afford. If one analyses an epidemic disease the effect on the psychology of people suffering from it can be found. Whether this effect is intentional ('God') or not intentional ('Darwin') is irrelevant for the homeopath, who simply needs to see the full picture to be successful in the treatment of the disease. AIDS is a good example. It is clear that in a society where love, respect, care and equality existed between sexual partners HIV would never spread. AIDS is a wake-up call to individuals to take responsibility within relationships, and those who do (for the other and themselves) can survive. In Africa this includes a change in tribal rules and beliefs with respect to the position of women. Intentional or not, that is what the disease does to the collective.

4.4 A new source

Since 2004 I have been increasingly involved with the treatment of epidemics in Africa. This started with AIDS, but gradually has come to include many more epidemic diseases as also representing manifestations of collective trauma. It was Peter Chappell's work with AIDS that made me decide to make the treatment of collective diseases my main focus (Chappell 2005).
I witnessed spectacular results with his remedy *PC1*, first in Malawi and later also in other African countries (Hiwat & van der Zee 2004).

I expect there are many ways, either based on spiritual practice or electro-magnetic technology, in which purposely designed remedies proceeding from a conscious understanding of 'what needs to be cured' (Hahnemann) can be made. My personal experience is limited to those prepared by Peter Chappell. In his search for a simillimum for AIDS in Africa, he couldn't find a suitable remedy in the existing Materia Medica and (luckily) was forced to find a way to design a Simillimum himself. He created a new technology to directly imprint healing information on water (see www.ARHF.nl). He named his first remedy PC1. What he initially may not have realised, but what he soon found out, was that with this new technology he could in principle create a resonance for any disease including trauma. So, following PC1, he developed many others, which together are referred to as PC Resonances. Although much more research is needed to show their efficacy, the data from clinical observations for a series of epidemic diseases until now is very promising. This new development bypasses the time-consuming and laborious process of Materia Medica development and makes it possible to instantly create a resonance/remedy for a disease for which the current Materia Medica has no satisfactory match. It combines the advantages of allopathy (one remedy for a diagnosis) with those of homeopathy (safe, no side-effects and cheap) into an effective treatment that can easily be applied by any health professional. Individualised homeopathic treatment can then be reserved for those cases where the collective approach is not indicated or is insufficient.

5 Collective trauma

5.1 Genocide in Rwanda

In 2005, when Peter Chappell was in Rwanda to treat AIDS, he realised that in addition to the AIDS burden people were still suffering from the effects of the genocide that had taken place eleven years before. He recognized this to be a collective trauma that should be dealt with using the Genus Epidemicus approach. He prepared a resonance that he called *PC War/Genocide Trauma* and gave that first to his patients: they responded remarkably well. All of the symptoms subsided rapidly, including the feeling as if it had happened yesterday, the flashbacks, nightmares and all other ways in which this traumatic miasm (PTSD) was being expressed in them (Chappell, web reference). This is what Chappell wrote on the topic:

> "This is built from the experiences of Bosnia and Rwanda and other war zones but it applies generally. In general PTSD includes flashbacks; this is the key symptom and the other symptoms seemed to me to be consequences of this. There are nightmares of great intensity, there is emotional shutdown and avoidance behaviour and there is hyper-arousal. The key thing in genocide was the tormenting memories after a sudden but premeditated, planned, savage, short-lasting, attack. Many similar such events occur

in war. For the survivors there are flashbacks of exact extremely scary, horrific moments during war or genocide that were really life-threatening, deeply painful, humiliating, guilt-inducing and lots more. These flashbacks are occurring daily, even hourly, even every minute of every day, and have lasted many years already. It is exact images of what happened flashing back all the time.

In consequence of these images, thoughts and responses:

- *They cannot get to sleep without tormenting images for a long period into the night.*
- *They cannot sleep properly at all, only getting light and partial sleep for these many years and they are not fully rested or refreshed after sleep.*
- *They cannot focus on any real daily problems as these get linked immediately to genocidal images, which they normally cannot blank out, and it is in the centre of their mind and any inner thinking goes directly to the 'TV goal-like replays. They cannot make rational decisions because they cannot think; in every thought they go into the genocide images and ruminate and get no further. They stay buried in these overwhelming processes.*
- *They cannot respond to the needs of others - typically their large family - and instead neglect them because they are unable to feel and think.*
- *They try to avoid anything that will stimulate the flashbacks and hyper-arousal; this can lead to extreme behaviour and sometimes they turn to drugs and alcohol or suicide/self-harming.*

Also:

- *They feel they could be killed at any moment, that any sudden sound frightens them to death day and night. Hyper-arousal is the term and it can occur from a child screaming, a loud bang or a stone dropped by a bird hitting the tin roof. There is the immediate expectation of being killed.*
- *They are very frightened as the killers are still at large, even living next door, even if the killers next door have tried to apologise. They cannot accept or contemplate the apologies.*
- *They are deeply disturbed by not having been able to bury their relatives. This lack of closure is a very common and serious PTSD in its own right.*

Also, as a consequence of their internalised fearful and deeply frightened state:

- *They fear the neighbours in the community who were the killers and generalise this and don't go socialising, don't go to church, don't engage in conversation, never get into laughing and joking, and instead stay at home, isolated from society. They even become speechless for long periods like years.*
- *They do not allow themselves to be helped by others.*
- *They feel it is impossible that anyone could even want to help them.*

They remain as dependent victims, having to beg for food, unable to even think of work, of restarting work, are instead living in dire poverty, starving (eating a small meal every few days), homeless, rootless yet often having to support large families of orphans. Children drop out of school due to the memories and the consequential inability to study. They can become homeless, criminals and addicted to cigarettes, not to mention drugs and alcohol.

Sometimes they do not realise that situation which is a state of denial. But the behaviour is completely out of normal after some traumatic events or being in a war etc. While I am sure this is not the full picture and that it represents mainly the victim's inner world, I am sure it's accurate for the many women and men I interviewed and replicated millions of times across the world in many variations."

So on the basis of his experience in Bosnia and Rwanda Peter created a PC Resonance for the trauma of war and genocide (PC304x) and applied it for the first time in Rwanda in 2005, eleven years after the genocide. The 30 people who took this PTSD resonance improved dramatically.

- *"The tormenting memories of genocide which were daily, even hourly, even every minute of every day, and had lasted 11 years, virtually disappeared overnight and they had many benefits from this.*
- *They could get to sleep without tormenting thoughts.*
- *They slept deeply, possibly the first time in 11 years.*
- *They could focus on daily problems without these being linked to genocidal thoughts and could then make rational decisions rather than stay buried in these overwhelming thoughts.*
- *They stopped fearing the neighbours in the community who were the killers in the genocide and started again socialising, chatting, going to church, laughing and joking.*
- *They stopped feeling they could be killed at any moment, that any sound would frighten them to death day and night.*
- *They felt the possibility that they could trust and allow others to help them.*
- *They felt able to begin the process of forgiveness and even actively encouraged it with those who killed their relatives.*
- *They could respond to the needs of others - typically their large extended family including orphans.*
- *They decided to stop being dependent and having to beg, and to start thinking about a small business and becoming independent.*
- *One child that had dropped out of school due to the memories and the consequential inability to study wanted to return.*
- *A businessman who took it because of high blood pressure and heart palpitations that occurred around the anniversary of the genocide found it resolved his symptoms, which is not surprising. This is just one of what must be millions of people who have a set of symptoms that belong in history to unresolved PTSD and this I suggest is the reason why the medical textbooks are full of comments about most chronic diseases where they say the cause is unknown and there is no known cure. These are the routine before-and-after comments you find in the bibles of medicine. And here is the cause and the cure."*

5.2 Second-generation Holocaust trauma: case of a 55-year-old woman with a deep pain

Working in Africa dealing with collective conditions like epidemic diseases and trauma I came to understand that in homeopathy we overemphasize the individuality of problems a patient presents. The majority, if not all, of so-called individual problems are expressions of universal themes, and the collective roots of these themes can often be traced back in the life of the individual and his/her family or culture. The expression in the individual person can be unique, requiring an individual simillimum, but there are many cases where if we look deep enough we can discover roots (miasms), that are collective. Let me give here as an example a case that really showed me the potential of addressing the collective traumatic roots of individual psychological problems.

H. starts by mentioning the troubles she has with her digestion, but shortly into the interview decides to talk about the real reason for her visit. By saying 'the digestion is something I can live with by taking natural medicines to prevent constipation', she closes the subject and comes to the core of her problem.

'My mother left the house when I was nine and I was looked after by housekeepers. My father was very ambitious and busy. I also spend months with family attending a different school. There was no basic security. I felt very lonely. All my sisters were placed at different addresses. I had to adjust to a different family and a different school.'

'My mother was depressed and institutionalised. If I saw her it felt as if I was with a dead person. In my puberty I started to release myself from my mother. I had a sort of allergic feeling to her passivity. To be touched by her was very difficult for me. She lived very much on her own. Only when she died was I able to love her again. Now I feel I have a more beautiful connection with her.'

'My parents had been hiding during the war and my mother's family has been completely wiped out in the concentration camps. That has been always there. It seeped through. I had the feeling I had to take care of my mother. I loved her a lot and missed her enormously. But the relationship with her changed. In her depression she could not be reached. My father remarried with a good woman but it was a very cerebral family. I felt insecure, not at ease. When I was eighteen I immigrated with my sister to Israel. I lived there for eighteen years, got married and had children.'

'My marriage was very difficult. Now that we have separated, the relationship is okay. I missed emotional support. When we were having a fight and I felt no understanding or contact I was sucked into very deep emotions that were beyond my control. Like a very old well of pain. As if I were losing grip. As if I were losing contact with reality. Going to a deep place where this was present. It is a completely different world, with strong emotions and loneliness. Being cut off. As if everything is useless. As if I can already see the end of things. The grief and pain there are so huge and I don't dare to feel the depth of it. I weep a lot.'

'Already at kindergarten I felt displaced. I didn't belong to the group, had no connection, even though I did have friends. Every morning I feel this heaviness when I need to confront the world again. By using my willpower I have done my work and looked after my children.'

'I have a very intense contact with my little sister and when she started to make herself loose from me that was very difficult for me. Each time I have to depart from people I get these feelings. Away from the connection, away from the security.'

'I tended to overeat and was fourteen kilos overweight. I loved cheese, ice-cream, chocolate and sweet dairy products. Then I would slim down drastically followed again by overeating. This is no longer so. Now I love salads and raw fish.'

'Ever since I started the relationship with my ex-husband I started having asthma. The attacks have always stayed. Very strong attacks. I get more and more asthmatic until it completely closes off. Very frightening. It is worse from wet weather, in autumn, from cats and dairy products.'

'I don't have nasty dreams, but can wake up in a panic, feeling the contact is gone, I no longer feel the relationship.'

'I'm the eldest of three daughters. Before me my mother had a miscarriage. Three months after I was born she was pregnant again. I have three children. In each pregnancy I would become depressed in the *seventh month. The last pregnancy was not planned and I felt my husband was not happy with it. Oh, I have been so depressed. I would leave the house in the middle of the night. No support. I felt like wanting to take it away using knitting needles. Because I felt so lonely. I was happy with the pregnancy at first but saw my husband's face change when I told him. My mother was an afterthought. Her mother was very cold and had manic episodes.'*

Analysis

What was most striking in the case for me was the pain and grief coming from a well deep in her that she did not dare to feel, that, as I felt it, was bigger than her. There are enough reasons in her personal life to have feelings of grief and of being alone, but this feeling of everything being useless and this notion of already seeing the end of things I could not fully connect with her personal history. It had a similarity to it, but the weight of her pain seemed to be so much more than her personal history would account for. I could understand it though from her mother's history and from the collective Jewish trauma of the Holocaust.

When she later mentioned that the whole family had been killed in the Nazi concentration camps, the depth of her pain became understandable. She was clearly suffering from something that was lying beyond her personal history, in the collective trauma of genocide.

I had read Chappell's report on treating genocide in Rwanda and asked the patient if I might prescribe an experimental remedy for her.

Prescription: PC304x (War/Genocide Trauma), 5 drops daily

Follow-up five weeks later

'I am very much surprised. There is a change I had never thought possible. I feel a completely different person. A dramatic change. For a short period I continued crying but since then it has not come back. It is a completely new period. I feel optimism, trust, love for life. It is miraculous. This weeping has travelled with me all of my life. The last couple of years it was constantly there. Before that in episodes.'

'I dream again, quite lucid, remember them better. My sleep is much deeper and I wake up less often. On waking up in the morning I am okay. No more panic or fear of being abandoned. I can continue with my life like this. I'm no longer afraid to move on, to be forsaken. A great trust has come. It is okay what happens or is about to happen. There is more peace inside. I can enjoy the simple things of life again. Before this all joy was lacking.'

'Before I started taking this remedy I had the feeling of being wiped out, taking no space. I might just as well not be there. Now I take a space and that has meaning.'

Prescription: continue with PC304x 5 drops daily.

Two months later

'A complete layer has been resolved, this layer of collective grief.'
'The insecurities I have now have to do with everyday practicalities. Like building my house. Then I feel a lack of stability and go back to the time our family was broken up. Like a sea without borders. I love the sea because it gives space, quiet and openness.'

'In the morning I have a bit of trouble starting the day, a little sadness. In the evenings I am feeling great. What I didn't tell you before is that I have a strong fear of spiders. For the last couple of months my menses have returned.'

Analysis
She is now completely free from this bottomless impersonal but collective pain and grief, and the complaints she has now she can relate to her own life. So now it is time to move on to a personal simillimum. With regard to her personal trauma, the broken relationship with her mother is the key element. She was disconnected from the source of security she was depending on, her mother, causing feelings of forsakenness and insecurity. This definitely happened at the age of nine when her mother could no longer cope, but also before that time her mother was depressed and not the source of warmth and comfort her daughter needed. Later in her life we see a tendency towards bulimia with a desire for sweet dairy products, including ice cream and chocolate.

Prescription: *Lac humanum* MK

Eleven weeks later
'I'm beautifully out of the dependency in my recent relationship (someone she met after her divorce). I'm on my own feet now. There have been no dips any more and my base has become firmer. All the symptoms that have improved on the first remedy never returned. Since this last remedy my asthma is a lot better, my stomach problems are gone and I no longer have abdominal pains.'

'I dream about my recent relationship. I dreamt of getting a clear view by literally putting on other glasses to be able to see further away.'

Three months later
'I'm totally fine and suggest we cancel the appointment. I'll contact you if anything new comes up.'

Two years later
Of course we do not know what would have happened if I had started with Lac humanum, but I honestly doubt whether she would have responded as she actually did. By fully clearing up the collective trauma, just one dose of her simillimum was enough to clear up all the remaining symptoms; to my knowledge a repetition of either remedy has never been indicated. This in itself is exceptional in homeopathic practice as relapses usually occur frequently; this indicates that clearing the collective trauma (miasm) first may greatly amplify the effect of the individual remedy that follows it.

5.3 Trauma and miasm
Homeopaths are used to individualising each individual case of psychological trauma, including those caused by collective events. The greater the distance in time between the trauma and the treatment of an individual expression of it, the more an individualised approach seems justified and the more difficult it may become to recognise the causative factor. As with collective trauma the number of patients involved may be huge; this in itself merits an investigation into whether an as-if-one-person approach to trauma (Genus Traumaticus) would be effective. Let us look at an example of collective trauma and the effect on psychological health in our time:

Kashmir (Washington Post, September 2008) "The number of patients seeking mental health services surged at the state psychiatric hospital, from 1,700 when the unrest began to more than 100,000... The patients have insomnia, learning disabilities, anxiety disorders and what Kashmiri therapists call the 'midnight-knock syndrome,' a fear stemming from the many pre-dawn raids by Indian security forces aimed at rooting out suspected insurgents...

Mental health groups estimate that 60,000 Kashmiris committed suicide last year, a record number, said Mushtaq Margoob, head of the Government Psychiatric Diseases Hospital in Srinagar...

More than 15 percent of Kashmiris are afflicted with post-traumatic stress disorder, according to a recent study by Margoob ... In January the army recruited 400 psychiatrists after more than 100 soldiers, including officers, killed themselves..."

The symptoms in each of these people described above may differ, but it seems very likely to me that an as-if-one-person approach would be very effective in the vast majority of the cases. And this is only Kashmir. I'm writing this part of the article on my way to Burundi and Eastern Congo, another area full of heavily traumatized people. Watching the news for some time is enough to convince anyone that many millions of people are suffering from collective trauma. It's the collective that is ill, out of balance, and it's the collective that needs to be treated. If we don't see that and act accordingly, we will never be able to heal these collective derangements. For in the time we need to treat one single traumatized patient using individualized treatment, ten new ones get traumatized. It is also a lot more practical to start with a Genus Epidemicus remedy (Genus Traumaticus in this case) and later to individualise those cases where the collective approach is not enough. Following such a strategy, we would be able to help many more patients and perhaps even be able to induce a real change in the collective.

Moreover, it seems as if unresolved trauma lies at the root of many chronic conditions. If we look at the language of *Vital Sensation* (the deepest way in which a patient experiences his state, for instance a sensation of being scattered to pieces - Sankaran) these are all expressions of trauma. These are sensations fitting a traumatic experience to a life form.

What follows are several key principles I have gleaned from my clinical work, observations in dealing with individual diseases in my private practice and in treating epidemic diseases and trauma in Africa. These represent a work in progress, but enough is already known for me to list the following key observations that have guided my work.

- *An Individual Trauma* can express itself in an *Individual Disease*. This is something we know from experience. For instance, an unresolved grief can be expressed in recurrent throat infections, or as a result of sexual abuse a woman can have recurrent bladder infections.

- Trauma is hereditary (miasmatic). See the case above. See also the work of Hellinger (www.hellinger.com). If we go back a few generations, there are lots of traumas that can be at the root of symptoms we come across in our patients. These include wars, periods of starvation, crashing stock markets, stillborn babies, rape, incest, and so on.

- A *Collective Disease can follow a Collective Trauma*. A good example is cholera following the horrors of war. It is interesting to see for instance that *Cuprum* is a remedy fitting both war (the typical Cuprum state is that of a soldier) and cholera. Of course there are also circumstances on the physical level, like lack of clean drinking water, that contribute to cholera epidemics, but that doesn't mean that trauma at the energetic level is not an essential part of the expression of the disease. By looking solely at material manifestations and circumstances, conventional medicine denies the role of energetic disturbances in many conditions. Let's not make that same mistake. Besides that, we know from research that traumatic events cause malfunctioning of the immune system (Segerstrom and Miller, 2004; Smith and Giannoudis, 1998), so circumstances and susceptibility come together to create disease.

- The language of the *Vital Sensation* is the language of *Trauma*. If we read all the different ways a vital sensation is expressed, this becomes very obvious. Whether it is being pressed together, falling to pieces, torn apart, exploded, scattered, and so forth, these are all very physical expressions of ways in which the integrity of an organism can be threatened. So the sensation of the deepest disturbance in an individual is trauma.

- There seems to be a chain reaction:
  1. (Collective) Trauma → Miasm
  2. Miasm → (Epidemic) Infections
  3. Infections → Genetic damage (genetic trauma) in individuals
  4. Genetic damage → Chronic disease

- Collective trauma →← Epidemic; a collective trauma can be both cause and effect of an epidemic; if for instance millions of people die from Avian Flu, this causes a trauma to many more millions of survivors. And, staying with that example, the fear and panic that comes up if such an epidemic is broadcast is the first symptom of the epidemic, the first way in which the collective shows signs and symptoms before or without the virus itself ever reaching the individual.

- Trauma seems to be primary. So in the chain of diseases and traumatic events - a limited two-dimensional path of cause and effect - it seems that the wheel starts turning with trauma. However, over the longer term, with accumulated miasms, the cause can be either miasm or trauma.

- Separation - the delusion that we are separated from each other and from the world around us, the mythological departure from Paradise – seems to be the Basic Trauma. (See above for details of the Psoric miasm, the departure from Paradise and the analogy in the birth experience as departure from the good womb and entering the birth process.) The way in which this trauma is experienced may differ per individual.

5.4 The trauma of war in Africa

After I had observed the dramatic effect of a Genus Traumaticus approach to a second-generation victim of the Holocaust (case above) I travelled to Burundi and Congo. The genocide in Rwanda made the headlines. In 1994 800,000 people were slaughtered in only ten days. In the region of Rwanda, Burundi and Congo it is estimated that more than 5 million people have been killed in ethnic wars and at the hands of rebels who try to get control over the precious resources. Even today many are still being killed or raped. Young children have been kidnapped from villages and have been forced to fight for rebels (child soldiers), or cook their meals and fulfil their sexual needs. In the whole region, hardly anyone has been spared from ethnic violence and many remain traumatised. Many people suffer from symptoms similar to those Peter Chappell observed in Rwanda. Adults often call this 'hypertension' as replays of trauma especially affect their heart. This manifests itself as anxiety with palpitation and hyperventilation and often fear of death. Children complain about difficulties concentrating at school.

Since the focus of this chapter is on collective issues, the impression may be given that the normal homeopathic remedies no longer matter. That is far from the truth and the following case shows how regular individually chosen remedies and PC Resonances addressing a collective issue can complement each other.

Case

Z. is diagnosed with cardiomyopathy and dilatation of the heart. It all started in 1997 in her fourth pregnancy, during the time that the war broke out. One day she woke up and found many dead bodies in the street and saw a dog eating from a dead body. That image has forever stayed with her. "Maybe," she says, "that caused my depression."
Prescription: PC304x (genocide / war trauma) once daily 5 drops.
Follow-up after six days: After the remedy she first had an aggravation with pain in her chest. That pain is now gone. She is still easily short of breath but the images of the war are gone.
After two months: When a few days ago the police were searching the house looking for illegal immigrants, the fear came back and she felt as if her heart were breaking in two. The images of the war never came back and she no longer dreams of the war. The heart symptoms are the same.
Prescription: Repeat PC304x daily for one week (for the revived trauma) and then start with *Cactus* 200K one dose per week (for the physical condition).

In these regions trauma is endemic or epidemic. Although the individual expression may differ a little from one patient to another, after listening to many of them it is clear to me that they are all speaking about a collective experience.

Traumatised children

60% of the 600 children at a primary school in Kiliba (DR Congo) were orphans. Many of them had lost parents in the war. Several had been recruited by rebels against their will (dragged from their parents' huts) to become child soldiers. Trauma is all over their faces, their eyes turned inside or staring into a void. These children were all treated with PC304x for the trauma of war and genocide. When I returned to the school two months later, I interviewed them and they told me how much they had improved. Their tormenting thoughts and dreams had stopped. Their teachers reported the children could concentrate now in class and looked so much brighter.

5.4 The trauma of rape in Africa

Another trauma that is very prominent around the world is that of rape. In my practice in the Netherlands I must have seen dozens of victims of rape and incest throughout the years. I used to treat them with individualised homeopathy, usually with good results. As with war trauma, though, as soon as one has seen more cases a pattern becomes obvious. Yes, there are individual expressions of how being raped is experienced and processed, but there is also great similarity between the cases. A clear expression of this is that most homeopaths will usually choose one from a limited amount of homeopathic remedies that they consider specific to the trauma of rape and sexual abuse. These are grouped under a repertory rubric 'Ailments from rape and sexual abuse'. This shows that what homeopaths have actually done is to create a Genus Traumaticus for rape consisting of a dozen remedies that will help in the majority of cases.

Once I got involved with the treatment of epidemics and trauma in Africa, I started using some of the PC Resonances in my private practice as well. I used PC435p for the trauma of rape and sexual abuse in a few cases and found they complemented my usual individual approach nicely. I had too little experience though to conclude that this would help in all cases of rape and sexual abuse.

The incidence of rape in Africa is staggeringly high. The sad reality is that in many parts of Africa a girl has a greater chance of being raped than of being taught to read and write. This means that the trauma of rape must be very strongly present in the collective subconscious of Africans. Raping civilians is a frequent practice for soldiers and rebels in war zones. In Congo, where I have treated rape trauma the most, thousands if not millions of women are traumatised by brutal rape. To divide the population into perpetrators and victims is too one-sided in my opinion. It takes a traumatised person to be able to inflict so much pain on another person. This is clear in DC Congo's Kivu province where the rebels from Rwanda, who kill and rape, are the selfsame young people who witnessed the atrocities of 1994.

5.4.1 A case of rape and gonorrhoea

M. is 38 years old. She was raped by two soldiers four years earlier and became pregnant. It was an extra-uterine pregnancy and the foetus was aborted. Now during intercourse she has a lot of pain, "as if they are trying to put a tree inside." She has frequent vaginal infections. Every time she has pain she thinks about the rape, and ever since the rape she is fearful on seeing a man. The joy of sex is gone, and instead she is afraid of it because of the pain. During intercourse anger is stimulated.

Prescription: PC435p (rape and sexual abuse) once daily 5 drops.

Follow-up after 10 weeks: "The thoughts about rape have disappeared. I have no longer an aversion to sex but desire it very much now. No more fear; I enjoy it now. When I see men, I'm no longer afraid. No more anger, even though having sex is still painful."
Nevertheless, there are still the physical problems of pain with intercourse and vaginal discharge. However, the pain no longer triggers anger and doesn't prevent her from enjoying intercourse. Most likely, the pain is caused by gonorrhoea as a result of the rape. Extra-uterine pregnancies are also regularly caused by gonorrhoea.

Prescription: PC180g (gonorrhoea) 5 drops daily until the complaints have disappeared.

Follow-up: a few weeks later she is completely well.

During my first trip to DR Congo, entering from Burundi into Kivu province, this woman was one of several people who had been raped that I treated, and all responded well. I have a DVD with this lady beaming with joy and to me it is still amazing to see how just a few drops of a remedy could rid her of this past trauma. I was very happy with this wonderful result. Not just because these women were so much better, actually completely better, but also because it meant that the approach of one remedy for rape was highly successful, and that by making the remedy available to any health professional in Africa, potentially millions of other raped women in Africa could benefit in the same way.

5.4.2 *The raped women of Bukavu*

On that first trip we were advised not go deeper into Congo, but on my second trip it seemed to be quieter and we went to Bukavu. Its population doubled when huge numbers of refugees tried to escape from the militias. Amongst them were thousands of raped women, chased away from their villages by their husbands or their husband's families.

In Bukavu I treated more women and with the help of a local organisation we set up a permanent Amma4Africa Clinic there (See www.ARHF.nl). The women who shared their experiences with me made me aware of how the act of rape is only part, sometimes even a smaller part, of their trauma.

Let me present a composite story of the raped women of Bukavu:

> *Rebels enter the house and demand that a woman undress. She refuses, after which they torture her with guns, knives and sticks. Many still carry scars from the severe wounds thus inflicted. Then several of them rape her in front of her children, or the children have escaped the house and try to hide in the woods. They may take older children with them and kill them later, or use them for their purposes as child soldiers or to satisfy their sexual needs. If the husband is there, they first kill him. One way they do this is to lock him in a hut and set fire to it and then rape his wife. If the husband was not there and later finds out about the situation, he usually chases his wife and the (remaining) children. She and her children walk to the city where she tries to find shelter and to earn some money by carrying heavy loads. She earns just enough to buy some food for herself and the children. But as she cannot afford school fees her children are expelled from school. Because of the rape she got infected with gonorrhoea or HIV, but cannot afford treatment. She is living in the past, experiences only hardship in the present and doesn't see a future for herself or her children.*

Three months later I received a follow-up report from Bukavu:

> *"We are happy to inform you that all the women treated for the trauma of war and rape are doing very well. Here are some quotes:*

> - *"I live free from the past now. The dreams and fears have gone."*
> - *"I can sleep well now. I have confidence in this remedy. It is helping me a lot."*
> - *"I am much better and I can work well now. I have no more fear and no feeling of being a victim any more. I accept the past."*
> - *"I am no longer the slave of my past. My thoughts are more oriented on the future now."*

> *The women are so much brighter than before. The only problem is that they are still facing a hard life that can bring more trauma to them."*
> *Nathalie and Angèle - Amma4Africa Clinic, Bukavu*

So many of these women experience trauma piled on trauma and end up doing the heaviest work for the lowest fee while their children roam the streets. Those not sent away by their husband are psychologically in a much better state and also live in better circumstances.

One could say that rape is endemic to most of Africa, making it a symptom of a collective derangement. The long-term effects are of course huge. AIDS is just one expression of the underlying trauma. To stop this we can contribute by treating all victims of these behaviours, rapists and raped alike. As the perpetration of rape is often an expression of a history of sexual violence in a family or nation, rapists have very frequently either been sexually abused themselves or carry the trauma of rape of their ancestors with them, very similar to the way infectious diseases of ancestors can cause miasmatic chronic diseases in their offspring.

6   Conclusion

6.1 Follow the river to its source

If we look at the role homeopathy can play in the world for the physical, mental, emotional and spiritual health of mankind, it makes sense to analyze what would be the most effective way of using our resources. Regrettably, in many parts of the world there are very few homeopathic practitioners. If chronic diseases (including mental diseases) originated from a miasmatic derangement of the Vital Force owing to (suppressed) infectious diseases, and if these in turn are responses to unresolved trauma, it seems logical to start by using our resources to deal with collective trauma, epidemics and collective endemic (cultural) diseases first. Luckily the treatment of collective disorders produces consistent results requiring very little skills. It was a strange realisation for me, that it took me years of study to be able to successfully treat a child with a running nose, while in only two hours I could teach a nurse or doctor who knew nothing about homeopathy how to provide effective, safe and cheap treatment for epidemics like AIDS and Malaria and the terrible trauma of genocide or rape. Having made several trips to Africa now and having treated many patients, I can no longer deny that this is the reality. The potential of homeopathy for treating collective disorders of any nature is huge and we have only started realising it.

Following the line of reasoning above, I feel that homeopathy needs to develop a practical approach to make the exploitation of its best asset a top priority. Treating the collective is what we do best and is what has a larger curative and prophylactic impact on humanity. Treating the collective is like using a wider filter that will take out the big chunks more effectively. The smaller chunks that it lets through can be filtered out using the more refined filter of individual treatment, be it homeopathic or otherwise, such as psychotherapy. By overemphasizing the individual expression of collective issues, our filters are clogged by a lot of collective debris and the effect of individual treatment is therefore often limited.

- The higher purpose of homeopathy on a global level is to know what needs to be cured in the world, a continent, country, society, or other such grouping of individuals.
- For this we need to be able to read the signs and symptoms of our time.
- An epidemic is an expression of a need for collective change.

- Treating today's trauma is preventing tomorrow's epidemics.
- Treating today's epidemics is preventing tomorrow's chronic diseases.
- Healing today's collective diseases is preventing tomorrow's individual diseases.

6.2 Impossible?

This sounds very ambitious, and it is. It may take decades to make this vision a reality. Impossible? Here are some famous predictions from the past that have been embarrassed by history:

- *"Heavier-than-air flying machines are impossible."*
  - Lord Kelvin, president of the Royal Society, 1895

- *"Unworthy of the attention of practical and scientific men."*
  - British Parliamentary Committee report on Edison's electric light bulb

- *"X-rays will prove to be a hoax."*
  - Lord Kelvin, president of the Royal Society, 1883

To use a more contemporary quote: "Yes we can" with the emphasis on *we*. This is what homeopathy can potentially contribute to the pallet of health care. To make this a reality will require dedication and action by homeopaths and cooperation with and from health professionals in other fields. In the field of mental health care, it is obvious that any form of therapy, that is not based on forceful suppression of the symptoms, will become more successful by integrating homeopathy into its protocol. For many cases, releasing past trauma with homeopathy will enhance the effects of psychotherapy. For clear causes one specific remedy covering the Genus Traumaticus can do this. Although ideally every patient besides a disease/trauma-specific remedy will also receive individualised treatment, this cannot be provided yet in many parts of the world, or may not be necessary as other professional skills can also be expected to complement the action of the homeopathic trauma remedy. Any professional in mental health care can learn how to use a Genus Traumaticus approach in a very short period of time and integrate it into an existing treatment protocol. My experience is limited in this respect to using PC Resonances, but I'm sure other homeopathic remedies can be identified that will be broadly as effective.

The easiest and most practical way of starting to address collective derangements of the vital force is by treating collective trauma and epidemics. There are lots of reasons why this is more than a good idea and why luckily several homeopaths are already practising this, especially in developing countries:

- It has no side-effects
- It is safe for pregnant women, babies and elderly people
- It is not expensive
- Production, storage and distribution are uncomplicated
- It does not induce therapy resistance
- It does not create more dangerous viruses and bacteria
- It has been effective in many epidemics in the past and is effective in today's epidemics
- Current experience indicates it to be also effective for collective trauma

We can hardly overestimate the positive impact on the health of humanity if, for instance, all Germans and Jews were to take a homeopathic resonance for the collective trauma of war and genocide, or all Jews and Palestinians involved in the replay of the Holocaust, all Hutus and Tutsis, all Cambodians, all Vietnamese and Vietnam veterans etc.

Similarly, the impact of releasing all victims of incest and rape (including raped and rapists) of their trauma can be expected to have a significant effect on the wellbeing of all of humanity.

As it is possible for any health professional to integrate this Genus Traumaticus approach into their daily practice and thus improve the success of their treatment, transcending the long-term effects of trauma can be within the grasp of many within a short span of time, or, as Hahnemann expressed it … in the *shortest, most reliable, and most harmless way.*

If we can imagine such a transformation … then we can also make it happen.

References

[1] Amma Resonance Healing Foundation – www.ARHF.nl and www.aidshealing.org

[2] Bedayn, Greg (1998) 'As If One Patient', *The American Homeopath* 1998

[3] Chappell, Peter (2005) *The Second Simillimum*, Haren (Netherlands): Homeolinks Publishers

[4] Chappell, Peter, www.peterchappell.com

[5] Dearborn, Frederick M. MD (1923) *American Homeopathy in the World War*. Chicago: American Institute of Homeopathy

[6] Dewey, W.A. (1923) Homeopathy in Influenza- A Chorus of Fifty in Harmony. *Journal of the American Institute of Homeopathy,* May 1921

[7] Hoover, Todd A. (2006) Homeopathic prophylaxis, *The American Homeopath*, October 2006

[8] Gebhardt, A. v. (1929) *Handbuch der Homöopathie*, Leipzig

[9] Grof, Stanislav and Halifax Grof, Joan (1995) *Realms of the human unconscious*, New York: Viking Press

[10] Hahnemann S. (1921) 6th edition of *Organon* translated by Boericke. New Delhi: B. Jain Publishers Pvt. Ltd, 1990 (reprint edition)

[11] Hahnemann, S. (1828) *The Chronic Diseases, their Peculiar Nature and their Homeopathic Cure*. Dresden, Germany: Arnoldischen Buchhandlung, Translated from the second enlarged German edition of 1835, by Prof. Louis H. Tafel.

[12] Hellinger B, www.hellinger.com

[13] Hiwat C & van der Zee H, PC1 – Answer to AIDS in Africa, *Homoeopathic Links*, Vol 17 (4): 264-269

[14] Humphreys, F. (1849) *Cholera and its homoeopathic treatment*, New York: William Radde Publisher

[15] Kent JT. (1900) *Lectures on homeopathic philosophy*, Lancaster, PA: Examiner Printing House

[16] Lazarou J, Pomeranz BH, Corey PN. (1998) Incidence of adverse drug reactions in hospitalized patients: a meta-analysis of prospective studies. *JAMA* 1998 Apr 15; 279(15): 1200-5

[17] Marani, Dr Lyndon, (Ministry of Health) (2007) Nairobi: *PlusNews*, 8 October 2007

[18] Null G, Dean C, Feldman M, Rasio D. (2005) Death by medicine. *Journal of Orthomolecular Medicine*, 2005 Vol 20, No 1, p 21-34. http://orthomolecular.org/library/jom/2005/pdf/2005-v20n01-p021.pdf ; Also at http://www.doctoryourself.com/deathmed.html

[19] Roberts, H.A. cited in Dearborn 1923 and Dewey 1921

[20] Saine, André, From its Roots Upwards', Interview with André Saine, N.D., *D.H.A.N.P.*, Vienna, January 1994

[21] Sankaren, Rajan (2007) *Sensation Refined*. Mumbai: Homeopathic Medical Publishers

[22] Segerstrom, Suzanne Ph.D., and Gregory Miller, Ph.D., *How Stress Affects the Immune System*, http://mentalhealth.about.com/od/stress/a/stressimmune604.htm

[23] Smith, R.M. and Giannoudis, P.V., *Trauma and the immune response*,
http://www.pubmedcentral.nih.gov/articlerender.fcgi?artid=1296840

[24] Stahl E., Hadulla M.M., Richter E. (2006) Homöopatische Behandlung der Influenza – Vogelgrippe, *Algemeine Homöopatische Zeitung*, 50: 15-22

[25] Winston, J. (2006) *Some history of the treatment of epidemics with Homeopathy*, www.whale.to/v/winston.html

[26] World Bank (2003) *Global HIV/AIDS Programme of the World Bank*, 17-18 June 2003

[27] Zee, Harry van der (2000) *Miasms in Labour*. Utrecht (Netherlands): Stichting Alonnissos

[28] Zee, Harry van der (2007) *Homeopathy for Birth Trauma*. Haren (Netherlands): Homeolinks Publishers

[29] Zee, Harry van der (2008), *Amma4Africa Manual – Basic Guide to Treating Infectious Diseases and Trauma*. Haren (Netherlands): Homeolinks Publishers

Chapter 9
Homeopathic Prescribing Strategy for Patients Taking Psychotropic Medications

Edward Shalts, MD DHt ABPN ABHT ABHM*

(*ABPN = American Board of Psychiatry and Neurology; ABHT = American Board of Homoeotherapeutics; ABHM = American Board of Holistic Medicine).

Edward Shalts, MD DHt
Museum West Medical
123 West, 79th Street, Suite PH4
New York, NY 10024
E-mail: dr.shalts@gmail.com
Website: www.HomeopathyNewYork.com

Abstract

We live in a polluted world. Besides the very obvious problem of pollution with poisons and drugs, our patients also take conventional medications and supplements in quantities far beyond reason. Many patients are given multiple drugs (polypharmacy) despite the best guidelines that exist in conventional medicine.

Homeopaths work in this environment every day and need to develop clinical approaches, which help to mitigate the impact of conventional medication on the accuracy of prescribing homeopathic remedies. One also needs to be able to detect the best time for and to develop a safe schedule of discontinuation of conventional medications as the patient improves. The chapter discusses strategic approaches to tackling these issues.

1   Introduction

We live in a world that consumes medications, supplements, vitamins, herbs and street drugs at an exponentially increasing rate. This is the reality that a homeopath cannot ignore. Almost every person in the so-called civilized world has taken some kind of a biologically active substance (frequently with psychotropic effects, too) at some point in his or her life. If there is a place in the modern world that is "uncivilized" in this sense (meaning drug- and medication-free), I would like someone to show it to me.

According to the EPA (Environmental Protection Agency), U.S. animal feedlots produce about 500 million tons of manure each year, more than three times the amount of human waste. This animal waste, (with antibiotics) also ends up in groundwater and surface water in huge quantities. In

China, 80 percent of the major rivers are so degraded that they no longer support fish. The Yangtze River is contaminated with 40 million tons of industrial waste and raw sewage every day, and the water in the Yellow River is so polluted that it cannot be used even for irrigation: http://www.webofcreation.org/Earth Problems/water.htm - _edn13#_edn13
The rainfall on the European continent is so full of toxic pesticides that much of it is too dangerous to drink [1].

Besides this very obvious problem of pollution with poisons and drugs, our patients also take conventional medications and supplements in quantities far beyond reason [2-4].

Some statistics on medication in the United States [2]:

- Nearly 2.7 billion retail prescriptions were dispensed in 1999, amounting to $110 billion in sales.
- Almost two-thirds of Americans currently use medicines: 49 percent use prescription drugs and 30 percent use non-prescription medications.
- Adverse drug reactions (ADRs) are reported to be the fourth-to-sixth leading cause of death. Serious ADRs occur in 6.7 percent of hospitalized patients.
- 32 million Americans are taking three or more medications daily.

The Department of Health and Human Services (HHS) released a report showing that at least half of all Americans take at least one prescription drug, with one in six taking three or more medications [3]. The report, "Health, United States 2004", shows that:

- Prescription drug use is rising among people of all ages, and use increases with age. Five out of six persons 65 and older are taking at least one medication and almost half the elderly take three or more.
- Adult use of antidepressants almost tripled between 1988-1994 and 1999-2000. Ten percent of women 18 and older and four percent of men now take antidepressants. Prescriptions for nonsteroidal anti-inflammatory drugs, antidepressants, blood glucose/sugar regulators and cholesterol-lowering statin drugs in particular, increased notably between 1996 and 2002.
- The National Health and Nutrition Examination Survey found a 13 percent increase between 1988-1994 and 1999-2000 in the proportion of Americans taking at least one drug and a 40 percent jump in the proportion taking three or more medicines. 44 percent reported taking at least one drug in the past month and 17 percent were taking three or more in the 2000 survey.

Over 60% of sexually active American females use birth control pills. Birth control pills have become very popular for "treatment" of the Post-Menopausal Syndrome (PMS). Marketed as "benign", these medications certainly alter functions of one of the most intricate integrative systems of the human body – the endocrine system. Some of the most common side-effects include migraines and depression.

A significant consequence resulting from polypharmacy, polyherbacy and nutritional supplement use is the potential for the occurrence of interactions among the various products [4].

The situation in the rest of the world is not much better. For example, in 2005 in France nearly four out of every ten adults (37%) had taken a psychotropic medicine at some point of their lives [5]. In another drug utilization pilot study conducted in Hong Kong [6]. One hundred Chinese adults were invited to participate. Structured interviews were used in the study. Drug utilization patterns of the subjects in the preceding two weeks were investigated. It was found that 44 adults took Western medications such as cough and cold remedies or analgesics.

Psychiatry has been notorious for utilizing polypharmacy (a situation when more drugs are prescribed than is clinically warranted). Even children and adolescents fall prey to this practice [7].

During the last twelve years of active practice in the US, I have seen only three adult psychiatric patients who were never treated with conventional medications. Two were females with Bi-Polar Disorder, who, interestingly, responded to the same remedy *Tarentula hispanica*. In both cases the presentation was very clear and the very first remedy prescribed had an amazing healing effect. One of the patients was a cab driver dressed like a 'biker chick'. She played drums at night, too. Another was a professional dancer who loved the Garry Glitter band (featuring loud drums). A particular fascination with rhythmic music and drums is a phenomenon very well-documented by homeopaths as common in patients who need this particular homeopathic remedy. Obviously they had other symptoms that led me to prescribe the remedy. I just find these similarities rather peculiar. Both of the women reported back to me over a period of a few years. As far as I know, they did not have to take any conventional antipsychotic medication.

The third patient was an 18-year-old white male with the first episode of Paranoid Schizophrenia. His mother was a nurse with a holistic background. She insisted on trying homeopathy first. The patient was significantly more concerned with getting rid of severe facial acne than with his bizarre delusions. The symptoms were very severe and had led him to break up with the girlfriend. The only reason he came to see me was a desire to serve in the FBI or the CIA. He knew that if he were to get treatment with conventional medication and use his health insurance for this, his dream would be shattered: not a very good and rather grandiose and delusional motivation for homeopathic treatment. The remedy was very clear (*Kali bromatum*). A combination of grandiose delusions with severe facial acne frequently points toward this homeopathic remedy.
To my great pleasure, and to the patient's great displeasure, the improvement in his mental and emotional state was accompanied by a significant aggravation of his acne. I had warned him about such a possibility. But this young man did not really care for Hering's law (Hering described that in a healing process the direction of cure is from inward out, that deeper pathology will be dealt with first by the Vital Force, and that an aggravation of an eruption is therefore a good sign). All he wanted was to get rid of his acne. Despite the great success in treating his mental illness with homeopathy, the young man went against the advice of his family and saw a general practitioner who prescribed Acutane (isotrotinoin) for severe nodular acne, and Zoloft (an antidepressant!). I have never heard from this patient again.

Unfortunately, the reality is that we live and work in a culture of fear. People are afraid that something bad is going to happen if they don't suppress the symptoms right away. And allopathic medicine offers this opportunity. It is very tempting: we cannot blame our patients for looking to get immediate relief. While we can easily provide not only temporary relief but a CURE for acute conditions right away, doing the same for chronic mental illness is not always possible. Patients "desert" homeopathy and come back disappointed with psychotropic medications. But they are on these medications anyway. What do we do? Or what do we do when a new patient comes asking for homeopathic treatment and we discover that (s)he is taking psychotropic medications? I am still learning, but certain answers to this problem have become clearer to me.

At this point it is worth correcting the misconception that patients on psychotropic medications cannot be treated successfully with homeopathy.
Yes, they can! And what follows will show how.

And, what illnesses are more treatable than others?

The answer is very simple. Any psychiatric illness except for mental retardation and severe dementia can be treated successfully with homeopathy. But simply finding a correct remedy is not good enough. We must be able to manage our patient's recovery. And that includes management of any conventional medications (s)he is on.

2   Management of conventional medications

In my opinion, understanding the selection of conventional medications in every particular case is very important. Good medicine (and bad medicine) can be practised within the limits of any system. There are good psychiatrists and bad psychiatrists; and there are good and bad homeopaths. Optimization of conventional treatment, with the emphasis on using minimum medications with minimal or no side-effects to gain maximum therapeutic effect, is crucial to the success of homeopathic treatment.

Partisan prescribing, whereby one dose of the miraculously found constitutional remedy solves all the problems, is a fantasy. Hard work is a reality. Both, the patient and the homeopath have to be prepared to opt for the latter while hoping for the former. No one has a 100% success rate, especially with the first prescription. And because we are dealing with mind and emotions, the risk of messing up the case and making things worse rather than better is too high to take a cavalier attitude.

Fortunately for me, and, hopefully, for my patients, I am a 'one-man-show' kind of a doctor. Board Certified in psychiatry, I am equipped with all the tools necessary to manage both conventional and homeopathic remedies. It is my understanding that there are very few psychiatrists who are well trained in homeopathy and vice versa. It means that one has to spend time creating a **treatment team** which includes the patient (very important!), the patient's family (if possible), a prescribing psychiatrist and a psychotherapist. Be prepared to meet resistance. Interestingly, psychotherapists can be very difficult - more difficult then physicians.

I once treated an elderly psychotherapist, who presented with symptoms of initial stages of dementia. She was no longer able to work with patients, mostly owing to an inability to make decisions and to forgetfulness. The remedy was not very difficult to find. Frankly, I did not have high expectations in a case of dementia, but the patient made a surprising recovery. Then I treated her husband who was a little bit older, a little bit more demented and a lot angrier. He also got better, was not angry any more and they lived happily thereafter. Impressed by these results, the psychotherapist referred a few patients to me. They also felt better. But the therapist got upset, because I "did not listen to her recommendations on what medications (conventional, of course) to prescribe." She just had to be in charge. I personally think she was also unhappy because the patients improved enough not to need her services any more.

The bottom line is – you need to be able to work together with everyone involved in the patient's care. The easiest way to do it is to establish a good working relationship with a psychiatrist and a psychotherapist. This way you will have a good working team. All that needs to happen after that is that the patient has to agree to switch to a new psychiatrist and a new psychotherapist.

I also believe that one should not introduce homeopathic remedies, unless the patient and the treating psychiatrist agree that the current treatment regimen is not going to change for the duration of the initial homeopathic treatment.
There also has to be agreement that the patient will not stop taking any of the current medications, unless instructed by the treatment team.

Once homeopathy begins to work its magic, the need to discontinue conventional medications will become obvious. It means that there has to be a clear plan of how psychotropic medications will be decreased and discontinued. This is not an easy task, however. Some medications are very difficult to discontinue. It is especially true in the case of short-acting antidepressants and benzodiazepines.

A few years ago, I treated a 17-year-old high school student who initially presented with what in the US are known as "anger issues". She was also unable to concentrate. She had psychotherapy and was prescribed Paxil (Paroxetine hydrochloride, sold as Seroxat in many countries). The medications did not make her or her parents' lives easier at all. The patient's mother who was a big fan of alternative medicine decided to stop the medication. But every attempt to reduce it even by a fraction of the initial dose made the patient experience severe anxiety. She also gained weight and became constipated. At that stage they came to see me. We agreed on a few things:

- no medication change will be made until we all feel that homeopathy is "working";
- I will change from Paxil to a significantly longer-acting Prozac (Fluoxetine Hydrochloride) before any homeopathic remedy is given and will make sure the patient tolerates it very well. This was done to allow a gradual discontinuation of conventional medication when the time comes. The plan had to be in place BEFORE homeopathy is introduced to provide a smooth transition to a medication-free life;
- no one else, not even the psychotherapist, will have any say in how conventional medication will be managed. This point can be brought in by agreeing that only the treating psychiatrist will manage the discontinuation of the medication he prescribed.

After a few attempts I did find the remedy. Actually it happened to be *Mancinella*. Only when the patient had become comfortable with me was she able to reveal that she feels controlled by some force she cannot resist. A relatively rare homeopathic remedy, Mancinella is frequently indicated for patients who present with a combination of feeling controlled by some foreign entity (or the Devil), combined with episodes of severe irritability and anger. When taken together with all other symptoms the remedy was clear. The patient recovered very well. Her anger went away. Her academic achievements were quite impressive. It then took me a full year to discontinue Prozac. The patient was very sensitive and after we arrived at the 5mg a day dose, I had to switch her to the liquid form (all of this was pre-meditated when the change to Prozac was made), and give her smaller and smaller amounts of medication.

In cases when the patient comes on multiple medications (this happens very frequently!) one needs to be able to decide what medication is discontinued first (that is, after homeopathy begins to work). I found that the wisdom of Nature helps to resolve this issue. Very frequently, after a successful constitutional prescription the patient starts experiencing new side-effects from medications.

For example, I treated a young man who had had a manic episode a few months before he came to see me. One day, he woke up convinced that his grandfather, who lived on the other side of the country, needed his help. The patient had to go there to become a leader of a large group of people to save his grandfather. He ran away from home and was found a few days later by police. He was immediately hospitalized, diagnosed with Bi-Polar Disorder and given certain medications. This young man did not believe in homeopathy at all. But, he also did not want to be on medication. So his parents convinced him to see me. Luckily, the remedy was pretty obvious. As in many (but unfortunately not all) occasions, a severe, complex psychiatric presentation did not require much in the way of sophisticated research homeopathically. The patient had nightmares, felt unfairly passed over on many occasions, craved salt (actually in the midst of his psychotic break-out he ate raw salt) and was extremely thirsty for ice-cold liquids. He was also quite restless despite being on sedatives. All these signs pointed towards the homeopathic remedy *Veratrum album*.

But he was on four conventional medications: an antidepressant, a mood stabilizer, a neuroleptic and a sleeping pill. We agreed that I would not suggest any changes until the patient felt he needed to stop one of the medications. Two weeks later the patient reported feeling unusually sleepy. We discontinued the sleeping pill. A month later the patient developed slight tremors in his hands (one of the typical side-effects of a neuroleptic). I decreased the dose of the neuroleptic very slowly and was able to stop it in six months. The patient remained in good spirits, and I was able to gradually discontinue the antidepressant. Despite all this success, the patient still did not believe homeopathy worked. He stayed on a mood stabilizer for over a year but then decided to gradually stop. It has been over five years and he is still doing very well.

3　　How to administer homeopathic remedies to patients on conventional medication

I adapted a model once suggested by Roger Morrison and Nancy Herrick: the initial dose of 200C (or higher) plus daily doses of 12C until all the conventional medication is gone.
The frequency of the repetition of high dilutions depends on many factors. One of them is the severity and the frequency of stressors the patient is exposed to. The other is the individual sensitivity of the patient. Some require more frequent repetitions than others. Some are very sensitive to coffee and alcohol, others not.

4　　Role of illicit drugs in treatment of mental illness

An unfortunate reality is that many people use drugs.

I spent four and a half years working at the Center for Health and Healing at the Beth Israel Medical Center, New York. Once I received a call from a physician from the hospital. She wanted me to see her son, who had been "very depressed", and because the "regular psychiatrists from the hospital weren't able to help him". After we had scheduled an appointment, the doctor told me that she might be 10-15 minutes late and I should start on time without waiting for her. A few days later I came out of the office to meet the patient. Just imagine a large beautiful waiting area, all feng shui with expensive plants, rugs and beautiful pictures and cabinets. It is winter in New York. And I come out to find a fully dressed young man lying on one of the expensive couches listening to his CD player. He was not drunk. So I concluded he was high. We came to my office, sat down, and then I told him that I knew he was using drugs. I just didn't know exactly what sort. And I wanted to find out before his poor mother came. Apparently this shocked him enough. And this young man admitted to me that he had been smoking pot and snorting Effexor (Venlafaxine, a phenylethylamine antidepressant) prescribed to him by a psychiatrist.
We quickly decided that he needed to stop. I worked with him very closely for a few months. Our agreement included his treatment at the outpatient rehab.

Again, not everyone worked on a dual diagnosis unit in one of the flagships of addictions psychiatry (Beth Israel Medical Center). My advice: take urine samples of your psychiatric patients routinely and test them for drug abuse. It does not have to be personal, just another routine test that can be done by a psychiatrist or a family physician.

The age of the patient does not really matter.

Many years ago I treated a middle-aged successful man with severe chronic sinusitis. I prescribed him a remedy and he improved quite dramatically. About three months later I received a call in my office. The patient called me from a business trip in Europe. All the symptoms had come back. The patient asked: "Doc, could it be from smoking a joint?" I forgot that my patient had spent the best years of his life in the late 60s - early 70s. After a brief (very brief) lecture on the risks of using drugs, I suggested that he repeat the remedy. Now the patient knows what to do and what not to do for his sinuses.

On a serious note, one should not underestimate the effects of illicit drugs in modern society. Drug addicts and alcoholics are difficult, sometimes impossible to treat owing to their resistance to sobriety.

5   Conclusion

Homeopathy can be used successfully to treat acute and chronic psychiatric illness. The key to success is the creation of the treatment team that includes the patient, a psychiatrist, a psychotherapist and a homeopath. Detailed understanding of psychiatry, psychology, psychopharmacology and addiction is a definite advantage.

References

[1] http://www.webofcreation.org/Earth%20Problems/water.htm

[2] http://www.americanheart.org/presenter.jhtml?identifier=107

[3] http://usgovinfo.about.com/od/healthcare/a/usmedicated.htm

[4] Loya AM, González-Stuart A, Rivera JO (2009) Prevalence of polypharmacy, polyherbacy, nutritional supplement use and potential product interactions among older adults living on the United States-Mexico border: a descriptive, questionnaire-based study. *Drugs Aging*. 2009; 26(5): 423-36

[5] http://www.ofdt.fr/BDD/publications/docs/eftafbm5.pdf

[6] Fok MS, Tsang WY (2005) The drug utilization patterns of Hong Kong Chinese adults. *Complement Ther Clin Pract*. 2005 Aug; 11(3): 190-9

[7] McIntyre RS, Jerrell JM (2009) Polypharmacy in children and adolescents treated for major depressive disorder: a claims database study. *J Clin Psychiatry*. 2009 Feb; 70(2): 240-6

Chapter 10
The Homeopathic Counsellor
Beyond the Remedy

Christopher K. Johannes, PhD DHM HD (RHom) MARH NCC LPC LMHC

Dr. Christopher K. Johannes
Tokunin Assistant Professor
Kansai Gaidai College/University
Program Director, Integral Health Studies, Akamai University
E-mail: cjohannes@akamaiuniversity.us
www.akamaiuniversity.us/IntegralHealthStudies.html

Abstract
Homeopaths are already providing a type of counselling which may be built upon to extend homeopathy's role in meeting the mental health care challenges of our times. A new 'Homeopathic Counsellor' professional credential granting the homeopath public and professional recognition as a mind-body mental health professional may be a way for homeopathy to realize its fuller potential in mental health care. This chapter examines that thesis with specific calls to collective membership, development and action.

1 Homeopathy's underutilized role in mental health care

In a previous work, a colleague and I discussed the viability of and basis for integrating counselling and homeopathy (Johannes & McNeill, 2005)[7]. After considering some of the theoretical and clinical compatibility of the two approaches based on our own clinical observations and citing others who have written on this successful integration in practice, we proposed the formation of a new professional credential—the 'Homeopathic Counsellor'. Given the emerging discussions and reports on how the integration was already being successfully practiced, we speculated on the possibility of formalizing the integration with an advanced training and/or continuing education curriculum towards the award of a Homeopathic Counsellor credential and an extended professional role.

Perhaps a majority of homeopathy consumers (hereinafter referred to as 'clients') enter the consultation with some goal of finding an alternative, natural, and safe means of relief from what they perceive to be mainly a physical problem; they do not tend to come to homeopathy for mental health counselling or to otherwise relieve an emotional or behavioural problem. Yet the homeopathic consultation and treatment process will frequently give these clients a profoundly insightful and unexpected type of therapeutic counselling with positive mental health outcomes beyond the presenting physical problem. As discussed below, the homeopathic consultation and treatment process can be considered and built upon as a form of counselling, and any review of the more than 400 distinctly different kinds of counselling and psychotherapy thus far identified and recognized (Kazdin, 1986)[8] by the mental health professions may lend some credibility to this assertion. Unfortunately, however, despite the enormous potential, homeopathy's role and value in mental health care has remained under-recognized, underestimated, and under-accessed. I believe there is a need for the general public and the health professions to recognize and exploit homeopathy's value in mental health care. The idea of the 'Homeopathic Counsellor' will therefore be further explored in this chapter towards the vision of expanding homeopathy's healing reach and potential through an already and potentially even more effective avenue of professional service.

2 The idea of the Homeopathic Counsellor

Are we ready to recognize an expanded or integrated role for the homeopath as a 'Homeopathic Counsellor"? Let me begin by further exploring the basis of this idea and suggest a few more underpinning commonalities (see Johannes & McNeil, 2005 for initial suggestions)[7] that may, at least in a conceivable sense, integrate counselling and homeopathy toward justifying this recognition. We may indeed by ready to discuss formal recognition through additional training towards a Homeopathic Counselling credential.

Outwardly, the public perception of homeopathy's therapeutic efficacy seems to hinge largely on its "mysterious" medicines (remedies) used in treating physical problems and does not fully recognize its role in mental health care or the counselling value of the consulting process. However, experience suggests that at least some clients prefer the 'counselling' value of the homeopathic consultations over conventional and, for many, inaccessible, culturally inappropriate, or stigmatized mental health services. Perhaps the homeopathy-consuming public's continued demand for homeopathy, despite popular media debates, does hint at an implicit acknowledgement of that value. However, if the public at large and homeopaths themselves are unaware of or tend to underrate the homeopathic consultation's counselling functions and significant mental health benefits and potential beyond the remedies themselves, we may be failing to address a larger and more important role for homeopathy in more affordably and efficiently meeting the enormous and increasingly serious mental health needs of our times.

Might it serve public mental health care needs if homeopaths were publicly recognized or formally acknowledged for their therapeutic abilities beyond the remedies themselves? Can the homeopathy profession formally extend and integrate its professional identity into the mental health arena without implying that its function is "just" a form of counselling around a placebo? Though many readers, understandably concerned about the implications of a professional identity crisis—or worse, a de facto admission of medicinal inefficacy—will give a negative answer, this discussion invites us to at least suspend those fears for a moment to entertain that possibility. It may be that the idea of an integrally trained homeopathic counselling professional is no more outlandish than that of a conventional psychiatrist trained to offer counselling and psychotherapy.

Why was the use of a "Homeopathic Counsellor" title suggested over another title? If some segments of the population have a problem with seeing a conventional counsellor, why not just stay close to base with "Homeopathic Consultant"? And why not "Counselling Homeopath"? If we use the first designation, the word choice emphasizes the homeopath's role as a counsellor whose approach to the work is informed by the discipline of homeopathy. It is a designation referring to integral professional training grounded in homeopathic principles that can make alliances and attempt to be on some dual footing with an established and recognized professional mental health discipline—the counselling and psychotherapy profession; in the "consultant" nothing is changed from the way things currently are; in the latter designation we would be referring primarily to a homeopath who has received the additional training to become qualified to provide counselling, which would still rest on a primary identification with the remedies. An integrative role under that title would be possible, but "adding on" often creates philosophical and synthesis dilemmas and may also sacrifice a greater professional recognition as more than "a homeopath plus". The choice of "Homeopathic Counsellor" title therefore seemed preferable.

Let's back up and again ask ourselves if it really justifiable to speak of a homeopath providing counselling analogous to, for example, a psychiatrist doing so. Even without the additional and advanced training the envisioned Homeopathic Counsellor would receive, we can answer affirmatively for the very obvious reasons that, firstly, the homeopathic treatment process already consists of a form of counselling (we will see why in the list that follows), and, secondly, homeopathic training programmes already incorporate some basic counselling skills in their curriculums. In other words, whether for case taking, psycho-educational practices of advising and information dissemination on health-promoting lifestyle and obstacles to cure, or the utilization of the homeopathic qualities of the client-practitioner relationship, the homeopathic treatment process already incorporates its own type of counselling approach. Again, one need only consider the more than 400 distinctly different kinds of counselling and psychotherapy thus far identified (Kazdin, 1986)[8] to understand why this argument seems justifiable.

The debate will continue about how and why homeopathy can work (or whether or not it is pronounced dead or alive in the popular press) when considered only on the basis of the efficacy of the remedies. The debate on the value of counselling is largely settled—it works! I know I need to be very careful here not to imply in any way that homeopathic remedies are not the issue when it comes to homeopathy, or to suggest that homeopathy is only a counselling approach that merely bestows a medicinal ritual space to a therapeutic placebo. Obviously this is not the case, as we know from clinical experience and the growing evidence base in the literature the reader will learn about in other chapters of this volume. However, it is also true that homeopathy can never be declared "dead" merely on the basis of whatever we continue to learn from clinical trials of the remedies themselves. Homeopaths do not simply prescribe medicines in the hurried and mechanized manner conventional allopaths often do. Something more occurs in the homeopathic consulting room—quite a bit more.

2.1 Something more: mental health benefits beyond the remedy

So what does that "something more" of the homeopathic consultation have in common with what we know works in a counselling relationship? Whether actual, speculative, or ideal, I suggest that the seven factors below may be some of these "something more" elements of therapeutic efficacy besides the remedies themselves that the formal homeopathic consultation process shares to varying degrees with professional counselling for positive outcomes:

1. The relationship between client and homeopath is a crucial factor in the healing process and outcome. The relationship "resonates" and opens a safe, supportive, and encouraging space within which to contain the client's experience and full expression toward organic healing outcomes. The homeopath provides an accepting and non-judgmental witnessing space that empathizes, shows care and regard for, elicits, reflects, and respects the client's process. Transference and counter-transference relationship dynamics during the consultation are taken into account and drawn on following homeopathic principles and the Law of Similars for the goal of healing. Seasoned homeopaths are finely attuned to how they experience the client, how the client experiences them, and the inter-subjective space that develops during the consultation. Homeopaths may incorporate some degree of self-disclosure and reflected observation within this relationship. Some measure of emotional catharsis or unburdening of suppressed and/or repressed material is not uncommon.

2. The homeopath provides a healing ritual toward the goals of restoring health and optimal functioning. The homeopathic process offers a particular methodology and process for the express intent of healing that relies on a unique and defined set of therapeutic procedures. This therapeutic methodology is consistently applied (more or less) and benefits from the healing effects of medicinal rituals known. The basic goals may include emotional healing, positive mental health, and healthy relationships.

3. The homeopath employs listening skills that encourage a complete and open-ended phenomenological "coming to terms" across mind-body-spirit dimensions of experience. The homeopath's active and reflective listening skills encourage the client's ability to put their experience (e.g. symptoms, reactions, dispositions) into words ("come to terms") thereby distilling and clarifying insight, order, structure, meaning, and some measures of acceptance, control, value, and/or distance from the experience to therapeutic effect.

4. The homeopathic process encourages the depiction, expression, and clarification of the client's "narrative" (their specific problem-related and contextualized overall life story as it developed over time in relation to others) across a range of experience of importance to the client and with special importance placed on the developmental sequence, unfolding, and important milestones of circumstances and events. This narrative assists in the homeopath's (as it assists the counsellor's) grasp of the client's constitutional and dispositional 'Sosein' (a term used in humanist-existential counselling) and in the 'perceiving of what has to be cured' (a phrase used in homeopathic case analysis). The client narratives and profile that result in the homeopathic treatment process encourage new insights, meaning, and an organizing and coherent "storying" of themselves to make sense of their experience—where they've been, where they are, and where they are going in relative surrender, acceptance, or renewed freedom and choice.

5. The homeopathic process provides a particular explanatory framework and model of concepts within which to make sense of the client's experience and narrative for healing effect. Within this framework, the client may be exposed to new ways of making sense of their experience, may arrive at new attributions, and may update certain belief and explanatory models on which to base current and future decisions. In this way, the homeopathic process may encourage a new way to adapt, cope, relate to self and others, or otherwise exercise relative will and

freedom of choice. The homeopathic framework's energetic, holistic, and transpersonal apects may facilitate subtle or significant shifts in how experience, self, others, and the world at large are related to and valued.

6. The phenomenological, developmental, individualized, and holistic aspects of the homeopathic process encourage a more "mindful", attentive, accepting, and integral perspective. Client self-monitoring, self-reflection, and accepting attentive awareness (e.g. Mindfulness, Focusing) are embedded throughout the homeopathic healing path. The individualizing of the homeopathic case is in line with humanistic counselling principles of regard and respect for the unique individual, their relative freedom, and inherent development and healing dynamics.

7. The homeopathic consultation often involves specific advice and education (e.g. providing information, self-care methods, dietary advice, stress management guidance) on matters of relevance to presenting concerns, to the deeper healing goals agreed upon, and the general welfare of the client.

We know from the counselling and psychotherapy literature (see, for example, Jerome Frank's review in *Healing and Persuasion*)[3] that virtually all of the various approaches share four common features which appear to underlie many of the similar positive outcomes among them: (a) a relationship between therapist and patient in which the therapist is seen by the patient as competent and caring, (b) a socially and culturally defined practice setting where this relationship intended for healing occurs, (c) a "story" or explanation accounting for the patient's suffering and how it may be resolved, and (d) a "method" or set of procedures that both therapist and patient place confidence in and agree to participate in for the intent of restoring the patient's health and wellbeing. Note also that the 400 or so distinct forms of counselling and psychotherapy differ in the time, frequency and duration of sessions (consultations) required within this four-fold confine, ranging from a single session of less than an hour to hourly sessions several days a week for years to marathon intensives.

If the above list of homeopathic consultation processes reflects even partially what occurs during these consultations, then homeopaths certainly offer a lot more than remedy provision to effect healing. The consistency with the four common features reported in the counselling and psychotherapy literature is obvious. The above list would appear to constitute enough of a common ground with the professional counselling process to say that counselling is inherent in and embedded in the homeopathic consultation process. Homeopaths are, therefore, already providing counselling whether they bill themselves that way or not. This is interesting, since at present, given that homeopaths are not specifically trained for roles as professional counsellors, these basic skills appear to issue mainly from the homeopathic training, methodology, and the discipline-specific process itself. Specific and formal integrated (or additional) training of between six months to two years in professional counselling and therapies for mental health toward the suggested Homeopathic Counsellor qualification would be building on a reasonably solid platform on which to build to refine and extend these capacities.

Is it conceivable that some people would be more inclined to go to a "Homeopathic Counsellor"? Is there anything else about homeopathy that might make it a desirable choice? Traditional mental health therapies are often criticized for their ethnocultural biases, and it is known that this is an important factor explaining why people from non-Western Euro-American cultures are less likely to access or benefit from needed mental health care (Johannes, C. K., & Erwin, P., 2005)[6]. Can homeopathy offer a more attractive and perhaps more culturally neutral position for this population? Reports from around the world of homeopathy's success in the treatment of mental health conditions, particularly where conventional counselling and psychiatric care is not available or poorly accessed, suggests that it can be. Perhaps there is even more to that "something more" homeopathy offers to make it an attractive option.

2.2 Even more: integrated mind-body-spirit health

Besides the above, homeopathy in mental health care also has something in common with its allopathic counterpart in conventional medicine, psychiatry, namely, the focus on the health of the body, psychosomatic and somatopsychic symptomatology, the embodied mind, and medicinal substances enlisted to help restore health or effect cure. However, the ultimate health-related outcome criteria of homeopathy and psychiatry have some important differences. It is not unheard of to consider a drug (allopathic)-dependent psychiatric patient suffering side effects, suppression, stigma, and heavy economic burdens who is deemed to be "successfully" treated by a conventional psychiatric drug that has restored "normal" functioning in an isolated area so that a psychiatric diagnosis is no longer applicable. This would be an unacceptable outcome for the homeopath.

Homeopathy goes beyond the focus it shares with conventional psychiatry in its holistic, humanistic, individualized, energetic, sometimes transpersonal, and nonlocal temporal conceptualizations and outcome criteria of human health and healing. Homeopathy provides an explanatory framework that acknowledges but can also transcend the psychosomatic and somatopsychic causal and descriptive frameworks of conventional psychiatry by incorporating nonlocal, temporally layered and nonlinear emergent frameworks—wherein the health condition that manifests is viewed as an individual qualitative expression resulting from systemic dynamics not reducible to psychosomatic or somatopsychic mechanisms (Johannes, C.K., 2002)[5]. In this way, the homeopathic process also provides a mind-body bridge to integrate the health of the body into any endeavour towards mental health.

We know that a large percentage of patients in primary care seek treatment for health conditions that defy clear diagnostic categories, that are poly-systemic mind-body conditions where causal pathways are not well understood, and that have been resistant to conventional medical approaches. We also know that the majority of drugs for mental health (e.g. SSRIs) are prescribed not by psychiatrists but by GPs, and that many GPs may be likely to view such ill-defined diagnostic conditions as stress-related or psychosomatic conditions in order to prescribe industry-recommended psychiatric medications. A study by Anderson et al (1989)[1] described the "necessary fallibility" and worrisome variations in accuracy of clinical diagnosis. To complicate matters even further, Flaherty et al (1989)[2], Schenkenberg (1999)[12], and Koranyi (1979)[10] found that a large percentage of psychiatric patients receiving medications for their 'mental health' troubles were later rediagnosed as having 'medical' disorders causing their psychiatric symptoms. We can speculate on the range of costs and burdens this "necessary fallibility" of conventional care entails. Homeopathy may have a clear role to play in such circumstances because it avoids these diagnostic knots and offers an alternative and cost-effective model of conceptualization and treatment that can be integrated with conventional care. The homeopathic approach can be readily incorporated into preventive, behavioural, and mind-body medicine programmes in which a Homeopathic Counsellor can be a vital member of an integrated treatment team.

Another fundamental part of the homeopathic treatment process may be its "mindfulness" supporting aspect. Basically, mindfulness can be defined as the ability to attend to and perceive with non-evaluative and accepting awareness one's present-moment experience. It is an ability to disidentify with and simply 'witness' the phenomenology of on-going moment-to-moment experience, whether inner sensations, thoughts, and feelings, or external events, in a non-attaching fashion. A substantial and growing body of evidence suggests that mindfulness is positively related to an increasing number of health-related parameters (Kohls, N., Sauer, S. & Walach, H. 2009)[9] and that emotional symptoms including anxiety, depression, and stress respond well to interventions based on mindfulness (Kohls, N., Sauer, S. & Walach, H., 2009[9]; Grossman, et al. 2004 [4]; Segal, Williams, & Teasdale, 2002 [11]). Mindfulness also supports spiritual health, poorly addressed in many conventional counselling traditions, and enlists the positive psychological benefits known to accrue from self-monitoring and self-acceptance. It is an ability that can be relatively simply taught and trained for therapeutic and healing benefit. The homeopathic consultation's focus on the phenomenology of symptoms and experience is very much in line with a mindfulness approach, and assists both homeopath and client in perceiving 'what has to be cured'.

The nature of the homeopathic consultation process requires keen abilities of attention on the phenomenology of symptoms across domains of being and experience. The phenomenological ability to attend to this holistic spectrum of functioning result in the awareness of connections, relationships, and meanings hitherto not consciously acknowledged—and usually the essence of the case that results in healing and cure. This quality of the homeopathic consultation already provides a certain kind of client introduction to mindfulness paving the way for further instruction in the kind of mindfulness interventions successfully used in mainstream treatment programs. So as mindfulness may be one of the most basic common factors besides the client-practitioner relationship in positive health outcomes, it is also a unique aspect already partially embedded in the homeopathic process that bridges its role and potential across mind-body health. Homeopaths' additional training in mindfulness-based interventions can be an added psycho-educational counselling tool to equip them for an even greater role as health professionals able to traverse mind-body experience.

3   Do we need a recognized Homeopathic Counsellor?

If homeopaths are already performing a counselling and mental health role with some success, why would we need yet another credential? Some homeopaths are separately becoming qualified in mental health therapies, just as some mental health professionals are becoming qualified in homeopathy. Doesn't their successful experience of integration mean that a new and integrated "homeopathic counsellor" professional credential is redundant or risky given the continuing debates? Since we now already have a desirable and increasing trend toward separately trained integrative professionals, the immediate answer for some readers may be yes, as this trend alone will undoubtedly do much to help realize homeopathy's role in mental health care. On the other hand, the practical shortcomings of separate training may not go far enough nor fast enough in meeting the needs of our times. Given the practical advantages an integrated training towards the new credential would provide, I believe the answer is 'no' - Homeopathic Counsellors can be trained more quickly, more cheaply, more efficiently, and in far greater numbers.

Separate training results in the establishment of one professional identity on which one then builds the philosophy, principles, and practices of another, leaving it much to the creative ability of the health professional to navigate. Done alone or even with like-minded colleagues, this is challenging, offers no integral framework and little guidance (though this book hopes to address that), and may result in a lot of missed insights and skills. The process can be extremely lengthy and not financially feasible for many that would like to go this route, with the result that the number of integrative professionals taking this route will remain relatively limited. Add-on training may face challenges in articulating an integrated professional identification and methodology to advance clinical practice. Developments in one field may be poorly aligned with developments in another. The role of a mental health therapist 'plus' or homeopath 'plus' identity may confuse potential client and public perception and a specialized approach to mental health care may be less readily identifiable. Homeopaths without the added qualification may have a greater struggle to advance homeopathy's role in mental health than those who have it. In short, the need to meet the greater mental health care needs of our times may be less well met than under an integrated training route.

What if, however, we had a longer integrated "homeopathic counsellor" programme as an option for a separate professional 'track' alongside traditional homeopathic training programmes? One that would scrupulously build any training in mental health therapies and counselling onto homeopathic philosophy, principles, and practice? One that would unite practitioners and research and development efforts? Wouldn't that save a lot of time and trouble, avoiding the shortcomings of separate training? Might that not create larger numbers of identifiable homeopathic professionals with a more identifiable and articulated mental health care role? Or, can any "add-on" training towards the qualification (e.g. six months to two years) be offered as an integral extension of the homeopathic training curriculum within homeopathic schools? As some independent therapeutic specialties for mental health such as the energy psychotherapies, hypnosis, or Neurolinguistic Programming have done, wouldn't it be possible for the homeopathic profession, given what it already does well, to recognize and define its own unique form of counselling, building upon that uniqueness to create an expanded role and designation for itself in mental health care? Can this distinct type of homeopathic mental health professional broaden and contribute to homeopathy's recognition, reach, and potential in mental health service provision, including a fuller grasp of the therapeutic validity and efficacy of homeopathy beyond the remedies alone? Instead of diluting its professional identity, might it not actually solidify and extend homeopathy's role in mental health care and mind-body medicine? Can it really create a recognized non-medically qualified counterpart professional role to the conventional psychiatrist? This article obviously takes a very Obama-campaign-like "yes it can!" position. When the idea was first offered in 2005 (see opening paragraph), we had a positive international response. The move from idea into action, however, may be challenging and will require a concerted effort.

4   Ideas into action

To realize the creation of a new cadre of Homeopathic Counselling professionals requires greater vision and practical resources than one or two individuals working alone. Therefore, I propose several steps to carry this idea forward and into action.

First, homeopathic and mental health professionals who are currently integrating the two approaches will need to join together to create a professional membership for this niche and hold annual conferences to collaborate to define, articulate, and realize their work into a cohesive whole.

Second, in addition to conferences, this membership body would publish newsletters and/or a journal on the integration of the two approaches. In addition to member readers, the journal could be made available to a wider audience. Like the conferences, the journal could report on research, development, clinical cases, theory, and advances in the field. Increasing media exposure may be likely.

Third, a committee within this membership body can be elected to draw up the professional training and curriculum requirements of varying levels of professional certification in Homeopathic Counselling (e.g. "R.C. Hom.—Registered Homeopathic Counsellor"). This committee would set out to define what a Homeopathic Counsellor is, what competencies and training background is to be expected, and what benefit to mental health care services this professional would offer. The committee would also adapt and create an additional code of professional ethics for this new professional. The committee would decide various levels of professional membership and certification for professionals holding different qualifications.

Fourth, homeopathic training schools would strive to collaborate with both college and university departments and professional societies relevant to mental health to establish the first professional training routes. Several training routes for different levels of certification may be established, ranging from existing training programmes that might broaden and extend their present curriculums, to various continuing education, intensive, and private professional certification trainings.

Fifth, research programmes, including qualitative research, clinical audit, quantitative outcome studies, pooled N=1 trials, and mixed methods research should be launched, preferably in collaboration with relevant university, private research, charity, or funding groups. Results would contribute to building a broad evidence base to inform practice, healthcare policy, training and continuing education, and expanded access to needed services.

Sixth, Homeopathic Counsellors, identifying with a broader role in mainstream integrative health care, would also seek to expand their services in behavioural medicine, applied health psychology, mind-body medicine, and primary care.

To summarize these action steps: we need to organize a professionally active membership group of Homeopathic Counsellors, articulate the professional role and the training paths to attain certification in this niche, apply the skills in reflective practice, and evaluate the results to improve services. This may be one further way homeopathy can achieve its fuller potential in providing safe, accessible, and affordable mental health care.

References

[1] Anderson, R. E., Hill, R. B. and Key, C. R. (1989). The sensitivity and specificity of clinical diagnostics during five decades. *Journal of the American Medical Association*, 261: 1610-1617

[2] Flaherty, J. A., Channon, R. A., and Davis, J. M. (1989). *Psychiatry: Diagnosis and Therapy*—A LANGE Clinical Manual. Connecticut: Appleton and Lange

[3] Frank, J. D. (1973, 2nd Edition). *Healing and Persuasion.* Johns Hopkins University Press, Baltimore

[4] Grossman, P., Schmidt, S., Niemann, L., and Walach, H. (2004). Mindfulness-based stress reduction and health: A meta-analysis. *Journal of Psychosomatic Research*, 37: 35-43

[5] Johannes, C. K. (2002). Somatopsychic conditions: medical conditions in psychological masquerade *Healthcare Counselling and Psychotherapy Journal*, 40 – 43, July, BACP, UK

[6] Johannes, C. K. & Erwin, P. (2005). Developing multicultural competence: perspectives on theory and practice. *Counselling Psychology Quarterly*, 17(3): 329-338

[7] Johannes, C. K. & McNeill (2005). A Vision of Comprehensive Care: The Integration of Homeopathy and Counselling. *Homeopathy in Practice: The Journal of the Alliance of Registered Homeopaths, Winter 2005*, 48-52

[8] Kazdin, A. E. (1986). The evaluation of psychotherapy: Historical perspectives. In Ponterotto, J. C., Casas, J. M., Suzuki, L. A., & Alexander, C. M. (Eds.), *Hand book of multicultural counseling*, pp. 3 – 16, Thousand Oaks, CA: Sage

[9] Kohls, N., Sauer, S. and Walach, H. (2009). Facets of Mindfulness—Results of an online study investigating the Freiburg mindfulness inventory. *Personality and Individual Differences*, 46: 224-230

[10] Koranyi, E. K. (1979). Morbidity and rate of undiagnosed physical illness in a psychiatric clinical population. *Archives of General Psychiatry*, 36: 414-19

[11] Segal, Z. V., Williams, J. M. G., and Teasdale, J. D. (2002). *Mindfulness-based cognitive therapy for depression: a new approach to preventive relapse.* New York: Guilford Press

[12] Schenkenberg, T. (1999). Neuropsychological issues in adult psychology. *Directions in Mental Health Counseling*, 9: 63-72

Chapter 11
From Unprejudiced Observer to Narrative Facilitator

Rogers' Person-Centred Approach and the Homeopathic Consultation

Ian Townsend, MA RSHom(ret'd)

Ian Townsend M.A., RSHom (ret'd)
Homeopathy Team, Complementary Medicine Unit, University of Central Lancaster
Greenbank 316
Preston, PR1 2HE
United Kingdom
E-mail: ian.townsend@yahoo.co.uk or itownsend@uclan.ac.uk

Abstract

The focus on case analysis and management is thoroughly established in homeopathic literature. Developments in homeopathic theory, different ways of viewing the patient's state and new provings are all expanding the richness of our insights. Yet the area of case *taking* has yet to show similar progress. This chapter reviews the relevant literature and acknowledges the potential contribution of other disciplines. The author draws on his long experience introducing both brand new students *and* seasoned practitioners to the therapeutic conversation and advocates Carl Rogers' Person-Centred Approach as *the* body of theory most closely fitting homeopathic case taking. He explains how a familiarity with this provides an unprecedented understanding of a missing element in the homeopathic undergraduate curriculum – the *how-to* of moving from student to unprejudiced observer to narrative facilitator. He concludes that such a familiarity would enhance the ability to relate to a wider range of mental health conditions, and give homeopaths a shared language with which to communicate with other health professionals.

1   Introduction

The fact that, independently, so many contributors to this anthology considered it important to address the integration of homeopathy and psychotherapy (Bell, Cichetti, Ferris, Johannes, Silvestri, Townsend) and to explore various models (Depth Psychology, Integrative, Jungian, Person-Centred) suggests that this is an idea whose time has finally come. Previous authors (Butehorn [1], Cichetti [2], Kaplan [3], Ossege [4], Twentyman [5], Whitmont [6, 7, 8]) considered the impact that specific psychologies could have on homeopathy. Indeed, Thompson and Weiss [9:6] go so far as to suggest the whole body of prior research on the therapeutics of interpersonal communication could be of potential relevance to us.

Kessler [10:5, 11] shows the extent of Hahnemann's awareness of what we would now call the therapeutic relationship:

Busche (2008) ... transcribed and analysed the original letters and journal entries of Hahnemann regarding the treatment of a family network of patients from 1831-1835 and was able to show that, in his practice, Hahnemann even anticipated essential elements of psychotherapy. He fostered an emotional and affective relationship with his patients, asked his patients to participate actively in the treatment by adopting a healthy lifestyle, and tolerated self-medication in critical situations.

My previous papers (Townsend and Lindley [12], Townsend [13, 14, 15, 16, 17, 18, 19, 20, 21]) explored the importance of the development of professional caring skills and attitudes, initially in nurse education and latterly for the beginning homeopath. They pointed out the emphasis placed on *analysing* cases to the detriment of the skills involved in the initial stages of obtaining them. They asked *how* this could be achieved in the face of the difficulty of learning the art of case taking. They noted a gap between exhortations to 'simply observe', 'be unprejudiced', 'take (or receive) the case' and a skills set [22] enabling this. Such a gap is illustrated, on the one hand, in Owen's chapter on *Receiving the Case* [23] which continues a long tradition of simply placing the subject within a homeopathic context, and on the other, by Norland's [24, 25] or Vithoulkas' [26] comments on the 'right frame of mind', inner preparation, detachment from all successes necessary for taking the case, concluding (unfortunately without helping the reader understand how these might be achieved and without acknowledging their precedents in, e.g. Freud [27], Shlien [28], Thorne [29]):

The homeopathic interview is a crucial meeting point and a very important one in the life not only of the patient but also of the physician. It is almost a love affair, a meeting of two beings at the right time at the right place for a purpose: to bring out the real "good" which is in both. Vithoulkas [26:xx]

Kaplan [30:6] remarked ...

The ability to listen well and say the right thing at the right moment is central to the homeopathic process. It is surprising that so little has been written about taking the case and the homeopath-patient relationship.

A range of earlier papers in our literature from (inter alia) Castro [31, 32], Lee [33], Pinto [34], Pool [35, 36], and Richardson [37] had called for greater understanding of our therapeutic endeavours, and often took an anecdotal, incident-based approach. Roberts [38] identified and explored a range of therapeutic skills which could be used by the homeopath, and Reilly [39:98] emphasised:

We need to begin to think of therapeutic history taking, the actual task of case taking being an act of therapy – not only a diagnostic tool but a therapeutic act – with intention and focus and respect and listening, and wonder, present.

Unfortunately, few authors have grounded their explorations in a coherent, clearly expressed knowledge base which might then have enabled ongoing debate and development of this area of our curriculum. Roberts took a vaguely integrative stance but inaccurately attaches skills and concepts described in his paper to transactional analysis. Reilly used hypnotherapy and the placebo response as metaphors for understanding therapeutic conversation and his excellent series of papers explored this area further [40, 41, 42].

Mackintosh [43, 44, 45] (in the 1980s) and Spring [46] (in the 1990s) briefly introduced Carl Rogers' pioneering work in psychotherapy to homeopathic audiences; but it was not until the publication of Kaplan's 'The Homeopathic Conversation – the art of taking the case' [30] in 2001 that his work became more widely known to us. Finally, Townsend [21] heeding the call of Johannes & McNeill [47:52] for *any integration of approaches (to) ideally have a consistent theoretical and clinical basis* established Rogers' *Person-Centred Approach* (hereinafter 'PCA') as the body of knowledge most closely paralleling the homeopathic process:

> *Rogers ... offers a powerful tool for helping students develop their caring skills, and there are striking similarities [explored briefly in Kaplan (2001) and Townsend (2002, 2004a)] between the writings of Hahnemann, Kaplan, Norland, Sankaran, Vithoulkas and many person-centred authors in terms of a general world view of man, health and disease which make it very attractive to homeopaths.* Townsend [21:4]

2   Rogers' PCA model

The work of Carl Rogers ranks in importance with that of Freud, Watson and Jung. In his time (roughly speaking, 1930s-1980s) he revolutionised the practice of psychotherapy and counselling and ultimately gave the entire field a focus which even today continues unseen to guide our practice in the homeopath-patient relationship. And like psychodynamic, behavioural and transpersonal psychologies, PCA continues to be developed and advanced by its proponents. What is even more surprising is the startling extent to which both homeopathy and the PCA share a radical outlook on health and disease.

Moving away from the authoritarian expert and diagnosis-based medical models common to the early 20th century, Rogers developed a non-directive psychotherapy. In doing so, he sounded a clarion call to those psychologists wanting to work *for and from the experience they were in*, rather than applying theory (or a model of theory) to practice. His 1961 book 'On Becoming a Person' [48] emerged as a landmark publication in the history of counselling and psychotherapy (see, e.g. http://www.carlrogers.info/aboutCarl-Barfield.html). Well known for almost half a century, he wrote in a way that made many readers feel he was writing *directly* to them, to their experience of the world, to their vague feelings that communication, inter-relationship, relations between human beings could be *significantly different*. Arising from his own considerable clinical experience (by the time the book was published Rogers had been a psychologist for more than 30 years, working in child welfare, psychiatric wards, and educational institutions) he suggested a set of six conditions (see Fig. 1) all of which need to exist in order for optimum therapeutic conversation to occur.

Figure 1: Rogers' Six Conditions (Townsend 2005, 2007 [49, 50])

> **1.** Psychological contact exists between client
>
> **2.** (who presents in a vulnerable state) and therapist, who offers:
>
> **3.** Unconditional positive regard and
>
> **4.** Empathic understanding and
>
> **5.** Congruence, all in such a way that the client is
>
> **6.** Aware of these elements.

The advantage for homeopaths of being aware of this work is that it supplies a language with which to talk about the therapeutic conversation (case taking) between ourselves and with other professionals. It provides a well-established set of concepts for considering what we are doing in that conversation, and it identifies an attainable set of skills and attitudes with which to advance the process. All of these are of considerable value in our training curriculum: just as being knowledgeable about homeopathic principles makes possible accurate case taking, analysis, and case management, so a facility with Rogers' six conditions potentiates the possibilities of the therapeutic conversation.

An individual homeopath's use of interpersonal skills contributes to the way in which she relates to her patients and understands their stories (observationally, intellectually, intuitively, emotionally and energetically) while communicating that understanding. The literature of psychology, counselling and psychotherapy is quite clear that this is achieved through a mix of active listening and adopting and maintaining the core conditions. (Haugh & Paul [51], Howe [52])

As Bhatia [53:3] comments:

> *Hahnemann put down many guidelines for the physician in his Organon of Medicine that resonate with the principles of Person-Centred Therapy. He mentioned the need for being unprejudiced (unconditional positive regard), listening attentively (active listening) and observing carefully, showing care to the patient (empathy), providing guidance to the patient to improve his health, using all the senses during the process of consultation (verbal and non-verbal communication), with the use of only tested medicines (medical ethics), avoiding medical jargon etc.*

Among person-centred authors, Dave Mearns & Mick Cooper [54] come the closest to our practice of case taking in their description of holistic listening. Other papers with an emphasis we would recognise are Rowan [55] and Friedman [56].

2.1 Rogers' six conditions

2.1.1 Making Psychological Contact

In the beginning lies in the importance of meeting: humans starting a therapeutic relationship need, to some extent, to be in psychological contact (aware of, communicating with) each other. This seems so obvious as to not be worth mentioning. Still, making that initial contact is an art in itself – for in those few seconds of early meeting we set the scene for the consultation to follow. We only have to compare instances where we (or our students) have been less than attentive with those where our patients have been met warmly and consciously to reflect on the impact these different experiences holds. The PCA has taken this idea, and shown its applicability even to those ...

> whose state . . . means they are rigid, remote and cut off from their emotions and from other people. Merry [57:45]

2.1.2 Vulnerable client, resourceful practitioner

Another truism is captured in Rogers' second condition. By virtue of the fact that they seek our help, patients are vulnerable: for they bring us their life concerns (from whatever level of health those concerns arise) at a time when those concerns are pressing and worrying. They come to us with the expectation we can help them, hoping they will be met with an expertise and professionalism which includes emotional and intellectual as well as technical resourcefulness. This reminds us of a truth and dynamic which all too often goes unremarked – the patient's vulnerability (uncertainty, concerns, fears, health issues) need to be received, respected and witnessed by a healthy and resourceful practitioner.

Of Rogers' six conditions, *three* are *core conditions*. A problem in the analysis of any subject lies in the identification, exploration and discussion of its separate parts: something which reduces its holistic application. Exploring Rogers' core conditions separately ignores his view that these occur as a *single configuration* (see below). Simply put, *these conditions are so interrelated that the presence of each one depends very intimately on the presence of the other two*. (Natiello [58:5])

2.1.3 Core condition 1: unconditional positive regard (UPR)

As homeopaths, we are already familiar with this condition under the label of *the unprejudiced observer*. Vithoulkas [59] used the phrase *non-judgemental acceptance* in regard to the patient's symptoms, and Kaplan [30] drawing from PCA (Thorne [29]) echoed Hahnemann (Kessler, ibid) in advocating a loving attitude or warmth towards the client. He also reminds us that a critical attitude (on our part) prevents patients from revealing important information needed for the homeopathic prescription - a fact which PCA research had established in 1957 [60]. Ross (2005), a graduate of the UCLan BSc (Hons) Homeopathic Medicine degree course, explored parallels between the unprejudiced observer and unconditional positive regard as the subject of her 3rd-year dissertation. [61]

Purton [62:25] remarks ...

> ... if the (practitioner) honestly respects the client absolutely, whatever feelings or attitudes the client has, then the client will no longer need to pretend to be other than they are, and will be released into being fully themselves, into being fully authentic.

"When you hear and accept ... her reasons" adds Janet Tolan [63:72] "so will she. Instead of worrying about your opinion of her, she will listen to herself."

While the homeopathic profession seems to be comfortable with the idea of non-judgemental acceptance, the disquiet felt by students on first meeting it has not often been reported in the literature. Does it, they wonder, mean there is no place for our own thoughts, feelings, opinions?

Watson [63:21] for example, has this to say:

> My experience in response to my patient's stories is to become moved; my conflict was that if I became emotionally involved I was no longer the objective/unprejudiced observer: effectively I become a participant. My observation is that becoming a participant is ok as long as I have an awareness of my own participation. I have abandoned the term unprejudiced observer in favour of the ideal of becoming a 'self-aware participant'.

So, yes, of course there is room for us. Appropriately, at the right time, and in the right place in the therapeutic meeting. We have a responsibility to be true to ourselves, our own understanding and experiencing (that's *congruence*, another of Rogers' core conditions) – but we also have the responsibility to perceive our patient as clearly as possible: for in that accurate perception lies the possibility of making the right (homeopathic) diagnosis. The attempt to understand the patient in her own life circumstances, her own frame of reference generates *empathic understanding*, Rogers' other core condition.

How we non-judgementally accept and understand others has an important result, for it depends entirely on how we hear and accept ourselves. Full circle – in order to offer UPR to our patients we accept and understand their experience via empathic understanding – and in order to be able to connect such understanding to unconditional positive regard we need to be congruent – as accepting and understanding of our own experience, beliefs, and actions as we hope to be of those of our patients:

> Such noteworthy observations on himself lead him to an understanding of his own sensations, the way he thinks and feels (the essence of all true wisdom – "know thyself"), furthermore – something no physician can dispense with – they make him an observer. Hahnemann [65: §141, fn.]

2.1.4 Core condition 2: empathy

Once again, empathy (the second of the three core conditions) is something homeopaths are already familiar with – despite the fact that our literature has only recently started to discuss it. (Fraser [66], Kaplan [30], Kuipers [67], Mercer, Watt, Reilly [68, 69], Muckenheim [70], Thompson & Weiss [9])

Rogers noticed that when client and practitioner met, the latter paying close attention to the former, congruently offering UPR and trying to comprehend the person's story, a phenomenon occurred which he came to call empathy or empathic understanding. He noticed that the attempt to be in another person's shoes, to have an *as if* experience [48] meant ...

> ... entering the private perceptual world of the other and becoming thoroughly at home in it ... It means temporarily living in the other's life, moving about in it delicately without making judgments; it means sensing meanings of which he or she is scarcely aware, but not trying to uncover totally unconscious fee-

lings, since this would be too threatening... To be with another in this way means that, for the time being, you lay aside your own views and values in order to enter another's world without prejudice. Rogers [71:142]

PCA practitioners are familiar with the idea that the act of focusing on the other person in this way, of trying to understand and be with her in her experience in an unprejudiced way, goes beyond intellectual clarity in allowing the observer sight [72] of unexpressed or only partly expressed parts of that person.

Homeopaths, too, seem familiar with the concept:

If you stay open to the case and realize the vital force is trying to teach you, you will learn the lessons. Often as the patient is in front of me I ask myself: what is the patient trying to tell me that I am not getting; what is the patient showing me by his/her actions that I haven't seen; what is the feeling that I'm getting from this patient that I haven't felt yet; how is the patient saying things that might give me a clue to what I need to understand? Often this will open up other senses that I've somehow closed off for the moment that will lead to new understanding of the case. Gruber [75]

This core condition - communicating in an empathic way - has two further benefits:

One is that the client elaborates, develops and reveals more of his or her phenomenal world to the therapist. The other is that clients tend to become more consistently and intently focused on, and express themselves from, the experiential source of what they are talking about. Brodley [76:26]

When Vithoulkas [59:169-189] compared the interviewer to a painter slowly and painstakingly bringing forth an image representing the essence of a particular patient's vision of reality, he was suggesting Hahnemann's detached observer become an active listener, ...

In listening actively to the patient, the homeopath's imagination and sensitivity must be highly involved. The homeopath must develop the capacity to live the experience of the patient. This is not merely a matter of putting oneself into the shoes of the patient, but rather one of perceiving the patient's experience in his or her own context. (ibid: 173)

... and when Bridger [77:17] advises ...

... the best way to be a good homeopath is not to adhere to any particular methodology – in fact to try to avoid them at all costs. Then forget that you are a practitioner and step into the shoes of a patient ...

... their recommendations seem so similar to Roger's original language that one wonders why his seminal works have been ignored by our profession. See also Vincent [78].

Sankaran's recent publications [79, 80] avoid identifying the features (empathic understanding, sensing) that PCA practitioners would be familiar with, although his brilliant development of them would come as no surprise:

In case taking, we might hear facts, emotions and stories. We sometimes get lost in stories. We need to go behind the story. The inner song, as I call it, expresses itself through gestures and non-human specific words in everyday conversations. It opens a secret door, and we explore a completely different world. In that world, we hear the source, the remedy speaking directly to us, as it were. [79:14]

2.1.5 Core condition 3: congruence

Homeopaths encountering person-centred theory have no problems with *'unconditional positive regard'*, and most who meet *'empathy'* for the first time understand that it has something to do with sensing the patient on a deeper-than-normal level. Rogers' third core condition – *congruence* - is more problematic for us (Yde, [81]), but no less important than the first two conditions, especially since psychotherapeutic outcome studies (e.g. Orlinsky, Grave & Parks [82], Watson & Geller [83]) have stressed the importance of each one of these.

For us, congruence links to the idea of self-awareness (Hahnemann [65], also in Dudgeon [84]); what Vithoulkas [59:170] refers to as the interviewer needing to become conscious of his or her own responses to the patient and Kaplan [30:101-106] extends to asking why patients would trust (and reveal their innermost feelings) to an inauthentic person, i.e. a person wearing a professional mask.

Congruence, as Merry [57:42] concludes, refers to a practitioner's state of integration, authenticity and 'realness' in the relationship, a state of ...

> *... realness, maturity and authenticity existing in persons who accurately perceive their self-experience. These persons are committed to being rather than seeming. They have attained a high level of self-awareness, self-acceptance, and self-trust. Such persons, naturally, are more open to their experience, feel less need for defensiveness, and have the desire and the ability to be emotionally and intellectually authentic in relationships. Natiello [58:6-7]*

> *... and in touch with himself. This includes daring to acknowledge flaws and vulnerabilities, positive and negative parts of oneself with a certain leniency, being capable of openness without defensiveness to what lives in oneself and being with it, having a solid identity and a strong enough sense of competence, being able to function efficaciously in personal and intimate relationships without interference of personal problems. Lietaer [85:37]*

The advantage of becoming more congruent, more self-aware, more in tune with our own self-experiencing is that the more familiar we are with ourselves, the more likely we are to be able to be unprejudiced and to be more empathic, being able to differentiate between our own personal reactions and our sensed reactions of others. Paradoxically, being self-aware makes it more likely we *will* be able to be unprejudiced, and becoming congruent is the exercise of such self-awareness. In the noticing from moment to moment of those attitudes, beliefs, thoughts, feelings, emotions with which we exist, in the simple paying attention to ourselves, we can find freedom from them. [86]

2.1.6 Communication: client awareness

The last of Rogers' six conditions proposes that in order to be effective the other five conditions should in some way be acknowledged by both parties in the therapeutic endeavour. It underlines the importance of mutuality in the communication process and makes the case for Conditions One to Five being present in an overt way, or, as Rogers puts it:

> It includes communicating your sensings of his world as you look, with fresh and unfrightened eyes, at elements of which he is fearful. It means frequently checking with him as to the accuracy of your sensings and being guided by his responses. Bernard [87]

2.2 Putting it all together: the idea of single configuration

Over the past twenty years, homeopathy students in more than ten institutions have shown me the folly of attempting to incorporate interpersonal or communication skills training into the undergraduate curriculum without first demonstrating its unique relevance to homeopathic theory and philosophy. They questioned its value, applicability, appropriateness and in particular found it difficult to relate individual skills-training exercises to what might happen within their consulting rooms. It was not until the direct links which exist between PCA theory and skills practice and then between *that* theory and homeopathy's holistic world view were demonstrated that such training began to be appreciated.

Rogers was the first person to make full-length recordings of practitioner-client interactions and subject them to careful critical analysis. He came to view the therapist's role as 'a midwife to change' (Rogers, [88]) rather than as an originator of change.

> It is the client who knows what hurts, what directions to go, what problems are crucial, what experiences have been deeply buried. It began to occur to me that unless I had need to demonstrate my own cleverness and learning, I would do better to rely upon the client for the direction of movement in the process. (Rogers: [88:11-12)

He was not only clear about the importance of relationship within the therapeutic process; he also advanced the idea that 'the essential conditions ... exist *within a single configuration.*' [89:230 - emphasis added].

This particular emphasis is lost when individual conditions are singled out for attention, something that is responsible for the confusion which exists around the positioning of conditions as 'skills', 'tools', 'attitudes', or 'values'. For example, Frankland & Saunders [90:150] describe Rogers' core conditions as 'fundamental relationship *tools*' whilst other writers focus on the six necessary and sufficient conditions existing *organically* within the *being* of the practitioner: Merry [57:40], Natiello [58:38], Mearns [91:xiii], Rogers [71]). Tudor [92] explains that, in the attempt to develop a general understanding of the therapeutic process, various authors identified specific change-facilitating behaviours within and across various approaches. He notes the term 'core conditions' was introduced by Carkhuff [93, 94], 'central therapeutic ingredients' by Truax & Carkhuff [95] and 'facilitative conditions' by Levant & Shlien [96]. More recently, authors have identified 'intervention categories' (Heron [97]) and 'communication skills' (Egan [98]).

Tudor (ibid) is very clear that Rogers regarded all six conditions as both primary and precise, a view echoed in Brazier:

We cannot doubt that Rogers was serious in his principles. He stated them again and again throughout his life with unambiguous clarity. Those who feel inspired by him cannot escape the struggle of coming to terms with the implications. Brazier [73:8]

As Natiello remarks:

There is no room for techniques here. This is a relationship between two real people, and it evolves as a conversation or dialogue evolves. Each therapeutic interaction is an unpredictable result of the spontaneous process between therapist and client ... You cannot fall back on techniques or expertise ... in order to be with clients in a person-centred way, you must be able to enter the relationship with absolute realness, with no agenda as to outcome, no need to control the client's therapeutic process, full openness to the experience that unfolds before you. Natiello [58:14-15]

The Bristol-based UK homeopath Mike Bridger captures this same person-centred sense when he writes:

We, as practitioners, are the patients' guides on a particular kind of pilgrimage. There are no relics, saints, holy waters or shrines at the end of their trip. There is nothing there but themselves. It is a unique pilgrimage and one which loses its magic if we reduce the process to categorisations, layers or methods. To be a good guide you need to know none of these things apart from who you are, where you are and in what direction you are heading. That way the patient will trust you for not trying to be too clever. Bridger [77:18]

3   Summary

Over twenty years ago, as a recently qualified homeopath, I remember being surprised by what the homeopathic consultation could achieve. I was astonished at the readiness of patients to reveal themselves and their lives. Reflecting on this then I was not able to explain it satisfactorily. It seemed that in the attempt to be unprejudiced, to understand the patient's story and to see the symptoms as clearly as I could, *something liberating* happened in the homeopathic consultation. More recently, developing a series of modules on therapeutic relationships (and writing this chapter), the explanation comes into focus. I had forgotten that before homeopathy I had a ten-year involvement in a radical countercultural psychiatric movement (Jackins [99]) which taught me the value of patience, of silence, of listening-without-interrupting, and showed me how humans could experience, manage, and survive in the face of the widest possible range of mental health pathologies. Training as a person-centred counsellor added further skills as well as a language with which to appreciate what happens in therapeutic relationships, and the stimulus to apply this to our profession.

If we ignore the riches of other disciplines [100] we run the risk of professional isolation and deny ourselves, our students and patients valuable attitudes, skills, lessons and explanations developed over decades of experience and research in those disciplines [102]. Recent examples of such riches sadly left unexplored are to be found in Smith's (2000) reflective account of what appears to be the use of congruence in practice incidents [104], Chauhan's (2006) discovery and application of a technique he calls focusing [105] – independent of its 50-year existence in experiential and person-centred psychology, Butehorn's (2007) comments on Sankaran's practice [1], and (to a lesser extent) Kuiper's (2008) account of empathy [67].

Winston [106:35] warns us of the danger of professional hubris, pointing out that

> ... contemporary with Kent was Freud and then Jung, and then followed the whole public acceptance of the mind and its unplumbed depths, and the tendency to over-psychologise. It overlapped into homeopathy. But most homeopaths are not trained psychologists, although they often act as if they are.

Bridger [107], reported in Ross [61:11], suggests that many trainee homeopaths do not fully understand the boundaries between psychotherapy and homeopathy and warns that this can lead to the consequent dangers of psychological harm, consultation-as-interrogation, or prescriptions becoming based on practitioner speculation. Throughout our history, authors have called for links to be made between psychology and homeopathy (Castro [31,32], Kreisberg [108], Mackintosh [43, 44], Pinto [34], Pool [36], Ross [61], Wansbrough [101]). Knowing more about these links would reliably inform our practice, and be especially helpful in those initial stages of learning to take the case in terms of enabling us and our students to talk about the therapeutic relationship and development of the therapeutic conversation in an informed way.

Comments from the students and experienced practitioners who have met Rogers' work both theoretically and experientially tend to support this:

> I completed a very intense Practitioner in Eating Disorders Training at the weekend. All the other participants were psychotherapists, nurses and person-centred counsellors. Without the reading for Therapeutic Relationships [113] I know I would have felt out of synch. As it was I jumped straight into the work with a shared language and an understanding of the therapeutic relationship which formed the core of the training. (Seth [110])

> The module on Therapeutic Relationships has a great impact on me in a subtle way, in that it seems to have crept into my psyche and settled there. I am very much more focused, sensitive and aware of my patients' needs in terms of feedback or counselling. I think the various concepts of PCA helped me become more aware of myself and who I am in the therapeutic relationship, especially in terms of the transpersonal elements at play, though I may not consciously involve them. (D'Souza-Francisco [111])

> A lot of what we learned throughout the Therapeutic Relationships module helped put words to the tacit knowledge I was holding after practising as a homeopath for 18 years. Helping me to better understand the processes involved in it and issues arising from it, in particular within the area of ethics ... set off some thinking processes on how students perceive us, what they actually pick up when we're teaching them homeopathy. Are they really learning (well enough) how to behave in the therapeutic setting? How they affect the patient and how the patient affects them? How their past affects their present? How the present may affect the future? (Viksveen [112])

> Most useful for me personally was the focus on the person-centred approach (PCA). Even though I had already read about and was aware of PCA, the Therapeutic Relationships module helped me put it even more into practice.(Viksveen [112])

Many aspects of TR and PCA were unknowingly touched upon during the process of consultation but a conscious effort to maximise the benefits that could be derived from the relationship was missing ... It was observed that having a technical understanding of these key concepts improved the patient-physician relationship in acute as well as chronic cases. You don't need lot of time to show warmth, understanding, compassion and empathy. The patient can often start feeling these qualities the moment she enters your consultation chamber. (Bhatia [113])

I suggest that the person-centred approach to understanding the complexities of human existence, and its unique mode of being with a person while she explores her concerns, best matches homeopathic endeavour. It certainly offers aspiring homeopaths an inspiring literature which talks to heart as well as mind, a template for making sense of the demands of the interpersonal relationship called into being during the homeopathic interview, and a methodology for developing the skills and attitudes necessary to our work. I would be more than happy to share curriculum plans and teaching materials and explore the topic further with anyone interested: please email me – ian.townsend@yahoo.co.uk or itownsend@uclan.ac.uk

This paper has focused on the implications of the Person-Centred Approach: how its powerful tools and concepts, particularly appropriate to those students encountering the challenges of case taking for the first time, can be introduced into homeopathy. The consequences of such integration are profound. Familiarity (the ability to identify, comprehend and work with its component parts) with a sister literature might well answer Winston's 2004 criticism. Being able to communicate an understanding of that literature provides a meeting place for and increases the likelihood of rapprochement with healthcare workers who themselves may be very unfamiliar with homeopathic theory and practice.

Whatever the mental health needs our patients present, ways of establishing and developing the therapeutic relationship originated in the work of the person-centred approach and are to be found in the majority of mental health practices irrespective of their current allegiance. Grounding our understanding of therapeutic conversation in the PCA provides us with a proven methodology for safe relating, enabling us to meet basic healthcare needs. Applying Rogers' necessary and sufficient conditions to taking the case while keeping our professional focus on this task guards against the temptation to slip over into 'therapising' patients, protecting them from any inappropriate attention. At the same time increasing our knowledge in this area might enable us to widen our remit, increasing our degree of comfort with a wider range of patients.

References

[1] Butehorn L. (2007) Homeopathy, Shamanism and Rajan Sankaran's Quest for the Vital Sensation. *Homoeopathic Links* 2007; Summer, 20 (2): 100-103

[2] Cichetti J. (2005) The Shadow of Homeopathy: An Analysis of the Current Situation in Homeopathy From a Jungian Perspective. *Homoeopathic Links* 2005; Summer, 18 (2): 75-78

[3] Kaplan B. (2006) Homeopathy, contrarianism and Provocative Therapy. *Homeopathy in Practice* 2006; Summer, 38-43

[4] Ossege, H. (2005) A Homeopathic Shadow Quest. *Homoeopathic Links* 2005; Summer, 18(2): 79-84

[5[Twentyman, R. (1989) *The science and art of healing*. Edinburgh: Floris Books

[6] Whitmont, E. (1991) *Psyche and substance: essays on homeopathy in the light of Jungian psychology*. Berkeley, CA: North Atlantic Books

[7] Whitmont, E (1991) *The symbolic quest: basic concepts of analytical psychology*. Princeton, N.J.: Princeton University Press

[8] Whitmont, E. (1993) *The Alchemy of Healing*. Berkeley, CA: North Atlantic Books

[9] Thompson, T., Weiss, M (2006) Homeopathy – what are the active ingredients? An exploratory study using the UK Medical Research Council's framework for the evaluation of complex interventions. BMC *Complementary and Alternative Medicine*, 2006:6 (electronic journal). http://www.biomedcentral.com/1472-6882/6/37 [last accessed 21/04/2009]

[10] Kessler, U. (2009) *Unleashing potential: Homeopathy and the therapeutic relationship*. Unpublished manuscript, Müllheim: University of Central Lancashire. 2009, cites Busche, J: Ein homöopathisches Patientennetzwerk im Herzogtum Anhalt-Bernburg. Die Familie von Kersten und ihr Umfeld in den Jahren, 2008: 1831-1835, Stuttgart: Haug Verlag

[11] Kessler, U. (2009) Potenzial freisetzen: Homoeopathie und die therapeutische Beziehung, *Allgemeine Homoeopathische Zeitung*. (2009: accepted for publication)

[12] Townsend, I., Lindley, W. (1980) Creating a Climate for Carers, *Nursing Times*, 1980: 03/07/80: 1188-1189.

[13] Townsend, I. (1980) *The Experiential Approach Explored*. Feedback, (2). Sheffield: NHS Learning Resources Unit. Mar/April 1980

[14] Townsend, I. (1982) *Communication Models*. Mimeo. Sheffield: NHS Learning Resources Unit. April 1982

[15] Townsend, I. (1982) *From Teacher to Facilitator*. Mimeo. Sheffield: NHS Learning Resources Unit. April 1982

[16] Townsend, I. (1983) *Approaches to Self-Awareness*. Sheffield: NHS Learning Resources Unit

[17] Townsend, I. (1996) *The Challenge of the Developing Practitioner*. Mimeo, 119 pps. Extended reading for Ethics & Communication Skills Module, Sheffield: Sheffield School of Homeopathy

[18] Townsend, I. (2002) Before the Actualising Tendency: Putting body into the person-centred process. *Person-Centred Practice*, 2002. 10 (2): 81-87

[19] Townsend, I. (2004) Ch.3: *Almost Nothing to Do: Homeopathic Supervision*. In Tudor, K. & Merry, T. (eds) Freedom to Practise: Person-Centred Approaches to Supervision. Hay-on-Wye: PCCS Books, pp335-430

[20] Townsend, I. (2004) *Bringing All of Ourselves to Supervision*. (Unpublished) presentation given at June 2004, UK Society of Homeopaths Supervision Conference, Sheffield: University of Sheffield

[21] Townsend, I (2009) *Developing the Therapeutic Conversation - A Personal Approach*. In ICH / ECCH Proceedings of the International Homeopathic Education Symposium, 23 – 24 April 2009. Leuven, Belgium. (2009 - in press)

[22] There is considerable debate in the psychotherapeutic literature, going back at least 50 years, on the most effective way of developing therapeutic skills. Proponents of micro-skills training hold that skills can be broken down into their component parts, explained, rehearsed, and learnt. Critics point to the artificiality of such approaches – for them, skilled therapeutic endeavour arises from a set of attitudes deeply held by the therapist. I use the phrase 'skills set' here to draw our attention to the need to think about how we might identify, encourage, develop, and refine both the skills and attitudes necessary for effective therapeutic communication.

[23] Owen, D. (2007) Ch. 13: *Receiving the Case*, in David Owen (2007) Principles and Practice of Homeopathy - The Therapeutic and Healing Process. China: Churchill-Livingstone Elsevier, pp163-175

[24] Norland M. (1998) A Few Thoughts on Receiving the Case. *The Homeopath*, 1998: 69: 10

[25] Norland M. (2008) Keeping doubt out of the healing room. *Society of Homeopaths Newsletter*, Autumn, 2008: 29

[26] Vithoulkas, G. (2005) The necessity for an inner preparation of the classical homeopath. *Simillimum*, 2005, 19: 117-122

[27] Freud, S. (1920/1955) *Beyond the Pleasure Principle*. Standard Edition: 18:1-144. London: Hogarth Press

[28] Shlien, J. M: A Countertheory of Transference. Person-Centred Review. February, (2), 1:93-119, in Pete Sanders (2003) To Lead and Honourable Life: Invitations to think about Client-Centred Therapy and the Person-Centred Approach. A collection of the work of John M. Shlien, Ross-On-Wye: PCCS Books, 1987/2003: 93-119

[29] Thorne, B. (1991) *Person-centred counselling: therapeutic and spiritual dimensions*. London: Whurr Publishers Limited

[30] Kaplan, B. (2001) *The Homeopathic Conversation – The Art of Taking the Case*. London: Natural Medicine Press

[31] Castro, M. (1989) Supervision: A Homoeopath's perspective. *The Homoeopath*. 8, 3: 108–127

[32] Castro, M. (1991) Sex in the Consulting Room. *The Homoeopath*. 11, 2: 39–44

[33] Lee, F. (1989) Homoeopathy and counselling: a worthwhile combination. *The Homeopath*. 8, 3: 128-131

[34] Pinto, G. (1995) In Practice: Psychotherapy. *Society of Homeopaths Newsletter*, September, 1995: 13-14

[35] Pool, N. (1991) Knowing Ourselves. *The Homeopath*, 11, 4:111-113

[36] Pool, N. (1995) Education and Training: Psychotherapeutics in the Curriculum. *Society of Homeopaths Newsletter*. 1995:30

[37] Richardson, S (1981) The patient: prescriber relationship. *The Homeopath*. 2, 2:61-63

[38] Roberts, E. (1998) The Relationship between Homoeopathy, Therapy and Counselling. *The Homeopath*, 70: 46–49

[39] Reilly, D. (2001) Ch. 6: *Some Reflections on creating therapeutic consultations*, in David Peters (ed), 2001. Understanding the Placebo Effect in Complementary Medicine, Edinburgh: Churchill Livingstone, pp89–110

[40] Reilly, D. (2001) Creative Consulting: Why Aim For It?, *Student BMJ*, (electronic journal), 9: 364–365, available at URL: www.studentbmj.com/back_issues/1001/education/364.html , last accessed 01-07-2007

[41] Reilly, D. (2001) Creative Consulting: How to Make the Room Disappear, *Student BMJ*, (electronic journal), 9: 413–414, available at URL: www.studentbmj.com/issues/01/11/education/413.php , last accessed 01-07-2007

[42] Reilly, D. (2001) Creative consulting: germinating recovery. What is a healing response? Student BMJ, (electronic journal), December, 9: 443-486, available at URL: www.studentbmj.com/issues/01/12/education/450.php , last accessed 02-07-2007

[43] Mackintosh, E. (1981) Exploring homoeopathy and modern psychotherapy - Part 1. *The Homeopath*, 2, 2: 55-60

[44] Mackintosh, E. (1982) Exploring homoeopathy and modern psychotherapy - Part 11. *The Homeopath*, 2, 3: 90-95

[45] Mackintosh, E. (1986) The Language of Homoeopathy. *The Homeopath*, 5, 4: 147-149

[46] Spring, B. (1990) Homeopathic Politics. *Society of Homeopaths Newsletter*, 1990: pp47-51

[47] Johannes, C. K. & McNeill, E. (2005) A Vision of comprehensive care: the integration of homeopathy and counselling, *Homeopathy in Practice*, Winter 2005, pp48-52

[48] Rogers, C. R. (1961) *On Becoming a Person – A therapist's view of psychotherapy*. London: Constable

[49] Townsend, I. (2005) CT2022: *Developing the Therapeutic Conversation* WebCT Module [Internet]. Preston: University of Central Lancashire Learning Development Unit.. URL: http://www.uclan.ac.uk/information/services/elearn/index.php, via eLearn https://elearn.uclan.ac.uk/webct/ [withdrawn 2008]

[50] Townsend, I. (2007) *HP4001: Therapeutic Relationships* WebCT Module [Internet]. Preston: University of Central Lancashire Learning Development Unit. URL: http://www.uclan.ac.uk/information/services/elearn/index.php via eLearn https://elearn.uclan.ac.uk/webct/ [Accessed 19 February, 2009]

[51] Haugh, S., Paul, S. (2008) *The Therapeutic Relationship: Perspectives and Themes*. Ross-on-Wye: PCCS Books

[52] Howe, D. (1993) *On Being a Client – understanding the process of counselling and psychotherapy*. London: Sage Publications Ltd.

[53] Bhatia, M. (2009) *An Analysis of the Use of Therapeutic Relationship and Person-Centred Approach during Homeopathic Treatment in an Indian Clinical Setup*. Unpublished manuscript, Jaipur, India: University of Central Lancashire

[54] Mearns, D., & Cooper, M. (2005) *Working at Relational Depth in Counselling and Psychotherapy*. London, Sage Publications Ltd., pp120-124

[55] Rowan, J. (1986) Holistic Listening. *Journal of Humanistic Psychology*. 26, 1: 3-102

[56] Friedman, N. (2005) Experiential Listening. *Journal of Humanistic Psychology*. 45, 2: 217–238

[57] Merry, T. (1999) *Learning & Being in Person-Centred Counselling*. Ross-on-Wye: PCCS Books Ltd.

[58] Natiello, P. (2001) *The Person-Centred Approach: A passionate presence*. Ross-on-Wye, PCCS Books

[59] Vithoulkas, G. (1980) *The Science of Homeopathy*. New York: Grove Press Inc.

[60] Dittes, J. E. (1957) Galvanic skin response as a measure of patient's reaction to therapist's permissiveness. *J. Abnorm. & Soc. Psychology*. 1957, 55: 295-303, cited in Kirshenbaum, H., Henderson, V. L. The Carl Rogers Reader, London: Constable and Company Limited. 1990: 113

[61] Ross, K. (2005) *Is the significance of becoming the 'Unprejudiced Observer' fully recognised specifically regarding the Homeopathic consultation?* Unpublished dissertation submitted for award of BSc. (Hons) Homeopathic Medicine, Preston: University of Central Lancashire

[62] Purton, C. (1998) *Unconditional Positive Regard and its Spiritual Implications*, in Thorne, B., Lambers, E. Person-Centred Therapy - A European Perspective. London: SAGE Publications, pp23-37

[63] Tolan, J. (2003) *Ch. 6: Unconditional Positive Regard*, in Skills in Person-Centred Counselling & Psychotherapy, London: Sage Publications Ltd, pp66–86

[64] Watson, I. (1991) Prescribing from an energetic perspective. *The Homeopath*. 72: 17-23

[65] Hahnemann, S. (1982) *Organon of Medicine*. (6th edition), translated by Jost Kunzli, MD, Alain Naude, and Peter Pendelton. Blaine, WA.: Cooper Publishing, footnote to §141

[66] Fraser P. (2003) Two ways of knowing: how language affects thoughts. *The Homeopath*. 2003, 91

[67] Kuipers, S. (2008) Empathy – friend or foe? Pros and cons. *The Homeopath*, Spring, 26, 4: 132-134

[68] Mercer, S.W., Reilly D., Watt G.C.M (2001) Empathy is important for enablement. *BMJ*, April 7; 322, (7290): 865

[69] Mercer, S.W., Reilly D., Watt G.C.M. (2002) The importance of empathy in the enablement of patients attending the Glasgow Homoeopathic Hospital. *British Journal of General Practice*, November, 52, 484: 901-905

[70] Muckenheim, M. (2007) Moving on - An Interview with Anne Schadde, *Homoeopathic Links*, 20, 3: 121-123

[71] Rogers, C. R. (1980) *Empathic: An Unappreciated Way of Being*, in A Way of Being. Boston, MA: Houghton-Mifflin Company, pp137-163

[72] 'Sight' is an unfortunate word to use here, suggesting this is a visual process. It can be; but empathic understanding arises from a wide variety of sources. Depending on our individual nature and the uniqueness of a particular homeopath-patient dynamic, it can emerge into any combination of the conceptual, metaphorical, imaginative, transpersonal, emotional, sensating or physiological awarenesses [20, 71, 74] Empathic understanding is to do with attending to the patient on every level: not just about listening to her words, but 'getting' her energy state, her non-verbal way of being, understanding her experience of herself and her life as if we were her, and in some way communicating that awareness back to her

[73] Brazier, D. (1993) *Beyond Carl Rogers*. London: Constable

[74] Cooper, M. (2001) *Embodied Empathy*, in Sheila Haugh & Tony Merry (Eds.), Rogers' Therapeutic Conditions: Evolution, Theory and Practice, Volume 2: Empathy, Ross-on-Wye: PCCS Books, pp218-229

[75] Gruber, F. W. (1999) Difficult Cases: Frustrating Ordeals or Learning Experiences? *New England Journal of Homeopathy*, (electronic journal). 1999, Fall/Winter, 8, 2, URL: http://www.nesh.com/main/nejh/samples/difficult_cases.html [last accessed 21/04/2009]

[76] Brodley, B. T. (1996) Empathic Understanding and Feelings in Client-Centred Therapy. *The Person-Centred Journal*, 3, 1: 22–30

[77] Bridger, M. (2008) The Minotaur's Maze. *Homeopathy in Practice*, Autumn: 16-18

[78] Vincent, S. (2005) *Being Empathic: A Companion for Counsellors and Therapists* (Carl Rogers' Core Conditions in Depth), Oxford: Radcliffe Publishing

[79] Sankaran, R. (2007) The Evolution of My Practice. *Homoeopathic Links*, 20, 1: 11–14

[80] Sankaran, R. (2008) *The Other Song – Discovering Your Parallel Self*. Mumbai: Homoeopathic Medical Publishers

[81] Yde, C. (2009) *Congruence – a necessary quality of the homeopath*. Unpublished manuscript, Copenhagen: University of Central Lancashire

[82] Orlinsky, D. E., Grave, K., & Parks, B. K. (1994) *Process and outcome in psychotherapy*. In A. E. Bergin & S. L. Garfield (Eds.), Handbook of psychotherapy and behavior change. New York: Wiley, pp257-310

[83] Watson, J. C., Geller, S.M. (2005) The relation among the relationship conditions, working alliance, and outcome in both process - experiential and cognitive – behavioural psychotherapy. *Psychotherapy Research*, 15, 1: 1-8

[84] Dudgeon, R.E. (1851/1995) *The Medical Observer*, in Dudgeon, R.E. (1995) The Lesser Writings of Samuel Hahnemann, translated by R.E. Dudgeon; India: B. Jain, pp724-728

[85] Lietaer, G. (2001) *Being Genuine as a Therapist: Congruence and Transparency*, in Wyatt G (Ed.) Rogers' Therapeutic Conditions: Evolution, Theory and Practice Volume 1: Congruence. Ross-on-Wye PCCS Books, pp36-54

[86] Of course, this is not such a simple endeavour. It's rather like the process of 'learning' to meditate – as anyone who has 'just' brought their attention to, for example, the 'simple' act of breathing might confirm

[87] Bernard, I. (1978) *Carl Rogers on Empathy* Pts 1 & 2. [Film, VHS], Corona Del Mar, Ca.: Psychological & Educational Films: Ipswich: Concord Video & Film Council Ltd

[88] Rogers, C. R. (1978) *On Personal Power*. London: Constable

[89] Rogers, C. R. (1957) The Necessary & Sufficient Conditions of Therapeutic Personality Change. *Journal of Consulting Psychology*, 21, 2: 95-103 in Kirschenbaum H & Henderson V L (Eds), The Carl Rogers Reader , London: Constable, pp219-235

[90] Frankland, A., Sanders, P. (1995) *Next Steps in Counselling*. Manchester: PCCS Books

[91] Mearns, D. (2003) *Developing Person-Centred Counselling*. London: SAGE Publications Ltd

[92] Tudor, K. (2000) The case of the lost conditions, *Counselling*, 2000, February: 33-37

[93] Carkhuff, R. R. (1969) *Helping & Human Relations Vol. I - Selection & Training*. New York: Holt, Rinehart & Winston

[94] Carkhuff, R. R. (1969) *Helping & Human Relations Vol. II - Practice & Research*. New York: Holt, Rinehart & Winston

[95] Truax, C. B., Carkhuff, R. R (1967) *Towards Effective Counselling and Psychotherapy: Training and Practice*. Hawthorne, New York: Aidne

[96] Levant, R. F., Shlien, M. (1984) *Client-Centered Therapy and the Person-Centered Approach: New Directions in Theory, Research and Practice*. New York: Praeger

[97] Heron, J. (2001) *Helping the Client – A Creative Practical Guide*. 5th. Ed. London: Sage Publications

[98] Egan, J. (2002) *The Skilled Helper: A Problem-Management and Opportunity-Development Approach to Helping*. 7th Ed. Pacific Grove: Brooks-Cole

[99] Jackins, H. (1975) *The Human Side of Human Beings: The Theory of Re-evaluation Counselling*. Seattle: Rational Island Publishers

[100] See, e.g. Wansbrough [101:122]: As homeopaths, we have limited time and knowledge, and few individuals in the community have the experience or knowledge of such eminent homeopaths as George Vithoulkas. Instead we must re-examine and cross-discipline to other domains, (in other words use different metaphors) to discover how we think and how we make decisions; it is not enough to continually pursue a particular way of thinking (i.e. classical homeopathy) when we are faced with what I would call 'a materia medica meltdown' as we try to constantly process information as though we still held dear the precepts of 'The Age of Enlightenment.'

[101] Wansbrough, C. J. (1996) Homeopathy and the unprejudiced observer. *The Homeopath*, 61. Available online at http://www.biolumanetics.net/tantalus/Homeopathy&Consciousness/homounprejudicedart.htm [last accessed April 14th 2009]

[102] Telling example of this can be found in Motschnig-Pitrik and Lux [103], whose work in computer science, education, and neuroscience helps strengthen Rogers' theories and to some extent anticipates Sankaran's work [80]

[103] Motschnig-Pitrik, R., Lux, M. (2007) The Person-Centered Approach Meets Neuroscience: Mutual Support for C. R. Rogers's and A. Damasio's Theories. *Journal of Humanistic Psychology*, 48; 287: 287-319. (electronic journal) 2008 available at URL: http://jhp.sagepub.com/cgi/content/abstract/48/3/287 [last accessed 22/04/2009]

[104] Smith J. (2000) The Practitioner's State. *Simillimum*, 13: 13-15

[105] Chauhan, D. (2006) Internal Focusing to explore the Vital Sensation. *Homoeopathic Links*, 19, 1:17-21

[106] Winston, J. (2004) Uh oh, Toto. I don't think we're in Kansas any more, *Homeopathy in Practice*, January: 32-37

[107] Bridger, M. (1998) Up the Swanee to Atlantis. *The Homeopath*, Winter 1998, 68: 835-839

[108] Kreisberg [109] is of the opinion that homeopathic courses should include the teaching of personal awareness techniques, meditation and reflection in order to stimulate the 'inner healer,' and promote the intuition and creative energy that encourage any healing interaction. (Ross [61:14])

[109] Kreisberg, J: *The stages of homeopathic education*. [online]. Available at: http://www.lyghtforce.com/HomeopathyOnline/Issue5/articles/kreisberg.html [05/03/05] cited in Ross (2005:14)

[110] Seth, P. (2009) Personal communication

[111] D'Souza-Francisco, L. (2009) Personal communication

[112] Viksveen, P. (2009) Personal communication

[113] Therapeutic Relationships is a required 2nd year, 12-week-long module which forms part of the University of Central Lancashire's innovative MSc Homeopathy by e-Learning. See http://www.uclan.ac.uk/information/courses/msc_homeopathy_by_elearning.php

[114] Bhatia, M. (2009) Personal communication

Chapter 12
Integrating Psychotherapy and Homeopathy

A Means of Determining the Needs of the Vital Force

Kenneth Silvestri, EdD CCH RSHom (NA)

Kenneth Silvestri, EdD CCH RSHom (NA)
268 Green Village Road, Suite #6
Green Village
NJ 07935 USA
E-mail: drkennethsilvestri@gmail.com
http://www.drkennethsilvestri.com

Abstract

In this chapter a conceptual framework is described that integrates psychotherapy and homeopathy. This includes a discussion of communication skills, supporting theory, the use of the "Genogram," (a multi-generational psychological tree) and the Stanford University Forgiveness Methodology that can help the practitioner determine the core "grievance" in selecting the simillimum and establishing a treatment plan.

1   Introduction

I would like to share a conceptual framework of how psychotherapy and homeopathy can work together to enhance the healing process. Psychotherapy (in its systemic essence) is defined here as the process where one is assisted in recognizing how problems and grievances are interconnected to past and present contexts, and resolution is the understanding of this pattern and being empowered to change for the better. Homeopathy is the second-most used healing method in the world according to the World Health Organization. It is based on the principle of "like cures like." Homeopathy's safe, non-toxic and regulated remedies stimulate one's immune system to follow its natural direction to heal the mind and body from recognized trauma. The correct remedy or "simillimum" is determined by its match with the gestalt of the presenting symptoms.

Thomas Kuhn (1967) in "The Structure of Scientific Revolutions," describes how change comes about when anomalies or mistunement are recognized. However, "change" will be co-opted and sabotaged if it is not supported and maintained in a new framework or "paradigm." Traditional psychotherapy has struggled with resistance and "back to business as usual." Homeopathy, although having a long history of clinical successes, has been plagued with the difficult process of determining the "simillimum." Together, psychotherapy and homeopathy offer complementary means to recognize the pattern of suffering and consequently strengthen and maintain the immune system to balance the body and mind.

In my practice, I regularly use an exercise consisting of a metaphorical "Stereoscopic Lens." I ask those seeking help to share with me *what it is that they are not getting in their life that causes pain*. I then ask them to imagine that they are seeing their current situation or "grievance" through a lens focused on the present, the view that we most often use each day. It's within this framed sense of perspective that we can mistakenly narrow and skew our sense of what may be happening. We can also, if we choose, begin to recognize mistakes, wrongs, and anomalies within this perspective, which can allow us profound insight into our current life situations, learning style, temperament and family legacies.

I initially suggest during this presently viewed framework that a few deep diaphragmatic breaths be taken that softly fill up the stomach, before moving up to the chest. Before exhaling, with a stress-releasing exhalation, I ask them, for a second or so, to widen their lens and see things in a peripheral vision, whether it is the distant corners of the room or the wider perspective of their physical and emotional environment. I then share a specific homeopathic-like induction consisting of an emotional simillimum i.e. a statement or narrative related to the change in the presenting problem or grievance that is desired. Within this statement, I suggest that it would be beneficial to focus on being grateful for something in their life. For example, a male patient who was 50 years old told me his grievance was that his mother never acknowledged or praised him. She was a single mother who worked long hours and never had time for him. I shared several stories with him about single mothers who made all kinds of sacrifices to raise their children. I also asked him to focus and be grateful for little things that his mother did for him that made him feel good, like shopping for food etc.

This, in most cases brings up from the subconscious a wider perspective about their originally viewed context; I then ask them to revisit this and share with me any revisions or feelings that they would like to make of that view. With very few exceptions, this simple exercise results in a new and positive response to their presenting problem. This process also elicits the core "grievance" or "tale of woe," that forms the basis of the imbalance in one's vital force (Luskin, 2002). I use this exercise progressively in treatment, especially relating it to information from the person's Genogram (explained below), which leads to more empathy and insight regarding remedy and psychotherapy directions over time as one articulates one's life.

My understanding of Hahnemann's case taking methods was that he readily recorded these systemic images by contextualizing how local befallments manifested themselves (*§86-89, refers to the sections in Hahnemann 2002, Organon of Medicine*). The "unprejudiced observer" was more than a mere recorder of verbal information. Today's enormous amount of information-sharing dictates that we politely dialogue and sensitively ask for clarification, especially since most communication experts agree that 90% of communication is non-verbal. This is eloquently demonstrated with examples of appropriate communication skills in Brian Kaplan's book *The Homeopathic Conversation* (2001). In the footnote to §96, Hahnemann states that, for instance, "the high pitch of the expression about their sufferings becomes, in itself, a significant symptom in the remaining set of symptoms from which the image is composed." He undoubtedly saw inter-personal communication as more than a linear recording of content.

As I experience the above each day, the following ingredients have emerged for me as a recipe in progress to integrate homeopathy and psychotherapy. Firstly, *celebrate interpersonal communication* with all its nuances of being connected. Secondly, *understand the interconnections of nature* so to have a peripheral vision in case taking. Thirdly, *explore psychology* as Hahnemann believed that "this pre-eminent importance of the emotional state holds good to such an extent that the patient's emotional state often tips the scale in the selection of the homeopathic remedy," and "can least remain hidden from the exactly observing physician (apt 210-11)." Fourthly, *respect constitution and temperament* to help understand symptoms and allow *collective connections* to assist in resolving them.

2   The ingredients to integrate homeopathy and psychotherapy

2.1 Celebrating interpersonal communication

Maintaining change necessitates not only an understanding of our systemic connections but also an understanding of interpersonal verbal and non-verbal communication (Keltner, 2009). When we communicate, there are superimposed rhythms that join humans. Participants synchronize their underlying biological rhythms. Implicit rules are part of communication although the process is out of the explicit awareness of the speakers. Listening involves rhythm matching which is also found in body movements. Communication is "the process by which any two pieces of the universe find their relationship to each other." It is thus important to see how humans "tune" into each other rather than seeing humans as "doing things to each other." Interpersonal rhythms lie between or across the biological and cultural, clear distinctions occur and conversations systemically correct themselves. This is similar to what Greg O'Connor (1998) says about Aikido, where "one dances in the flash and flow of 'win-win' energy." Flaws in this process can cause and identify pathology.

The frame or context equals the rules of communication. This allows, encourages or penalizes behaviours. Without context that is shared by the speaker and hearer, meaning is unclear. It is the sharing of frames or contexts that allows for the recognition of anomalies to be changed. By understanding how multi-level frames work, we can avoid "right-wrong" labels. When sharing states you can, as Paul Beyers (1985) States, tune into the "love, sacred, ecstatic, transcendent, aesthetic, peak, turned on, art, music, dance etc."

Hahnemann knew that tuning into content alone only contributes to disharmony as it leads to a chase through the repertory without the needed context to match a remedy. When enacting change within a larger holistic or communicational frame, the vital force can be freed to help articulate feelings and give rise to the striking, unique and peculiar symptoms. Hahnemann, in §7, points this out in that the essential nature (*Inbegriff*) of the symptoms is the outward reflected image of the inner essence (*Wesen*) of the disease, that is, of the suffering of the life force."

This shared time frame is like a hologram, in that we all share fixed biological rhythm and a subjective modulated one. The aesthetic is possibly the largest available frame. When we recognize its reflection, we can feel it. Paul Byers (1985) believed that "tuning to content contributes to disharmony - when i.e. evil is enacted within a larger aesthetic frame, the inner, natural ideal can shape our feelings and frame our attempts at a solution." The "aesthetic is the name of the ideal human game." If we can understand change in larger and larger frames, we can find ourselves sustaining it in the natural flow of things.

2.1.1 *Implications*

It is important to "join" those seeking our assistance. A comfortable interpersonal environment is essential as we synchronize and form shared rhythms. The unprejudiced observer needs to go to the next level and see things in "context" in order to truly understand the essence of one's inner existence. This can only be accomplished as the homeopath becomes an active participant-observer.

2.2 Understanding context and systemic treatment

In developing an understanding of someone who is seeking assistance, we have been taught by Hahnemann and Boenninghausen to listen to the narrative that fills the person's presenting context. The open questioning ("as if") brings forth information regarding the location, sensation, quantity, time, circumstances, modalities and concomitants. My preference for using the family **Genogram** (see part '3. Genogram format') allows me to have a peripheral vision in case taking. Each bit of narrative information can be seen not as facts and content but as being simultaneously part of the interconnected levels of the wider lens.

In the ecological movement of the past few decades, it was shown how the chemical DDT was able to kill the predators of certain damaged agricultural crops. In this context there were cheers and accolades especially as crop values increased. However, within a few years DDT was found to have entered the food chain, soon entering human mothers' milk. Many species of insects and animals either became extinct or were soon to be so.

It became apparent that something that seemed good in one context might not be good in a simultaneously connected wider context. Similarly, using corporal punishment on a child in one context may alleviate the presenting problem, yet on a wider psychological level it can do harm. It turned out that marigolds (*Calendula*) could have healed (and did heal) the crops, keeping their natural predators safe and restoring that particular ecological pattern. What we learned from ecology is that the patterns of these contexts connect to form our "Gaia" (Silvestri, 2007).

The beginners' mind of case taking is the ecology of the mind. The mind-body narrative that is seen within this context allows for the emergence of unique stories. The strange, extraordinary, unusual and odd, is the kind of 'every snowflake being different' theory. The nature and essence of a person can only be determined from this framework if we are to truly sustain the change we are looking to promote. The alternative is to have the 'dog chasing its tail' syndrome.

Since homeopathy is the only healing form that so extensively records the mental and emotional patterns of its remedies, it stands to reason that contextualizing case taking can better help find the simillimum. "These [patterns] above all, must correspond to the very similar ones in the symptoms set of the medicines sought" (§153). Other common symptoms also need the defining context of sensations, modalities and accompanying symptoms to become useful in this framework. Stepping outside of content and organization of the facts is to recognize the anomaly that Kuhn mentions, and helps us to perceive the "mistuning of the psyche" and the "instinctual nature" of the pattern that needs to be changed to restore the "*vigor vitae.*"

Hahnemann developed a holistic view of human nature. It was the "conscious spirit," the psyche and its consequent functioning; "instinctive vital force," the essence (inner Wesen); and the "physical organism," the essential nature (Inbegriff), that worked together to become more powerful than the disease that was mistuning the vital force. The mistuned energy (innate and acquired) is the subconscious language of the vital force. To effect change, the anomaly is articulated from that inner voice. To hear it necessitates recognizing how "emotions circle like satellites around archetypal complexes. Every person is a mixture of feeling and thinking, every symptom has a circle of possible related symptoms. By knowing how the concentric circles of the symptoms fit together in the individuals we come to understand the essence and the totality" (Little, 2001). This is how patterns can be described as systemic, holistic or ecological. One has to tune into this inner voice and empathize with the contextual connections that qualify the totality. This means using whatever variations, be it the stereoscopic exercise mentioned earlier or the various repertorising methods stressing mentals (Kent) in some cases; physical generals and particulars of Boger; the more clinical and organic pathology that may be more suited to Boenninghausen's methods and/or others. If the recognition of the change that is needed is not supported by a combination of systemic means to address the fundamental, exciting and maintaining causes, the patterns of business-as-usual will sabotage any possibilities of sustaining such change.

The framework I use to record a case and to look for solutions to someone's problems and hurt is a three-generation relationship family tree called a "Genogram," (M. McGoldrick, et, .al, 1999) which is used regularly in systemic psychotherapy. This allows me to understand the emotional and physical descriptions of a person's life, legacy, and presenting grievance. A Genogram is a transgenerational depiction of one's family pattern and legacy. It is a tangible and visual means of mapping large amounts of information in a concise manner. At a glance, one can see the complexity of a family context and its connections to past emotional issues. It allows a clear introduction and way to get to know someone's life patterns. Providing a sense of history and psychological attri-butes, the Genogram portrays the ongoing evolutionary journey and interconnections to larger contexts of education, employment, race, culture, ethnicity, class, religion, and health and many other structures and issues.

The wider perspective of the Genogram (see Fig. 2 in part '3. Genogram format' for Genogram symbols) also reveals hidden information and magical connections creating a perspective that frees the individual in many cases from blame or a deviant label. The theoretical basis of the Genogram is from *Family Systems Theory* (McGoldrick, 1995) which describes how the family system moves to maintain and adapt to input within a given context that is simultaneously part-to-whole connected to wider contexts. Within this framework, I have added another dimension that to my mind is the foundation for successful psychotherapy: "Forgiveness." It is here that I emphasize how one deals with patients' "grievances'" or " tales of woe'" which is when people do not get what they may want. Usually, this is the window to how one manages stress, creates demands, and attempts to change what may not be in one's power to change.

2.2.1 Implications

Understanding how our world works in part-to-whole connections is understanding nature. By recognizing that Homeopathy is in tune with how nature works, using a wider ecological framework such as the Genogram can depict multi-levels in a person's legacy. It is within this map that unique patterns, miasms and coping skills emerge and are learned and determined to match with needed remedies and subsequent lifestyle changes.

2.3 Explore psychology

Hahnemann supported the use of humanistic psychology in treatment. "In all the so-called somatic diseases as well, the mental and emotional frame of mind is always altered (§210)." In §211 he comments that "this pre-eminent importance of the emotional state holds good to such an extent that the patient's emotional state often tips the scale in the selection of the homeopathic remedy. This is a decidedly peculiar sign, which, among all the signs of disease can least remain hidden from the exactly observing physician." Homeopathy's context includes detailed information of psychological states produced and cured by its remedies.

The importance of using homeopathic psychology is further supported by how physical symptoms disappear as mental illnesses appear. Documented cases demonstrate how serious physical disease can suddenly turn into deep one-sided mental and emotional dysfunction (§216). In many cases the physical symptoms improve while the mental situation becomes worse, as the vital force deals with the most presenting and immediate problems (§220). Hahnemann used crisis remedies when physical or mental symptoms worsened, then returned to the chronic remedy when appropriate to sustain his treatment. In §221, he recommends acute intercurrents when a flare-up of an acute crisis occurs. At this point, retaking the case and using Boenninghausen's concordance and relationship of remedies is very helpful in continuing psychological assessment and ongoing treatment. The differential assessment of psychological symptoms can point to old habitual patterns of unhealthy lifestyle and can be assisted by psychotherapy. In §228, Hahnemann writes that psychology is "diet for the soul" and that the use of "honesty" and "empathy" is essential in joining with a patient and ensuring continuing trust. David Little (2001) points out that being sympathetic to the suffering of others is part of our own healing process and that the power behind cure is compassion.

Homeopathic mind cure must be homogeneous to the symptoms and in the context of the individual. The "disease mistunements can be caused by imagination and therefore similar remedies can cure them" (footnote to §26). Because strong similar powers extinguish a weaker similar power "both physical affections and moral maladies are cured this way" i.e. grief cured by hearing another greater grief even if fictitious. Hering, for instanc,e resolved his emotional grief while seeing a ballet based on a Greek tragedy that was similar to the origin of his situation. J.T. Kent in his *Lectures on Homeopathic Philosophy* talks of being empathetic: "Sympathy and similar can go a long way in the realms of the psyche." The blending of homeopathic psychology and mind/body patterns represent a largely unexplored region of the *Organon* and can be used effectively when following homeopathic principles of being similar and in a minimal dose (Silvestri, 2002).

Fred Luskin (2002) in "Forgive For Good: A Proven Prescription For Health and Happiness" emphasizes a forgiveness methodology based on rigorous research that documents the effects of unresolved grievances on one's emotional and physical health. Forgiveness is not condoning or minimizing one's hurt. It is for oneself to be in the present and not allow one's grievance or pain to take up unnecessary space in one's head. When a grievance is embedded and shows no resolution, the sympathetic or "fight-or-flight" revved up part of our nervous system becomes overused. This part of our nervous system is great for reacting to a life-threatening situation, but injurious to our mental and physical health if overused. When we have unresolved pain there is a tendency to become the victim and create demands that are "unenforceable." Statements of "how could this happen to me," do not recognize that the world says "no." However, we can have choices and wishes to change our framework and utilize our parasympathetic nervous system (the "calm down" part). This can be accomplished by mindfully focusing on and being grateful for the good in the world. It is here that homeopathy can help the immune system to recognize any mistunement and allow it to continue its natural direction to heal the mind/body (Silvestri, 2009). For Luskin's nine steps for forgiveness see Fig. 1.

The forgiveness framework (see next page) articulates causation/solution in conjunction with the Genogram, which provides context/information, and produces an integrative process for determining the sensation, modalities, location and other associated symptoms needed for determining remedy and counselling directions.

2.4 Mindfulness, forgiveness, and health

In my own practice I employ and teach mind-body techniques with "mindfulness" at their core. My clients are willing and eager to explore the benefits of using these techniques, but for many of them it is easier said than done. Our complex and fallible nature often needs assistance in overcoming unhealthy patterns. This is where homeopathy's role in getting us "unstuck" is so evident. The main tenet of being mindful or of having a "beginner's mind" is to pause and focus while viewing the world as a part-to-whole interconnected process. The consequence of not recognizing our mutual interdependence with nature and others can lead to stress and "fight or flight" patterns, all of which have been linked to compromised immune systems and other health threats. Thich Nhat Hanh, a Vietnamese Buddhist monk who has helped popularize mindfulness, urges us "to be fully alive" and to "look at living beings with the eyes of compassion." This sounds simple but it can be very difficult to enact. Forgiving the past – oneself and others – is a key step in fostering this kind of mindfulness as well as improving health. Fred Luskin (2002), as mentioned above, further describes how we form "grievances" as a result of not getting something we desire. When it becomes "personalized" ("why me?"), the grievance has enormous power to distort our perceptions and harm us both mentally and physically.

We cannot erase the marks that our wounds leave on us, but we do have a choice between uncomplicated grief that is put into perspective and complicated grief that stays connected to the past. The grievance or tale of woe keeps the connection. Luskin's main point is that the "offender" need not be the hero of the story at our expense. Continuing to live in the story keeps us in "fight or flight" mode, whose constant overuse can cause physical damage as well as mental and emotional problems. Forgiveness is a mindful process that can disconnect us from the past and empower us to heal, but it is not easily accomplished without help and nurture.

Fig. 1: Fred Luskin's "nine steps for forgiveness"

1 *Know what you feel* so you can allow empathy to produce a "non-denial" of feelings. Soul sickness is lack of perspective. Widen the lens to view what is the "wrong" that hurts you. Our good side, persona, is constantly overtaken by our shadow side when we lose perspective.

2 *Forgiveness is for you* and it is a process to make peace with yourself.

3 *Forgiveness is not about minimizing the hurt*; it is about changing your grievance story. Forgiveness does not necessarily mean reconciling with the person who upset you or condoning their action. It is to set a goal to let yourself go to a spiritual side that does not blame or hinder your well-being. It is in a sense a way to stop relieving the grievance and stop unnecessary dwelling on the negative.

4 *Choosing to forgive.* Is choosing health as opposed to being a victim. Get the right perspective on what is happening. Recognize that your primary distress is coming from the hurt feelings, thoughts, and physical upset you are suffering now, not what offended you or hurt you two minutes or even ten years ago. Uncomplicated grief is easy to handle, i.e. you missed your movie or the grocer was out of your favorite food. Complicated grief is when you credit your bitter bank and become a millionaire in bitterness. The tale of woe gets bigger and keeps you connected to negativity in the past. The gap between what you want and what you got is an important gauge as to your health. Life says "no" in so many ways; it is part of the natural suffering we encounter every day. As Richard Carlson wrote "don't sweat the small stuff." How serious we take ourselves manifests in how we balance our mind and body. We need to make peace with the "no." This is not to minimize your hurt but to realize that the grievance story may not be reality. The map is not the territory but our 'flight or fight' mechanism will nevertheless react to the map. If the threat is gone, don't continue to have your body injured. Think of the grievance, take a deep breath and create a loving image of your positive possibilities.

5 *Have positive emotions* as you cope with confidence. At the moment you feel upset, practice the Positive Emotion Refocusing Technique (PERT) to soothe your body's 'flight or fight' response. You can choose the TV channel that you wish to see. Why not choose the life view that you want to live within.

6 *Give up expecting things from those who will not give them to you.* There are certain unenforcable rules that strengthen the grievance story. If we cling to a grievance we will live the grievance. We cannot demand a return to desire. Let go and soften yourself. You may become more vulnerable but you will be more human. Learn to forgive yourself: smart people can do stupid things. My friend John Welshons writes in his recent book *When Prayers Aren't Answered*, (Novato, California: New World Library: 2007) that "... the acceptance of things as they are in this context does not imply complacency...the acceptance of things as they are is merely intended to alleviate suffering we habitually create in our minds with the desire to change things we simply cannot change (p.151)."

7 *Put your energy in a positive place.* Have self-compassion. It is what we learn from suffering. Embrace positive intention. We cannot write off the other who hurt us. It may have just not worked out or the other had karma beyond your control. If you apply your intent in a non-demanding way your interactions will synchronize if the other is willing to join you in an honest win-win volley. Acceptance of who you are and your evolving growth is love. We are all fallible and we have choices to have noble intent.

8 *Remember that a life well lived is your best revenge.* Instead of focusing on your wounded feelings, and thereby giving the person who hurt you power over you, learn to look for the love, beauty, and kindness around you. When you look inside your enemies you see their pain. When there is no revenge you are forgiving and a life well lived is your response. If you seek revenge you are digging two graves and we become what we don't forgive. It is our choice not to define ourselves by the others who have hurt us.

9 *Amend your grievance story to remind yourself of the heroic choice to forgive.*

Between the lines of the above description of grievance and forgiveness are the clinical experiences of generations of homeopaths using homeopathic remedies to awaken self-awareness and balance the immune system after all kinds of trauma. The homeopathic repertory (a reference work that lists symptoms and the remedies that are known to address them) contains a host of information about mental-emotional symptoms related to "grievances" such as; brooding, disappointment, grief, anxiety, anger, humiliation, reproach, resentment, hatred, and holding on to the past. We also know that certain remedies address physical ailments that can result from withheld grievances, such as exhaustion, nervous affections, heart problems, immune system problems, and hypertension.

Many homeopathic remedies have the potential to address nearly all of the traumas one may encounter. I have found, however, that the framework of the forgiveness methodology facilitates the recognition of the needed "constitutional" remedy when one is holding on to a "grievance." The remedies shown below are examples of just a few that might be indicated for any particular individual in need of forgiveness and psychotherapy (Silvestri 2008).

2.4.1 Selected "forgiveness remedies"

Aurum metallicum (pure gold, a mineral remedy) can help people who are full of self-reproach and blame and may address depression that arises from this. People who need Aurum set very high standards for themselves, so they tend to feel failure and guilt keenly. Their sadness is intense and can be suicidal, usually as a result of not achieving their high goals. Aurum is indicated when a sense of loneliness is prevalent and there is a tendency to be very quarrelsome. The temperament of people needing this remedy shows strong duty-bound and workaholic tendencies. There is much self-reproach, despair and shame within their tale of woe. They feel worse from cold and boredom and usually feel better with music. This remedy can be called for when someone has difficulty expressing anger because of their depressive state, whereas people who need *Staphysagria* (see below) will still function and outwardly express their dissatisfaction. Other Aurum remedies may be more specific for certain differentiating symptoms, such as when there is enormous anger when thinking of one's ailments, especially after mortification (*Aurum muriaticum*; chloride of gold). *Aurum muriaticum natronatum* (double chloride of sodium and gold) would be indicated when there is extreme unrest and impatience and *Aurum sulphuricum* (sulphide of gold) when there is a strong sense of despair regarding recovery from a trauma.

Ignatia amara (Ignatia bean, a plant remedy) can help people who exhibit hysteria and a sense of being stuck in grief. In people needing Ignatia, bitter and longstanding disappointment manifests itself in deep brooding and despair. The grievance pattern is supported by a worsening with criticism and being alone. There can be suspicion about what others think of them, and they are prone to contradict even though they crave attention. The sentimental yet quarrelsome nature of people needing Ignatia makes them vulnerable to taking affront. When they have a grievance, they come across as being beside themselves as they hold on to their insult. They may have a sensation of a lump in the throat. The person needing Ignatia feels better with heat, cries easily and improves from eating unlike a *Natrum muriaticum* person who is aggravated by heat, suppresses tears and is worse from eating.

Nitricum acidum (Nitric acid) is indicated when the inability to forgive is characterized by anxious, complaining, irritable behaviour and strong resistance to resolving their tale of woe. People needing this remedy can be very abrupt, unforgiving and vindictive with aversion to any conflict which produces strong resentment. Negativity, peevishness and nasty behaviour can be traits leading to this remedy. They are prone to hold on to their grievances in a grudging manner. They can be restless and dissatisfied with everything. Anxiety about health is a keynote as well as not admitting to any obvious improvement to their health. There is a strong oversensitivity to what people may think about them, which supports their holding on to hurts and blaming others for taking the joy out of their life. Food cravings revolve around fats and salts, they are chilly by nature and complain of splinter-like pains. They have a strong sensation of inner uneasiness or constriction throughout their body and are usually better when lying down.

Natrum muriaticum (common salt) may help those who are romantic, responsible, somewhat fastidious, introverted and prone to cultivate grievances based on their great sensitivity in relationships. The grief and the tendency to take things very personally keep their tale of woe very silent and suppressed. They are better for solitude, worse for consolation, yet with extreme dwelling on past offenses, reminiscent of the story of the biblical wife of Lot, who on looking back turned into a pillar of salt. There is a clear vulnerability, with fears of rejection and affects of loss, separation, resentment and humiliation. There is a liking for salt, symbolic of the dried-up tears of long-term grief, and other characteristics of dryness. There is much exhaustion but usually amelioration with fasting when this remedy is indicated.

Phosphoricum acidum is indicated when there is an overwhelming sense of disappointment and loss, especially of loved ones. They become negative and long for acceptance. There is a flat indifference, doubt and a weak, apathetic quality to their grievance story which differentiates them from the other remedies. The need for this remedy is also indicated when there is a collapse and forgetful state. There is a yielding and slow disposition with a silent holding on to their grief.

Staphysagria (Stavesacre) is warranted when there is difficulty expressing the grievance clearly. There is much anger and apathy about all things, yet there is an underlying sense of being mild and sweet which can confuse their sense of expression. Constant dwelling on unpleasant thoughts with low self-confidence is evident. A sense of betrayal with indignation and an irritable temperament are characteristics of this remedy. Horrible and sad stories affect those in need of this remedy and they can easily throw things as a substitute for verbally expressing their anger. There is an aversion to physical exertion, being touched, and confrontation.

2.4.2 Implications
Psychology is the framework where solutions are found. Using the forgiveness methodology can produce the means and information to create solutions. Rubrics appear in the articulation of "grievances" and relevant mindfulness skills, which, in conjunction with homeopathic treatment, takes the healing process to new levels.

2.5 Respect constitution and temperament
In homeopathy we are taught that causation, constitution, and the totality of symptoms are three critical factors. Boenninghausen writes about the importance of understanding who, what, why, with what modes, when. He also emphasizes the need to understand causation and how imbalance in a person's make-up opens the door to the need for change. David Little (2001) describes how remedies have a multi-polar nature having been tested on a wide variety of people. Constitution and temperament are what we view first in the patient. This helps contextualize symptoms that are similar and places them in the perspective of, for instance, the thin and dry constitutions (the twin biles of melancholic and choleric) or the heavy and wet constitutions (the sanguine and phlegmatic metabolisms).

How one feels, radiates and adapts are further cues about their ways of gathering information and handling their evolving contexts. Their family legacy and life cycle narration play a part in this determination. Learned communication and somatic foundation is the basis for confirming complex emotions "that circulate around the centre like satellites." Reactions from dialogue can lead to exploring essential patterns that define striking, extraordinary, unusual and outstanding symptoms. Respecting constitution and temperament allows the observer to participate in patients overlapping states i.e. nervo-choleric, sanguine-phlegmatic etc. and through homeopathy's wonderful case narratives and provings point to remedy resolutions and lifestyle changes.

2.5.1 Implications

In continuing the homeopathic treatment, understanding one's temperament and constitution provides resources to maintain improvement. Psychotherapy, especially using the forgiveness methodology, can help create lifestyle and mind/body skills to support and adjust the changes (including complementary remedies) that accompany the healing process.

2.6 Allow collective connections

The final considerations in sustaining change deals with a deeper understanding of how our patients construct their world. Reconciling subjective and objective experience is one of the ongoing challenges within our human fallibility. Jung believed that the subjective part gets its information from symbols of inherent instincts, ancestral connections and universal archetypes. "The collective unconscious communicates from the timeless space that is the source of all religious, myths, visions, dreams, fantasies, altered states, fairy tales and folk stories." It is a holding place for all the experiences of humanity and a means to wholeness. As ignorance can misguide us, the grasping of one's potential as well as constraints can enlighten us. "When we confront the mythological core of our experience it offers transcendental meaningfulness to our lives" (Silvestri, 2002). The objective psyche is an energetic field of experience lived through these archetypes. Edward Whitmont, who himself was a psychiatrist and homeopath, further elaborates that psychological happenings are processed and manifested in the language of symbols. This is a demonstration of the "purposeful direction of movement that expands that which is deficient and balances what is exaggerated." This natural movement toward wholeness is what Jung called the "self." If this is the case, "then all psychosomatic phenomena can be given meaning, intent, and provide information about the state of the unconscious if interpreted symbolically" (Silvestri 2002, 2008). It can also be the source for articulating one's grievance story or "tale of woe" which perpetuates the "fight or flight" part of our sympathetic nervous system. It is in this realm that Fred Luskin (2002) demonstrated the injurious effects of unresolved grievances to one's emotional and physical health.

As humans we have a nature that moves inherently toward collaboration. Neurosurgeon Karl Pribram describes how our brain acts holographically within a holographic wider context of our world (Byers, 1977). This can easily demonstrate the archetypal development and accessibility to our interconnectedness (i.e. yin-yang, I-Thou etc.) that all of us need in order to be awakened from ignorance. Jung demonstrated how the ego provides our conscious with content, yet the shadow, our compensatory subconscious, provides subliminal experiences.

The collective unconscious and the self are information sources that go far beyond personal experiences. The blend of the conscious and unconscious dialogue is constant and the symbols that arise in consequent dreams are the language of the unconsciousness, and could be a medium of inspiration and art. It is this process that can also be the driving force behind psychosomatic problems.

Being out of "sync" is an indication of imbalance. Although we never see the invisible pure form of the archetypal thing, we can strive to harmonize with its manifestation pattern and essence. The awareness of these simultaneous connections, the "Ah" experience, is the spontaneous automatic reaction that does not follow the rules of the rational mind. Jane Cicchetti (2001), in an interview, said that "Jung felt that symbols were the best possible expression of a reality and wholeness that is greater than the intellect can conceive; that symbols point the way to a greater reality." She also points out that when we open our minds to this reality we are able to make connections and see the wholeness of a homeopathic case more readily."

2.6.1 Implications

Being aware of connections and how symbols give us understanding of life's paradoxes and potential creativity is the basis for moving toward wholeness. Homeopathic remedies resonate with nature's plan and they can be identified and matched with the emerging articulated "self." Homeopathy and psychotherapy when integrated provides ongoing assistance to this process.

3   Genogram format (McGoldrick, 1995)

The Genogram is a transgenerational and psychological family tree. Using the symbols (see fig. 2) one can depict an individual's relationships, family patterns and influences. Factual information about illnesses etc., help determine miasmatic patterns and legacy. Parental traits and communication (i.e. open, closed, nurturing, controlling, abusive etc.) from the patient's own narrative allow for an understanding of how they were raised and reared relevant to developing communication and cultural traits. Constant recording of "grievances," sensations, modalities, locations, and other related ailments will produce an ongoing narrative and openings for striking and unique symptoms applicable to determining homeopathic remedies and psychotherapy directions.

Some initial questions:
- How do family members think about one another? (Look for characteristic labels that are brought up i.e. the loudmouth, spendthrift, softie etc.). This provides articulation of joys and pains. Patterns of enmeshment and cut-offs can be the "not-well-since" beginnings of past and present aggravations, resentments and grievances leading to symptoms found in homeopathic repertories.
- Who was named for whom in your family? (Look for how names reveal roles, hidden meanings, historic connections and psychological patterns).
- Were there coincidences between the births of family members and moves or migrations, illnesses or death, changes in family finances, etc.?
- How closely did the family conform to gender stereotypes of their culture and era, which members did not conform, how were they viewed and how did the family demonstrate flexibility (or inflexibility)?
- How did the family deal with rituals, stress, rules, leisure, beliefs, and explaining or telling stories of death, money, education, betrayal etc.?
- What kind of relationships did the patient's parents have with their parents? How did they relate to their parents, the good, the bad, any grievances, traumas, life cycle and developmental issues etc.?
- How did they relate to their siblings? How were siblings expected to behave? What roles did they and their siblings have in the family?

- What are the patterns of couples relationships in their family? Divorce, power struggles, gender roles, employment, attraction, strengths, weaknesses, and how did this effect their development etc.?
- Class, culture and diversity questions can include narratives of ethnic background, celebrations, stress management etc.

Fig.2: Genogram Format

A genogram is created with simple symbols representing gender, with various lines to illustrate family relationships. The figure below illustrates basic genogram symbols with various types of individuals. Some genogram users also put circles around members who live in the same living spaces. Genograms can be prepared by using a complex word processor, or a computer drawing program. There are also computer programs that are custom designed for genograms.

(Symbols: e.g. male, female, unknown gender, pet, adopted child etc.)

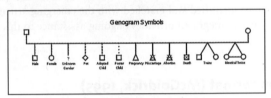

Genogram symbols will usually have the date of birth (and date of death if applicable) above, and the name of the individual underneath. The inside of the symbol will hold the person's current age or various codes for genetic diseases or user-defined properties: abortions, still-births, SIDS (Sudden Infant Death Syndrome), cohabitations, etc.

One of the advantages of a genogram is the ability to use colour-coded lines to define different types of relationships such as family relationships, emotional relationships and social relationships. Within family relationships, you can illustrate if a couple is married, divorced, common-law, engaged, etc. The figure below illustrates the symbols commonly used for family relationships.

(E.g. marriage, separation in fact, legal separation, divorce, etc.)

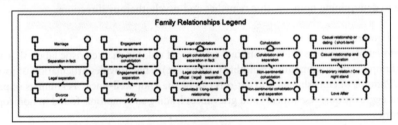

Genograms usually also include emotional relationships. These provide an in-depth analysis of how individuals relate to one another. Colour-coded lines represent various emotional relationships that bond individuals together. The next figure illustrates the symbols commonly used for emotional relationships.

(E.g. indifferent, harmony, hostile, violence, abuse etc.)

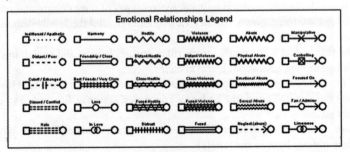

3.1 Implications

The questions suggested above provide background and support for assessing the presenting problems, grievances (what one is not getting), unenforceable rules (see the Nine Steps in the forgiveness methodology), coping skills, and stress management. This allows for more concise ways of describing sensations, modalities, location and other related symptoms. The recorded narrative, information and behavioural patterns can then be used to determine a constitutional remedy and through the forgiveness methodology (explained above), a therapeutic framework.

Using the forgiveness methodology and the Genogram format provides relevant additional information that will help determine the core grievance and differentiate between indicated remedies (see selected forgiveness remedies above).

3.2 Case example

A condensed case example was a woman in her early thirties who presented with a *Phosphorus* persona. She was very intuitive, extroverted, open and impressionable. There was a sense of self-importance and desire to be the centre of attraction. She however was very concerned about her sense of physical weakness (chief complaint) especially when things were not going her way.

She had been treated previously by a homeopath with Phosphorus, but felt there was little change in her symptoms and disposition. Her family of origin depicted in her Genogram indicated many stories about the lack of structure, encouragement and affection received from her parents. She felt she could not succeed at her job (retail/sales) and told of trouble organizing herself. However her evaluations and performance were acceptable to her employers. She mentioned being criticized by her parents for her choice of employment. Her narration of her early family dynamics stressed that she was never "good enough," and even when she was motivated or excited about doing something her parents and older sibling would "bring her down."

She was not able to express this or show disagreement since this was unacceptable. Asked how she dealt with this, she explained how she would become very introverted and held her anger inside when at home but would constantly discuss her sense of dissatisfaction (not anger) with her life with anyone who would listen (a strong Phosphorus trait). When asked what it was that she was not getting in life, she expressed it as wanting "her integrity," that her parents destroyed. She thought of this daily and blamed her parents for her dissatisfaction with work and life. She would become exhausted whenever she focused on this feeling or was involved with her parents. When she was sad and tired she would become yielding and feared losing her integrity and "self-control." What emerged from her family narratives and her grievance story was someone who had clear extroverted intuitive traits who would move to an angry introverted state. This would be what Carl Jung described as one moving from an outgoing sanguine state to her inferior side which was an inward choleric state. Her outgoing "persona" was one of being impressionable, artistic, intuitive, and the centre of attention. The "shadow" side or inferior trait (usually where the strange, peculiar and unique symptoms needing attention are located) was characterized by false pride, self-pity, and dwelling on her problems. This resulted in an inability to finish her objectives and compromised her sense of integrity.

Repertory rubrics that came to the surface revolved around her "loss of position," shame regarding her parents and sibling dynamics, loss of control, and a distorted sense of self-importance. The remedy *Staphysagria* was further confirmed by her aversion to being touched when she was exhausted, desire to throw things when angered and her recent articulation of indignation toward her parents' behaviour.

She was given the remedy in a 30C medicinal solution, followed by a Q1 potency, with striking improvement. Her follow-up sessions focused on her changing her "grievance story," using relaxation exercises and having positive intent following the forgiveness steps. After six weeks she began taking Phosphorus (solution of the Q1 potency) which was now clearly indicated as the Staphysagria symptoms dissipated. She reported continued improvement in her total well-being and felt "invigorated and confident."

4   Conclusion

I have always believed that the process of psychotherapy or, for that matter, life itself, is to recognize and "differentiate" between injurious patterns that compromise a person's optimal health. We cannot isolate ourselves from the many contexts of life, but we can keep our integrity and simultaneously see the larger picture that we are part of and within. When homeopathy is combined with psychotherapy, the process of becoming "whole' is much more attainable. Understanding one's role in a family system can for example unveil dynamics connected to grievances and consequent symptoms that represent universal archetypes, opening up new avenues for understanding what is needed for cure. If the goal of classical homeopathy is to intervene with remedies representative of the whole person, then homeopathy can benefit from psychological assessments which can indicate how the family/community contexts can foster or hinder better health.

Anthropologist Paul Byers (1977), when explaining how systems worked, used the metaphor of a watch with its many parts placed on a table. It showed little resemblance to a timepiece. Yet when put together it could either tell the "correct" or the "wrong" time. Like a thermostat regulating a heating system, it is the input of setting and maintaining that allows a system to avoid the ever-present forces of entropy (movement to disorder). The human system, with its regulating forces of communication, temperaments, ethos and other homeostatic elements can be the source of conflict warranted by our fallibility but also exciting grist for creativity and joy. Being in touch with this map can help in understanding possible avenues of change and the resources to sustain that direction.

I am not suggesting the replacement of existing case analysis methods in homeopathy; however, using a visual map of family dynamics leads to a richer yield for the questions of *who, what, where,* with *when, why, what* modalities of the homeopathic assessment. This in turn demonstrates how homeopathy helps provide new solutions and understanding for lifestyle changes and other psychological interventions. Looking at the part-to-whole connections allows for depth of analysis and avoids self-defeating negative consequences. The qualifying interactions and chronological data in such a process put into context the qualitative attributes of the individual and their system. David Little (1998) describes this process as how "conceptual thought is a manifestation of the archetypal drive toward order and meaning." The format that I am suggesting helps depict this "meaning." All the institutions and contexts that have influenced a person's development can be understood in their part-to-whole connections. In this framework, the chief complaint for instance can be a portal to the essence of the case, as can be gestures and themes; however, using a wider lens allows for the multiple layers to unfold and to temper or avoid superficial diagnosis.

Using the Genogram and probing for "grievance formations" allows a participant observer (homeopath) to trace and interact with the different types of temperaments and their psychic manifestations (i.e. visual, auditory, feeling etc.). The energy of the person's legacy literally and figuratively "jumps out." If the self and the collective conscience are more than conditioned reactions, then this mapping of interactions and relationships can be part of the larger archetypal drive for balance. Sometimes a map which is really not "the thing" can still help visualize the manifestations of a person's "Wesen." Responses to how the person feels ("as if ..."), are the interplay of the unconscious mind's associative functions and the rationality of the conscious quest for explanations. In this map, the invisible energy of the archetype emerges as form. Feelings and tones can give many messages, as well as silence and tears. All this can be used to assist the self's innate move toward wholeness, and the symbols of the system are a key to understanding and changing any psychosomatic dysfunction, which can be achieved by homeopathy's clinical provings.

The integration and reciprocity of psychotherapy and homeopathy encourages a guided narrative of the person's self-identification in the context of their significant relationships and developmental stages. It provides a familiar backdrop (not always comfortable) to answer all of the questions suggested in Hahnemann's *Organon*. Hahnemann regularly investigated entire family trees to better determine the befallment of issues affecting the vital force and chronic miasms (§82-99) because for him "the cause of a thing or an event can never be at the same time the thing or event itself" (*Organon*, introduction, p. 10).

This is relevant today since we are constantly influenced by cultural and language constraints, what Martin Buber (1970) called the "I-it," which is antithetical to the "I-Thou" of optimal health. For me the Genogram offers a wider format to join with another and avoid the "name is the thing" trap by understanding patterns that point to a constitutional state through the person's own description and perspectives. There are an infinite number of visualisations similar to what I described above; my point is that, for homeopathy, the "widening" of its lens can provide more opportunity for the identification of fundamental beginnings, awareness of exciting (causative) influences and the altering of disease states from the life context of the individual.

The process of homeopathy is more akin to interpersonal relations and communication skills than it is to the "medical model." The ongoing conversation or dialogue with those seeking help is what constitutes the essence of homeopathic remedies and the many possibilities of seeing them in different and updated contexts. Learning good communication skills is also the vehicle for learning more about ourselves as humans with our own fallibility. This enhances not only our role as homeopaths but also the biological connection we have access to when we tune into and "be" together rather than "do" things to each other.

References

[1] Byers, P. (1977) A personal view of nonverbal communication. *Theory Into Practice*. Vol. XVI, Number 3: 134-40

[2] Byers, P. (1985) Communication: cooperation or negotiation? *Theory Into Practice*. Vol. XXIV, Number 1: 71-76

[3] Buber, M. (1970) *I and Thou*. New York: Charles Scribner

[4] Ciccchetti, Jane (2001) Symbolism, Dreams and Homeopathy: A Discussion With Jane Cicchetti and Barbara Osawa, *Simillimum*, Fall, Vol. XIII: 22-23

[5] Hahnemann, Samuel (2002) *Organon of the Medical Art*, 6th edition, edited by Wenda Brenster O'Reilly, Palo Alto, Calif.: Birdcage Books

[6] Luskin, Fred (2002) *Forgive for Good: A proven Prescription for Health and Happiness*. New York: Harper

[7] Kaplan, Brian. (2001) *The Homeopathic Conversation*. London: Natural Medicine Press

[8] Keltner, Dacher (2009) *Born to be Good: The Science of a Meaningful Life*. New York: Norton

[9] Kuhn, Thomas (1967) *The Structure of Scientific Revolutions*. Chicago, Ill.: University of Chicago Press

[10] Little, David (2001) Hahnemann Online Education, V. 4, (www.simillimum.com)

[11] McGoldrick, M., Gerson R. & Shellenberger S. (1999) *Genograms in family assessment*. New York: Norton

[12] O'Connor, Greg (1998) *The Elements of Aikido*. Boston, Mass: Element Books

[13] Silvestri, Kenneth (2002)The Art of Sustaining Change: A Personal Framework for Homeopathic Emotional Healing, *Simillimum*, summer, Vol. XIV: 85-98

[14] Silvestri, Kenneth (2005) Homeopathic case taking from a communication perspective. *The American Homeopath*. Vol. 11: 77-78

[15] Silvestri, Kenneth (2007) The Joy and Wisdom of Systemic Thinking: Teaching and Understanding the Aesthetic, *The Journal of Systemic therapies*, Spring 2007, Vol.26, 1: 11-22

[16] Silvestri, Kenneth (2008) Steps to an Ecology of Self: implications for homeopathy, *Homoeopathic Links*, Summer 2008, Vol. 21, 2: 67-71

[17] Silvestri, Kenneth (2009) Remedies for Forgiveness, *Homeopathy Today*, Vol.29, 1: 21-22

218

Chapter 13

Unlocking the Door to Human Potential

A Jungian Perspective on the Treatment of Emotional Disorders with Homeopathy

Jane Tara Cicchetti, RSHom(NA) CCH

Jane Tara Cicchetti, RSHom(NA) CCH
26 Springwood Drive
Asheville NC 28805
USA
E-mail: janetara@janecicchetti.com

Abstract

A clinical case with commentary showing the process of profound healing from emotional trauma using homeopathy and Jungian dream analysis. It illustrates how dreams can express the deepest levels of the psyche and reveal the curative remedy and the changes this remedy brings about once it is administered.

1   Introduction

This chapter will attempt to illustrate how homeopathy, when used in conjunction with Jungian dream analysis, can help alleviate mental and emotional disturbances, shorten the time needed to heal these problems, and stimulate transpersonal development. It will also reveal how a respectful alliance between patient and therapist can stimulate dreams, recollections, and symbolic language that disclose the inner core of suffering in an individual. These symbols are valuable gifts that point the way towards the unfolding of health and wholeness, and are the key to the appropriate homeopathic remedy. We will begin this exploration with a dream.

2   An early childhood dream

"A group of Native American people took me to a white sand beach and put crystals in my body. Quartz crystals. They told me they were doing this so I would always remember that this was my medicine."

This is an early childhood dream of a courageous and sensitive 60-year-old woman who, from a very young age, realized that the crystals in this dream were symbolic of her ability as a healer, "it was like having a crystal ball inside of me." The dream also taught her that it was important to speak of her many clairvoyant experiences as dreams so that people wouldn't think she was strange.

The dreamer, Maggie, had a very difficult childhood. With a mother who suffered from periodic mental breakdowns, and an abusive, alcoholic father, she was sent to live with different relatives as an infant.

When she was three years old she started seeing spirits - good spirits - "they were there for me." Shortly after that time, she was sent back to live with her parents, where she witnessed her father physically and verbally abusing her mother.

Both parents said she was "too sensitive" and physically beat her, but she felt an inner concern for others and did her best to care for her siblings and parents. She said that she always felt that she had to earn a place in her family and that the lack of support felt so awful that she wanted to die.

Being open to all of the possibilities within the individual's life story is essential in homeopathy as it is in psychotherapy. Often, it is the most unusual, conventionally overlooked aspects of a person's life that are useful in the therapeutic situation. They are the gold nuggets which are easily ignored by the homeopath and suppressed by the patient. We tend to filter out whatever doesn't make sense to us, what we cannot understand with the rational mind. Acknowledging the whole person and the expression of his or her most unique self requires that the clinician accept possibilities of reality that are beyond what is conventionally acceptable.

Carl Jung wrote about the importance of listening to the wholly personal story of the individual:

> "In many cases in psychiatry, the patient who comes to us has a story that is not told, and which as a rule no one knows of. To my mind, therapy only really begins after the investigation of the wholly personal story. It is the patient's secret, the rock against which he is shattered. If I know his secret story, I have a key to the treatment. In most cases exploration of the conscious material is insufficient."
> P. 117 MDR [1]

Carl Jung is well known for his contribution to transpersonal psychology. What is less well known is that he was successful in treating individuals with severe psychiatric disorders. His early work in psychiatric institutions served as a basis for many of his theories and attitudes towards mental health and led to his formulation of the concept of the collective unconscious.

By listening to patients in a compassionate and unprejudiced manner, he was able to help those who were thought to be incurable. This open-minded attitude towards the individual enabled him not only to help a wide variety of individuals but to begin to understand something of the workings of the human psyche. He did this not with theories or by categorizing diseases of the mind - although he considered this to be important - but through careful and caring observation. With this in mind, let's return to Maggie's story.

In her late thirties, after years of working as a social worker, Maggie suffered from what she now calls a nervous breakthrough. She put together a lethal cocktail of drugs and was going to drink it. But instead she smoked marijuana and went into a deep sleep. "Something shook me awake," she said, "and I saw that the room was filled with thousands of spirits who asked if I was ready. "Ready for what," she thought. Then they disappeared. She didn't take the poison.

Maggie now feels that, at this time, she had been delusional. She knew that she had seen spirits her whole life, but at that point she was paranoid. She couldn't trust anyone. She was put into a state mental hospital and was later released because the psychiatrists said there was nothing wrong with her. Her mental and physical health continued to deteriorate. She became homeless and was suffering from severe malnutrition. Maggie was finally put into a state mental hospital where she was badly mistreated:

> "They handcuffed me to a bed, pumped me full of thorazine, and left me alone. I had to scream to get someone to let me go to the bathroom. They said that because I was indigent I had to stay there. At this point I was 89 pounds. I couldn't eat, I had dentures since I was sixteen, my teeth had been crumbly and soft. You could just break them off. Now I had ulcers in my mouth.
> It was terrifying for me, they gave me injections and I'm scared to death of needles. They thought I was a street person. They wouldn't let me go unless someone agreed to be responsible for me. Finally, a girl-friend agreed to take responsibility for me and I was released".
> "I weaned myself off the drugs - went for therapy. I worked in a doctor's office as a receptionist. I had a good experience with massage helping a pinched nerve in my neck so I decided to go to massage school. That's what I do now."

Over two hundred years ago, *Samuel Hahnemann*, the German physician who founded homeopathy, wrote about the need to treat mental patients with respect. He was acutely aware that their disease was made worse by mistreatment:

> "Above all, these patients are embittered, and their disease is worsened, through scorn, deceit, and noticeable deceptions. **The physician and attendants must always appear as if they credit such patients with reason.**" (Author's emphasis)

He was also adamant that homeopathic treatment was the most effective form of therapy in these cases:

> "In the cases of mental or emotional disease (which are incredibly various), if the selected remedy for a particular case is entirely appropriate for the truly sketched image of the disease state, then the smallest possible doses are often sufficient to produce the most striking improvement, which is often quite rapid. This is never achieved by medicating the patient to death with huge, frequent doses of all other unsuitable (allopathic) medicines." [3]

Homeopathy has a long history of working with mental and emotional diseases by treating the whole person. It is very easy to see only pathology. A psychologist, for example, will often focus on mental symptoms and not consider the physical state. Or a psychiatrist who is committed to treating with medication may think primarily about brain chemistry and appropriate pharmaceuticals.

One of the values of homeopathy is that it considers all of the symptoms that are characteristic of the individual.

Homeopathic philosophy of healing has from its inception recognized that all symptoms, mental and emotional as well as physical, are guideposts to the fundamental imbalance in an organism. Hahnemann wrote about the need to treat the whole person, body, mind, and emotions, without forming theories or prejudices:

> *"The unprejudiced observer, even the most sharp-witted one -- knowing the nullity of supersensible spe-*
> *culations which are not born out of experience -- perceives nothing in each single case of disease other*
> *than the alterations in the condition of the body and soul, disease signs, befallments, symptoms, which*
> *are outwardly discernable through the senses. That is, the unprejudiced observer only perceives the devi-*
> *ations from the former healthy state of the now sick patient, which are:*
> *1. felt by the patient himself,*
> *2. perceived by those around him, and*
> *3. observed by the physician.*
> *All these perceptible signs represent the disease in its entire extent, that is, together they form*
> *the true and only conceivable gestalt of the disease." [4]*

In Maggie's case, along with her history of mental symptoms, there is a unique physical symptom; teeth that were so soft that they crumbled and could be easily broken off. This was so severe that she had lost all of her teeth by the time she was sixteen. From the homeopathic perspective, this is an important indication of her constitution. She also has had a strong fear of needles; she uses the word "terrified" when referring to having been given injections. When we consider these symptoms, along with her intense feeling of not having support as a child and her tendency towards clairvoyance, we see indications for a homeopathic remedy that contains silica.

By the time Maggie shows up for homeopathic treatment, she has been struggling with "waves of depression", is having financial problems, and is still feeling a terrible lack of support. She's about 30 pounds overweight, wants to stop smoking, and to start taking better care of herself. At 60, she still has some menopausal insomnia:

> *"I wake up depressed and my whole body feels heavy. When I'm down, I get this feeling, like a big stone,*
> *I can feel the weight of it. It's a real heaviness. I feel defeated, like there's nothing I can do about it."*
> *"I pick at my skin - I have spots from this all over me. I pick at wherever I can reach. I cry but it doesn't*
> *make me feel any better. Sometimes it makes me feel worse."*
> *She says that she has a history of endometriosis for which she has had many surgeries. She also has some*
> *bone loss in her lower jaw.*

2.1 Case analysis

The homeopathic remedy Maggie is given is chosen after careful consideration of all her present symptoms, history, and, the symbols contained in the childhood dream that showed her "her medicine". She is given a *Quartz Crystal* prepared into a homeopathic remedy in the 200C potency, to be taken one time. Quartz Crystal is primarily silica and, as was noted previously, she has many symptoms that indicate the need for homeopathic silica. [5] But Quartz Crystal is a closer match to the symbol that appeared in the powerful dream from her childhood. In considering the symbols from the dream as well as her emotional and physical symptoms, we are honouring her as a whole person. We are giving credence to the symbols that are messages from her psyche. This allows us to find a remedy that is the closest match to all aspects of her being.

2.2 Follow-up

In a series of monthly follow-up visits over a period of fifteen months Maggie's health improves. She has a renewed sense of purpose, feels more grounded, and is much less depressed. She has stopped smoking and has made a change in her diet resulting in the loss of fifteen pounds. The compulsive skin picking has almost disappeared. During this period, the Quartz Crystal was repeated three times in the 200C and then given in a higher potency, 1M.

After sixteen months of treatment another set of symptoms emerged. She began to experience deep sadness and loneliness about not having a partner. She very much wanted to be in a relationship but exhibited deep fears based on her past experience. In previous relationships, she had done a lot to support the man who she lived with at the expense of her own integrity. She feels that this pattern began with her father:

> "Everything was done for the man. That's cultural for me. Dad always received the most food. The women in the house did everything for him. I remember really loving him as a young child, but when I got older I couldn't get that love. He became abusive. I think that that has affected my ability to have a loving relationship with a man."

We are now entering a different phase in the healing process. Most of the physical and compulsive symptoms have disappeared or are greatly improved. The compulsive skin picking is no longer an issue. What is now revealed is the underlying heartbreak, so common to the human condition. This is where we move from what is often referred to as pathology to the development of the full personality, or, as it is called in Jungian psychology, the process of individuation. Homeopathy has since its inception recognized that health is much more than the absence of disease; it is the ability to live one's life fully on all levels. In order to achieve even deeper healing, it is important to find the appropriate homeopathic remedy for this stage of Maggie's journey.

Without veering from the original dream symbol of the quartz crystal, the prescription is tailored even more precisely to her needs. *Amethyst Immersion* 200C is chosen. We know from the extensive research done on the homeopathic remedy made from this gem by P. Tumminello et al [6], that it is indicated where the individual has a strong desire for love relationships but has great difficulty with boundary issues. Those who benefit from the remedy tend to put their loved ones ahead of themselves, to their own detriment. It is also a form of quartz, a silica compound with the addition of a small amount of iron giving the purple colour so typical of this mineral. It is a remedy that suits her present needs but is still consistent with her structural symptoms, earlier physical symptoms, and the symbolism in the childhood dream.

Over the next few months she begins to feel very well. One month after the Amethyst she gives the following report:

> "I realize that my heart is breaking open. The armour is falling away." She has the following dream:

"A male friend of mine came up to me and leaned his body gently against my back. He laced my fingers in his and kissed me gently. He rocked me gently, like a baby. It was so sweet and delicious that I didn't want to wake up out of it."

"For at least a week, I have had positive, caring dreams about men. I think this is a very good sign."

This series of dreams of men nurturing and caring for her shows a deep level of healing. From a Jungian perspective, it is the conscious emergence and healing of the male side of herself: the *animus*. The animus in a woman is an internal manifestation of both societal and personal attitudes of men towards women. It is an inner dynamic that is projected outward into the world and affects a woman's relationship with men. Because the animus is formed at least partially by a woman's early experience of her father, it is no surprise that Maggie would need to go through a transformation of this part of her psyche in order to have a healthy relationship with men.

The inner knowing, the intelligence inherent in the psyche, is beginning to express its needs. At this point it is not unusual for memories of important material to be recollected but the psyche begins to express itself through dreams and even synchronistic events that indicate what remedy is needed. Patient and therapist become witnesses to the unfolding of a heretofore unimagined process of healing into wholeness.

The healing deepens even further and we see some very interesting developments in the next month's follow-up session:

"My emotions are much more stable. I definitely want love in my life but I don't feel sad or melancholy about not having a partner. I'm learning to put myself first and am getting lots of acknowledgement from others. I am having a great social life. Often, I weep with gratitude about how well I feel. I never thought that I could get to where I am now."

She has the following dream:

"I was on a road and along the side of the road were bicyclists. They had been in accidents and some of them may have been dead. I started giving them remedies.

Then, I was at my grandmother's house; I was surprised that her old Studebaker was in the driveway. I went into the house and there were many people inside. I was very surprised that Grandma gave me the keys to her car and said I could drive it. When I'm driving it, I realize that there are not brakes and I can't control the steering. But then I understand that I can't control the steering with my hands; I have to do it with my attention."

When using dreams for homeopathic treatment, it is important to have the dreamer give his or her own view of the dream. That way we avoid superimposing our own opinions on this very intimate expression. This is Maggie's analysis of the dream:

"The bikes are, I think, cycles of my life that are finished. I've passed through them. My grandmother was really quite a socialite and very artistic. She was stern but a good teacher for me. She represents the wisdom of the elders for me.

In reality her black and white Studebaker was her prized possession. I was stunned that she gave me the keys. I didn't get afraid when the brakes and the steering didn't work because I knew that I could direct the car with my attention."

We now see the process of healing accelerate and deepen. The patient becomes much happier, more social, and her dreams indicate a movement towards individuation. While her own interpretation of the dream is of greatest importance, it is useful to add that vehicles in dreams, especially automobiles and airplanes that are being driven by the dreamer, are often signs of the transpersonal self. The connection with and allowing oneself to be guided by this larger inner wisdom is an important part of the individuation process.

The car in this dream is black and white, representing the opposites, the ever present reality of life. The black and white car that is steered by her own intention represents her ability to manoeuvre through these polarities. She is beginning to realize that there is a force that is beyond "hands-on" effort that propels her through her life.

Awareness of a positive force that guides an individual through their life is an experience of great value and comfort. One could say that it is the basis of mental health. Hahnemann related it to a state of health, where the life force of an individual was flowing freely.

> *"In the healthy human state, the spirit-like life force (autocracy) that enlivens the material organism as dynamis, governs without restriction and keeps all parts of the organism in admirable, harmonious, vital operation, as regards to both feelings and functions, so that our indwelling, rational spirit can freely avail itself of this living, healthy instrument for the higher purpose of our existence."* [7]

Maggie had, at the time of the Studebaker dream, been treated with homeopathy for just under two years. She has continued ongoing treatment in order to maximize her potential and to bring her gifts to the world. She is very excited about sharing her story with others so they might benefit from it.

3   Conclusion

When a homeopath is open to hearing and considering all that the patient says, then he or she will discover the previously hidden and unspoken truth that leads to effective therapy. This may include the nuances and sensations of physical symptoms, early childhood emotions, fears and anxieties. The symbolic expressions of the psyche that are usually not allowed to surface begin to emerge. These symbolic expressions are sometimes seen in physical symptoms or in waking fantasies and delusions, but they are most often found in dreams.

As we have seen, dreams can be an important part of homeopathic therapy. When homeopathic remedies are used we do not need to rely only on the therapeutic alliance itself -- we have medicines that will act in accord with the deepest expression of the psyche. In this way, homeopathy can help to shorten the period of time required for healing of mental and emotional disorders. It contains the possibility of helping those who may not be able to be helped by other forms of therapy, and is able to go beyond the treatment of symptoms into transpersonal development.

Given the value of dreams in homeopathic treatment, homeopaths would do well to study Jung's method of dream analysis. Along with learning the technique of dream analysis it would also be helpful for the homeopath to journal and analyze his or her dreams by these methods, as familiarization with one's own psyche is an essential step in working with dreams. The ideal would be for those with training in Jungian psychology to teach these methods in greater depth in homeopathic seminars.

It would also be useful for Jungian analysts to understand more about homeopathy and how it can help someone in analysis break through to deeper levels of healing and, in some cases, allow for healing that would be otherwise unlikely. In general, communication between the professions of homeopathy and Jungian psychology would greatly enhance the benefits of these therapies in the treatment of mental illness.

References

[1] Jung C. G. (1989) *Memories, Dreams, Reflections*, New York: Vintage Books: p117

[2] Hahnemann, Samuel (1996) *Organon of the Medical Art*, Ed. Wenda B. O'Reilly. Washington: Birdcage Books: p204

[3] Ibid. p205

[4] Ibid. p62

[5] Vermeulen, Frans (2002) *Prisma, The Arcana of Materia Medica Illuminated*. Haarlem: Emryss bv Publishers: pp1232-1243

[6] Tumminello, Peter (2005) *Twelve Jewels*. Bondi Junction: The Medicine Way: pp13-53

[7] Hahnemann, Samuel (1996) *Organon of the Medical Art*, Ed. Wenda B. O'Reilly. Washington: Birdcage Books: p65

Chapter 14
Homeopathy as a Tool for Personal Evolution

Hannah Albert, ND

Hannah Albert, ND
Fertile Ground Homeopathy
USA
E-mail: DrAlbert@HannahAlbertND.com
www.HannahAlbertND.com.

Abstract

This chapter discusses ways that homeopathic treatment can enhance personal growth, ease resolution of trauma, and promote creativity and self-expression as a complement to psychotherapeutic treatment. It also touches on the incidence of cancer as a symbol of thwarted self-expression.

1   Introduction

In my role as a Naturopathic Physician and homeopath, I treat teens to people into their sixties for a wide range of mostly chronic health concerns. My approach as a healer is always to identify "in what way is this person expressing his/her dis-ease?" aside from specific physical symptoms. Choice of words, body language, and style of dress can provide a plethora of information - even within the first five minutes of a visit. By allowing each person to reveal her "story" at her own pace, I'm able to perceive how she has characteristically responded to the challenges of life. By the time our visit concludes, I've listened to many significant aspects of the patient's life from birth to the present moment. Embedded in that unique landscape are patterns and symbols that lend clues to the "essence of cure."

2   Methodology

I will attempt to distinguish my method from the psychotherapist's, which often includes inquiry into "why" the patient is unhappy, confused, or anxious [1] followed by many sessions of discovery over weeks and months. The psychotherapist's goal might be to guide the patient towards understanding herself through choices made at various stages of life, for example. An area of conflict such as role, relationship, or work might be addressed in a variety of ways such as speaking and reflecting, art or sandplay therapy, Jungian archetypal investigation, or some other methodology. The patient then achieves a greater sense of self and heals through understanding and acceptance, goal-setting, and/or various creative techniques.

My intention in the first visit is to tread lightly – to leave no footprints whenever possible - while watching for the patient's "brand" and identifying core patterns. Rather than act as teacher or guide of new behaviours or habits, my primary technique is listening. My role as a compassionate witness allows the patient to feel safe letting her guard down and share what underlies her chief complaint. I find the patient will tell me precisely what needs to be cured as long as I allow her to "run the show."

2.1 What I seek in the interview

My mentor, Louis Klein, uses the term "inbegriff" [2] or impression to describe what is sought in the interview process. By using intuition and observatory skills, I'm able to identify the underlying essence of what needs to be healed. While patients are not always aware of what that might be, my job is to perceive it without the patient feeling invaded or pressured. My prescription will need to match the tone, texture, and totality of each patient's expression. If the medicine does not resonate with the patient's energetic matrix, no response occurs. If the prescription is only partially accurate, whatever is being overlooked tends to make itself more pronounced. In this way the patient either consciously or unconsciously presents further clues towards an accurate prescription.

2.2 What happens with treatment

What homeopathy accomplishes is a kind of "reorganization of the vital force" by presenting information to the energy field. The treatment acts profoundly on the physical, mental, emotional, and spiritual levels of the individual's being for months and even years. As in psychotherapy, layers of transformation occur over time and a series of prescriptions might be needed. Homeopathy can promote the shedding of old skins; the start of an inner blossoming; an unfolding of clarity. The resulting changes of state help the patient move towards self-discovery, inner harmony, and greater authenticity.

The beauty of homeopathy is that it is not just a vehicle for physical healing, mental maturation, or emotional and spiritual growth. Homeopathic treatment is all of the above: a modality for personal evolution on all levels. In this way it enhances and complements many modes of language-focused psychotherapy. Cognitive and emotional lessons from psychotherapy can be accessed newly, promoting a more rapid yet gentle progress for the patient. I would like to use a case to illustrate these introductory comments, below.

3 Case Study

G is a pleasant 29-year-old height-weight proportionate Caucasian female who comes to see me for "help with self-care." She works with children and is in a monogamous, stable relationship. She complains of chronic migraines that began in childhood and recurrent UTIs (urinary tract infections) that in the past had progressed into kidney infections. Her menses have always been exhausting, erratic and unpredictable. She finds it difficult to feed herself, not ever fully being aware of what is "good" for her body. She is prone to constipation, has a touchy stomach, and experiments with many diets. She feels unbalanced, and often reaches for something to stimulate or relax in order to get through each day. Her sleep is marked with vivid, disruptive dreams and her days are often filled with anxiety.

G describes her childhood as chaotic. Both parents were overextended and often unavailable, literally and figuratively. Her mother had undergone invasive surgery for a mysterious cancer two months before G was conceived, and my patient remembered her mother always being in "some kind of cancer treatment" until her untimely death ten years now past. Along the way her father was also treated for testicular cancer, the details of which were not discussed. Denial of the parents' health and its impact on the patient and her sister was consistent with the suppression of emotions that guided all family "communication." She remembered feeling "zoned out" and extremely moody as a child. By high school she was used to having "no boundaries" yet also being under strict prohibitions: she was not allowed to cut her hair, which was long enough to sit on.

The family moved mid-school-year when she was nine, at which time a family friend sexually molested her (G kept this secret). G describes some of her past relationships as being with abusive or drug-addicted partners. Her current housemate is a friend with alcoholic tendencies for whom she caretakes. She had explored art psychotherapy and delved into yoga in more recent years as a means of resolving some of her past traumas. In spite of the above experiences and her chaotic family life, the patient reported being "pretty even keeled", having only "surface-level mood swings, and pretty even temperament." She sought my help to leave behind a legacy of erratic and ungrounded choices and to "build sustainability" in her life.

G's delivery of her story was rambling, non-chronological, and interrupted by random thoughts as they floated into her mind. She was wearing a dark shirt and pants with no makeup and little adornment of any kind. Her hair was pulled back with an elastic band. Eye contact was direct when she wasn't looking down at the floor or up at the ceiling. She chose a plain white cup for her tea.

3.1 Assessment

My observation of G was of a cautious, sensitive woman with an inner chaos she struggled to keep beneath the surface but whose symptoms belied the calm exterior. Her physical attractiveness was subdued, ostensibly so she could more easily stay in the background and embrace the role of caretaker - to her family, the children she worked with, and many of the relationships in her past. Her skills for self-care were grossly underdeveloped, and I assessed the gravity of her symptoms to be substantial for a 29-year-old woman. I assessed this patient to have a high chance of developing cancer at an early age, so deeply was she imprinted by both her family history of cancer, her lack of willingness to take basic care of herself, lack of boundaries with others, and her own unresolved traumas around sexuality and identity, as well as displaying an obvious endocrinological imbalance. Many studies in the science of psycho-neuro-immunology have demonstrated the relationship of trauma, abnormal immunology, and imbalances in the neuro-endocrine system [3]. I assessed this patient's state as being "in the cancer miasm."

3.2 About miasms

In homeopathic language, one way we can describe a person's state of being is to use the word "miasm." This term refers to the energetic and/or physical imprints of a disease process or organism that remain after a person has received treatment or has had an experience that exposed him or her repeatedly to that substance. The remaining residual influence can persist energetically as part of a pattern of functioning that becomes grafted onto a person [4]. For example, having a family history of heart disease or cancer; being treated repeatedly with antibiotics; exposure to bacteria or viruses during travel or through sexual contact; or even living in close proximity to someone that has a serious or chronic condition caused by some type of infectious agent. In some cases it could be that a viral agent remains in the body while no longer expressing symptoms for long periods of time, such as Human Papilloma Virus or Herpes Simplex. We now know that some viruses and bacteria can be causative agents of DNA damage leading to cancer. The viral or bacterial agent itself is expressing its evolutionary agenda through symptoms.

Homeopaths Louis Klein [4,5], Dr. Jan Scholten [6], and Dr. Rajan Sankaran [8,9] among others have contributed to my understanding of the mental/emotional state of the cancer miasm: that of one who has an impossible task to achieve - requiring a kind of superhuman effort - to avoid a feeling of failure. The source of these feelings might come from a childhood of being overly controlled, having very high parental expectations, or from experiencing denial, disrespect, or suppression at a formative age of one's own ego development.

Klein has discussed the cancer theme around the idea of having taken on someone else's agenda or idea of how to live, leading to confusion and an inauthentically lived life. The ensuing inner chaos that develops over many years coincides with a need to maintain tight control over the impression one makes on the partner, parent, or teacher the patient is trying to please. The need to present a pleasing impression to everyone can develop into a perfectionism, a tendency to doubt one's self and "give too much."

This behaviour is an exhausting pursuit leading to a refined yet erratic energy level characteristic of this type of patient. Klein uses the analogy of the automobile governor that helps to maintain the smooth functioning of its engine; in the patient the governor is broken, leading to wildly shifting levels of energy, cognition, and symptomatology.

Scholten sees a relationship between creativity (various artistic and ideological pursuits), sexuality, and cancer, each of which concern individuation and expression of the self.
"The strongest creative power in a body (is) found in the ovaries and testes... the sperm and egg are capable of growing into a complete body." [6] On the microcosmic level the cancer cell itself has lost its way; has stopped differentiating and doesn't mature. The themes of perfectionism, artistic nature, and suppressed personality central to the remedy *Carcinosinum* are echoed in the group of remedies related to problems with performance and creativity.

Sankaran sees the situation as of a person having an upbringing of prolonged fear or unhappiness, where "one's survival depends upon performing tasks which one feels incapable of performing. There is a need to be something that is almost beyond one's capacity. The patients stretch themselves to the utmost in the hope of success, because to them failure means death and destruction ... The need for control over oneself and over one's surroundings is tremendous, as is the need to keep order in the midst of chaos. The disease cancer itself represents a breakdown of all control mechanisms within the body, with chaotic behaviour of the cells." [7]

It is interesting to note how, in U.S. culture, patients are often lauded for their bravery, cooperation without complaint, willingness to "battle" with a smile, and avoid showing any weakness or suffering. There is the popular "Livestrong" branding of the cancer industry brought to us by Lance

Armstrong; pink ribbons, hair ornaments worn by sweet little girls, have become the symbol for the "fight against breast cancer."

3.3 Homeopathic prescribing

In homeopathy, a person's uniqueness is everything. Compared with conventional medicine in which unique or unusual symptoms are typically ignored, homeopathy is all about how each patient presents her "dis-ease" in a characteristic manner. In this paradigm, the particular way in which a person expresses her physical symptoms also reflects the "totality" of a core belief system. Scholten suggests that disease symptoms could be seen as a strategy for expressing ourselves. A good homeopath sees how everything "in the system" resonates with a specific pattern and then matches those elements with a homeopathic remedy embodying those qualities.

During the process of homeopathic treatment, patients may need medicines that contain the energetic imprint of a bacteria or virus, or plant, animal, mineral, or other substances. Prescriptions are chosen based on a number of factors. There may be history of injury or trauma, often indicating an initial plant medicine; one or more miasms related to personal or family history of disease, or "constitution" which represents what could be described as the patient's core, basic state unimpeded by trauma or miasm.

The order in which these layers are treated is based upon presenting symptoms. Homeopaths vary in their approaches and philosophies as to the validity and efficacy of the ideas presented above.

In the above case, I saw this patient as actually lacking an identity to a certain degree. Both her physical presentation and the way she described her life resonated with the idea of cancer, the unexpressed and over-controlled. In contrast to the many patients I see that express strong opinions, dress with a particular style or "brand," and exude a presence born of life experiences that include failures and successes, this patient was like a canvas waiting to be painted. Her family history contained cancer, and she presented with many hormonally-related symptoms, so I prescribed one dose of Carcinosinum 200C. This remedy (nosode) is prepared homeopathically from breast cancer tissue, and the results of giving it in this case were dramatic.

3.4 Follow-up

First follow-up

One month later, the patient arrived unsure if the remedy had changed anything. She wore a bright green shirt and large earrings and beamed as she sat down.

She reported after taking the remedy of "feeling the presence of (her) mother", and of realizing it was time to live her own life. She told her mother in an internal dialogue it was time to get off her back and let her be. "I don't feel like I have to be the one in control," she added. She went on to report having met for dinner with her father for the first time in ten years and had an honest conversation about her mother's death and discussed how they could spread her mother's ashes.

Her period had come within 30 days for the first time since menarche. She reported having extremely bad cramps for one day with repeated vomiting, like she was "purging." She realized the next day how toxic she had been feeling all the time.

She had continued to shift towards a nourishing diet and prepare meals for the week with her partner's help. The planning felt like a huge task, and there was internal conflict with which she felt uncomfortable. It brought up memories of being fed Pop Tarts for breakfast and anger came with it. She had memories of been discouraged from eating healthy foods.

She felt strong emotions and noticed she was "really in (her) body." She was quite agitated about that, recognizing she often fought to get out of her body. Her partner actually told her that she was calmer, and asked "I don't know what that doctor gave you - but can I have one of those Yoda pills?"

After she shared all of the above, we agreed that the remedy "may have done something." The plan was to wait another three weeks and return for bodywork to help integrate the feelings, sensations, and emotions of her shifting state.

Second follow-up
She said she had gone for an acupuncture session because she was constipated, felt anxiety, couldn't put herself to bed and was "amped" like she used to be at sixteen. The practitioner suggested she was having manic symptoms.

Another period had come and gone, and in contrast to the previous month, she had the most minimal PMS, breast tenderness, and cramping that she could remember.

In the last month, she recalled the insanity that ensued when she and her family moved to a new home in the middle of her fourth grade year. The home was shared with a family that had nine cats and a child with brain cancer. Previous to the move she had tested as gifted in school; after the move she couldn't remember her multiplication tables. As emotions came up she said, "I'm starting to tell myself I DO have the capacity to do many things."

She remembered being on vacation as a young child, being fed a lot of sugar and not sleeping, after which she would be vomiting and needed to stay in a dark room all day. This pattern was repeated for almost 20 years. She expressed some discomfort at her current weight - which is a healthy one - because she was "not used to taking up space as an adult." In the past her weight had fluctuated from 115 to 160 pounds and back.

I noticed after giving her an osteopathic-type treatment she experienced a new kind of comfort with the way she moved and held herself.

Third follow-up
G wore a black dress with ruffles and lace and several pieces of jewellery.
She reported some itching in her ears and a bit of constipation related to her periods. Her general energy level was so much better, very consistent. She was excited to read books about nutrition and explore subjects using logic as she embraced her resurfacing cognitive skills. It was as if a light had gone on.

Her sleep was good although she said it was hard to wind down because of the environment with her alcoholic roommate. She reported that as she'd started to care more about her own needs and focus on healing her body, the roommate had grown resentful and belligerent and the tension was high. The roommate was to move out in three weeks and G's partner would be moving in. She felt lucky to have a partner who appreciated her not for how she sacrificed herself but rather as someone to have fun with and learn and grow together.

In the past, she "would have disengaged if uncomfortable situations arose" but she was no longer using avoidance as a strategy. She felt a lot of grief around her father's lack of communication but persisted in sharing her feelings with him. She noticed in many ways she was drawing the line in order to take care of herself first. Being selfish, as she called it, was starting to feel good instead of provoking anxiety and guilt. She was starting to notice how extremely demanding she had been of herself.

G is experiencing an awakening I would describe as a personal evolution. Her internal life has radically shifted in the four months since she began treatment, and her external world is reacting to those changes. It is not all positive feedback, and G is feeling challenged. But she expresses excitement about her future and the possibilities for living a more satisfying and balanced life that holds space for real feelings, the forgiveness of mistakes, and joy that comes from just being herself. This patient has been treated for six months as of late September 2009.

4   Conclusion

As suggested above, homeopathy has the potential to assist the patient's progress in psychotherapy while treating physical pathology. By recognizing the underlying cause of distress and symptoms, a homeopath can establish and enhance healing by prescribing a series of homeopathic medicines. These medicines act as a kind of resonant energy field to catalyze a change of state. Because homeopathic medicines do not cause side effects, they do not require cessation of pharmaceutical prescriptions. Treatment is complementary to other methods, yet also stands alone in its efficacy. Because many disease states begin through exposure to viral and bacterial agents programmed with an evolutionary agenda, homeopathy can treat the mind and body together through a miasmatic approach. In this way, generations of healing can occur in one lifetime.

References

[1] Not all psychotherapists focus on the question of "why" or practise lengthy courses of treatment, but for the sake of differentiating my method I have chosen to focus on a common experience

[2] 'Inbegriff' - http://translation.babylon.com/German; n. embodiment, concrete manifestation, personification in concrete form, epitome, exemplar

[3] In clinical practice patients with emotional distress and reproductive system imbalances commonly present with a history of compromised immunity and thyroid/ HPA axis disorders

[4] Klein, Louis (2009) *Miasms and Nosodes; Origins of Disease Volume 1*, Kandern (Germany): Narayana Publishers, pp. 9-40

[5] Klein, Louis (2001-2009) Class notes from the Homeopathic Master Clinician Course and additional seminars

[6] Jan Scholten (1996) *Homeopathy and the Elements*, Utrecht (Netherlands): Stichting Alonnissos, pp. 525-530

[7] Rajan Sankaran, Nosodes Notes: Carsinosin, ReferenceWorks software, San Rafael CA: KHA

[8] Rajan Sankaran (1994) *The Substance of Homeopathy*. Mumbai: Homeopathic Medical Publishers, p. 55

[9] Rajan Sankaran (1991) *The Spirit of Homeopathy*. Mumbai: Homeopathic Medical Publishers, pp. 274-276

Chapter 15
Treatment of Mental Diseases, A Clinical Diary

Dr. Seema, BHMS MD Hom [dip IACH Greece]

Dr. Seema, BHMS MD Hom [dip IACH Greece]
Centre for Classical Homeopathy
#3446, 1st F Cross, next to Bunts Sangha
Vijayanagar, Bangalore
560040 Karnataka
India
E-mail: info@centreforclassicalhomeopathy.com, bhatseema@hotmail.com
Website: www.centreforclassicalhomeopathy.com

Abstract
This chapter is an excerpt from a busy clinical practice in Bangalore and illustrates the variety in presentation of psychiatric cases and the scope of homeopathy in truly identifying and solving these problems. The cases are presented in a diary like fashion so the reader understands the flow of thought of the physician and can arrive at the correct analysis of the case themselves.

1 Introduction

All living beings in this world are unique in their form and function. The human is unique because he possesses a reasoning mind as well as highly evolved emotions. His existence involves the exercise of these components and his thoughts and feelings make him the epitome of evolution. Yet, even these highly abstract organs of the human organism are susceptible to derangement as is his earthly body. This derangement comes at a great cost: life is compromised at the highest level and living becomes mere existence.

Man has sought to alleviate his suffering in the human mind through various means. Many methods of rearranging the mind have been devised. The claim of homeopathy to be able to "cure" when compared to the "rearrangement" of other methods deserves a hearing from humanity.

My first association with **mental disorders** came when I was still a student at the university. I worked as a volunteer in a school for autistic children. Since then I have explored different means for helping the mentally disturbed and challenged individuals. Eventually I realized that the best answer for most of these people was the very system that I was learning: **homeopathy**. Over the years, my personal experience along with that of my colleagues and that of my teachers have shown me that homeopathy gets to the root of the cause and brings about a change in the very depths of the person. I have studied patients who are on homeopathic treatment and others who only received regular psychiatric treatment. The difference in most cases is that those on homeopathic treatment respond immediately, with no remnant side effects or dulling of the senses. In other words, the result was harmony throughout and return of their original creativity as well as clarity. This observation motivated me to document cases on video or paper for scientific study. Today, even though far from claiming to have a complete answer, I can say with conviction that homeopathy can often offer a far better solution than the regular system of psychiatric health care.

2 Excerpts from the case diary

Here, I present some cases that have shown exceptional improvement under homeopathic treatment. These cases have been treated by my husband Dr. Mahesh and myself at the Centre for Classical Homeopathy, Bangalore, India. It is intended that these examples serve the purpose of understanding and analyzing the psychiatric cases as well as to demonstrate the scope of homeopathy in such conditions.

[The symptoms that help in repertorisation are highlighted in **bold** and the essence of the case is written in ***bold italics***, wherever applicable; the repertory used in all these cases is Synthesis repertory 7.1]

Case 1

I first saw this woman in 2002. She had been residing in a mental asylum for over twenty years. She had been diagnosed with paranoid schizophrenia that began towards the end of her pregnancy. Her family first noticed she was indifferent to her baby and this situation advanced to full fledged schizophrenia. The product of this pregnancy was a son who was then twenty years old when he brought her to the centre. When the case was taken, she was very **indifferent** to the whole situation. She muttered to herself and was quite oblivious to the surroundings. Other than this she **wept** incessantly with no provocation. She had little else to say except that she had recurrent **headaches in the left forehead, just above the eyes.** She asked for no particular food and did not talk much to others. On interviewing the family, there was no other information except that she had ceased to communicate and cried a lot.

Sepia 200C and later 1M (single dose each) were prescribed on the basis of this presentation and within seven months she was able to do her household chores. She was well except for a headache (over the left eyebrow) that troubled her often. This also went away after another six months. She did not require any other remedy while in her mentally disordered state. The understanding in this case was that she had entered a state of indifference to her environment and did not emotionally transact with anyone. But, at the same time she would cry for hours and this indicated that the emotions were not dry or hard yet but did not flow easily. Her headache was also characteristic of Sepia. The prescription of Sepia was not based on repertorisation but on the essence of the case. There was *stasis* in her emotionality and she wept for reasons she did not know [Vithoulkas, 1988]. Yet there are some rubrics that we may consider for academic purpose here:

- Mind, indifference, children to her
- Mind, weeping, causeless
- Head, pain, forehead in, left side

The above case brings to my mind another case of Sepia where the lady suddenly showed **no interest** in her work and became aloof from her family. She also wept without cause and became very **rude to her family**. During the consultation, she answered no questions but only **wept**.

Case 2

This man suffered with chronic fatigue and was even hospitalized because of extreme **exhaustion** but no further diagnosis could account for his state. In addition to his physical exhaustion, the man made no effort mentally or emotionally. He seemed exhausted on those levels as well and in fact seemed more exhausted on the emotional level than any other. He was not even interested in getting well.

Phosphoricum acidum 1M was prescribed and he miraculously recovered from this state. He is presently well and has not required any other remedy after this. As in the previous case, it is the essence that directs us towards Phosphoricum acidum. The man had no strength mentally, emotionally or physically. In addition, there was not even the interest to get well. Such **apathy** and exhaustion points to Phosphoricum acidum [Vithoulkas, 1988].

Case 3

The daughter brought this woman for an appointment for **cellulitis** of her forearm. She had been in the hospital due to an acute illness and was given intravenous antibiotics. The area of the intravenous catheter had inflamed and spread to the whole forearm. She was a diabetic, taking insulin and her blood sugar was quite high. After I spoke to the daughter I asked the patient to come in. She came and sat in the consultation for about five minutes, the whole time resting her head on the table and not bothering to answer any of my questions. After five minutes she told her daughter that she would wait in the car and subsequently walked off. The daughter told me that the lady had been like this for several years now and did not respond much to their care and concern. She spoke very little and was exhausted all the time.

We considered the following rubrics for this case:

- Mind, answering, aversion to
- Urine, sugar
- Mind, indifference, apathy

Phosphoricum acidum 30C was prescribed, repeating once a day for one week (followed by increasing with two potencies at intervals of a month – 32C, 34C etc also once daily for a week), and she came out of her apathy. But an interesting phenomenon occurred with this lady. Every time we gave her a dose of Phosphoricum acidum, her sugar would drop and she would come out of her apathy and be happy but after some time she would have severe haemorrhage in the urine. At such time she would either be hospitalized or we would prescribe another remedy and she would relapse back into the apathy. This went on for quite some time before we realized that her haemorrhage was being suppressed.

Then, the next time the Phosphoricum acidum brought her out of apathy and the haemorrhage set in, *Erigeron* 30C once a day for five days was prescribed. Here the pure haemorrhage from the urinary bladder with no associated symptoms led us to prescribe a remedy based on pathology rather than on symptoms.

This time she did not relapse back into apathy and the haemorrhage did not recur. We must wait and see what level gets affected next. It has been three months after Erigeron now, in total about three years of follow up of the case.

The extent and character of apathy in this case were responsible for selecting Phosphoricum acidum, coupled with the fact that the diabetes was progressed, which is a pathology covered by Phosphoricum acidum [Murphy, 1994].

Case 4

This boy was brought when he was three and a half years old. He was diagnosed with Autism Spectrum Disorder. On taking his case it was revealed that the features suggestive of the disorder increased **after** his booster dose of Hepatitis B **vaccination**. The boy made eye contact but did not sustain it. He spoke irrelevantly and was **hyperactive**. He was so difficult to manage that if they left the door ajar even for a little time he would run into the street. He had **violent impulses** at times and would hurt anybody around him. He liked **salty food and sweets**. His thirst was moderate and he was **restless during sleep**. He **perspired heavily** and his mother complained that his urine was **offensive**. His motor milestones seemed normal except for **speech**, which was **delayed**. There was also **bedwetting**.

These indicated *Mercurius solubilis* especially since it was speech that was delayed and he had violent impulses at times when he seemed blinded by rage. The restlessness was also severe. He received Mercurius solubilis 200C one dose almost every month for over three years during which time he steadily improved in terms of speech and writing. His hyperactivity lessened and he was permitted to attend a normal school. The bedwetting also stopped. He slowly began showing features such as possessiveness about his things and was hysterical to some extent in between. He mingled easily at school and was responsive to emotional transactions at home. The boy first came in 2004 and is doing well now in 2009. After Mercurius solubilis he became very independent and was able to go shopping by himself.

After some time there was a change in his presentation and he began to crave oranges a lot. *Medorrhinum* 200C was then given. Medorrhinum is the gonorrhoea nosode and a strong carving for **oranges** is one of the keynotes leading to its prescription. The changes became even more established as the facial grimaces went away and his interaction became totally normal. After Medorrhinum he also developed a thick yellow discharge from his nose that continued for some time. Later he entered a phase during which he craved onions and was given *Thuja* 200C based on the following rubrics:

- Nose, discharge, thick
- Nose, discharge, yellow
- Generals, food and drinks, onion, desires

Thuja brought out fears in him, which had not been pronounced before. He now feared the dark and dogs and was having nightmares. He had become very talkative and wanted the light on to sleep. He was given *Stramonium* 200C, one dose, based on the following rubrics:

- Mind, Fear, dark
- Mind, Light, desire for
- Mind, Fear, animals, dogs
- Dreams, nightmares
- Mind, Loquacity

A month later, he came out with very high fever accompanied by difficulty in walking. This suggested not just a fever but cerebellitis. He was unable to walk in a straight line and we videoed this state to compare a day later. He asked for **lemonade** during the fever and hence was given *Belladonna* 200C. The fever came down immediately. We had to video the boy three days later just to record the drastic changes in him. He walked freely now. But after this phase was over he relapsed back into the *Stramonium* phase and was given a dose of *Stramonium* 200C again. Presently he is keeping well and we have not heard of any more complaints. It has been over a year since the last remedy was given. The boy has been treated for about five years altogether.

Case 5

There come some times in one's life when one wonders about the dark side of the human being. This happened to me when this lady, complaining of **sleeplessness** and some **obsessive negative thoughts**, sought my consultation. She was suffering a lot and was dissatisfied with the kind of answers or counselling that she received anywhere else. She then came across an article of mine on the Internet and approached me for treatment. It was quite a difficult case to take because she knew her diagnosis of Obsessive Compulsive Disorder and told me only symptoms of the diagnosis. Then, after some time, when she realized that I was not interested in the diagnosis as much as I was interested in her, she began to tell me her story. She was abused sexually when she was only five years old by a close relative. Even now she has very bad reactions and turmoil within her whenever she has to face him. She has a loving husband and a wonderful family and yet she could not come out of this abyss. She kept having **nightmares** about bathrooms (where she was abused) and felt a total wreck.

She said that everyone she spoke to concerning this problem, be it a psychiatrist or a homeopath, told her that she had to let go of her negative thoughts and should take life positively. This she just could not do. Then, when I told her that she must stop attempting to do such things and let the remedy take course, she was heartened. While taking the case, she also said that she was **scared to sleep alone** because she would **wake up with terror** in the night. So she went with her husband wherever his work took him. This was the clinching point for me to prescribe *Stramonium* 10M, one dose [Vithoulkas 1988].

The rubrics that helped in this prescription were:

- Mind, ailments from, fright
- Mind, fears, dark of
- Dreams, nightmares

- Mind, thoughts, repetition of
- Mind, fears, alone being, night
- Mind, clinging

She called me the next day and said that for the first time in her life she had fulfilling sleep without the aid of any tranquilizers. She continued to improve over the next six months, and slowly a new picture surfaced. She now did not suffer because of sleeplessness or from her memories but was now caught in a **moral dilemma** [Vithoulkas 1997] which involved feelings of guilt and righteousness, and a strong feeling that she was doing something very wrong. She also exhibited severe headaches and felt that her **brain was moving** within [Vithoulkas 1997].

At this point I prescribed *Cyclamen* 200C one dose, based on the keynote of a moving sensation in the brain and also the essence of a moral dilemma. For seven days after *Cyclamen*, she wept for hours without reason. She even felt exhausted and wanted to leave all work and take rest. I was happy with this reaction and asked her to wait. A week later, she was free from her suffering and now complains mostly of physical problems. It has been two months now after *Cyclamen* and a total of about eight months of treatment.

This sort of reaction is the best that a homeopath can get in a psychiatric case. Many times when the right remedy is given the patients complain of a desire to weep without reason, to withdraw from all the work and to sleep. The emotions are healed this way. After this phase is over, they come out with (often severe) physical problems and this indicates to us that the problems have left the psyche and have shifted to a more superficial level. This is the only way that real cure can take place.

Case 6

This man was thirty three years old and did nothing. He did not even get out of the house. He could not go to the shop that was at the corner of the block. He refused to take up any kind of responsibility or go to work. He had tried doing many things initially but had eventually given up everything and just stayed at home. The observation was that he **could not stand to leave the house** [Vithoulkas 1988] (agoraphobia). He could not go away from his territory. He would suffer panic attacks and even fainted in such situations when he was forced to go a little further. With this indication, and on delving further, it was revealed that he had received anti-rabies vaccination after a dog bite in childhood. This confirmed the prescription.

Lyssinum 200C (rabies nosode) was prescribed. One week later, he went to visit his brother who lived twenty kilometres away. He also started taking up responsibilities and now goes about independently. Lyssinum has this tremendous phobia to leave the house or familiar surroundings and go outside (agoraphobia). It is over one year now since the prescription and he continues to do well.

Case 7

Then there was this case that one of the students had taken and brought as a paper case to the centre. The lady had severe suicidal depression and was on regular antidepressants. Despite the medications, she was not well enough to be left alone for any amount of time. If left alone, she would immediately resort to some sort of suicidal act. There was no consistency in the mode she sought for executing this. On enquiring deeper, there were not any symptoms to rely on except that the student had elicited the symptom that the lady **did not feel pain easily** [Kent 1996] when hurt physically. She narrated few instances where the lady should have had severe pain but did not complain.

On this basis, *Opium* 1M was prescribed as painlessness is a keynote of Opium and in this case there were no other symptoms to form a better picture.

Within a month, the lady began to do her household chores and was doing well. After two months, she complained of an earache and discharge from her ear. The student who had initially brought the case prescribed *Natrum sulphuricum* for this. The following day the lady ran off and attempted suicide on the railway track. Somebody saw her and brought her home. Then it became even more difficult to control her suicidal depression than before. Opium had to be prescribed again to bring her back to normal. Of course she later had many more physical symptoms that had to be dealt with very carefully in order to avoid the relapse of depression. This case especially demonstrates the problem of over prescribing. We must assess at every change as to what is happening and whether the situation calls for the next prescription or not. If we falter, the best we can do is cause a relapse. At the worst, a change of symptoms occurs, going on complicating the case even further.

Case 8

This gentleman came for treatment of **diabetes mellitus**, which had been diagnosed one year ago. He had tried homeopathy elsewhere during this time, but with no results and his blood sugar continued to rise. He was told that if he could not get his glucose to come down he would have to take allopathic drugs, which he wanted to avoid. When I took his case, I was baffled; there were no symptoms at all. He had high blood sugar and that was it. The daughter who accompanied him told me that there had been some emotional problems between them during the past year. She thought he **felt he was losing her,** because he sometimes acted very **hysterical**. She even narrated an incident that happened a few days prior: he had fainted after an argument with her and she had to agree to his terms. She wanted to marry and he was not happy about it. He did not say this directly but made it evident with his behaviour. This brought to my mind the possibility of *Ignatia* or *Pulsatilla*. On delving further, there were no symptoms to support Pulsatilla but he had aversion to fruits, which is a confirmative keynote for Ignatia.

Rubrics that further confirmed Ignatia are:

- Mind, consolation aggravates
- Generals, fainting, hysterical

Ignatia 200C was prescribed and he came down with an acute cold and fever which he did not remember having in recent years. After that the blood sugar dropped and stayed normal. A fortnight later he complained of severe pan in the right hypochondrium. I knew he had been diagnosed with cholelithiasis earlier and that this was a good sign. I put him on placebo and the next day he passed stones in his stools. So just one remedy had taken him this far from the original diabetes that he came with. This case is an example of how depression can present as a corporeal disease and how it is upon us to find the real pathology in the person.

Case 9

This is one of my most recent cases. The lady was around forty years old. She complained of some joint pains and vague body aches. Her main problem however was her tormenting thoughts. She always felt that **something bad was going to happen**. She was always depressed and down and had episodes of not wanting to do anything. She had lost her son twelve years ago and still suffered from this as if it were yesterday. There was no hardness in her emotionality or any difficulty in emotional expression. Her problem was that she could sense that something was going to happen to someone and became even more terrified when those things did happen. **She asked me if she was going mad**. I assured her, 'not yet'. She was an **obese** person as well. But this was not enough yet to confirm the prescription I had in mind. On enquiring she revealed that she was very **sympathetic** indeed. The character of her sympathy was that she could not even stand to hear bad or gory things happening to others. This helped me prescribe *Calcarea carbonica* 200C, one dose, though I was sure she would need *Carcinosinum* sooner or later with her clairvoyant abilities and history of cancer in the immediate family.

Rubrics:

* Fear, insanity
* Generalities, obesity
* Mind, ailments from bad news

Calcarea carbonica brought out an insect bite like rash all over the body in one week's time. Her daughter reported that for the first time in all these years her mother had not suffered so much on the anniversary of the death of her son. She finally seemed to have accepted the fact. Also when I saw her the following month, she looked free of her own suffering, which she had been full of earlier. A total of three months have lapsed since she first approached me and now I only have to deal with her joint pains and skin rashes.

3   Conclusion

These cases are the most dramatic of the lot. The others, and they are in majority, show slow but steady improvement over the years. In the above cases, we may observe a few things. When the number of remedies indicated is less, the case has the capacity to be cured even if it is autism. This also means that the health level of such a person is better and responds very quickly to treatment. Secondly, even though counselling and training play a part in psychiatric cases, homeopathic remedies can bring about changes from very deep and the results are almost miraculous.

Today the world is wrought with practices and influences that divide the mind of man into many pieces. Nobody is sure anymore as to what is right and what is wrong. We have diluted all our morals and confused our mind in the name of modernization and freedom. But are we truly modern and free today? We are held by our own negativities as never before in the history of mankind. We have come far away from the being that nature intended us to be...we have come far away from nature itself.

This situation cannot last long, because it goes against nature. It is time we realized that there are rights and there are wrongs in everything we do. We must collect ourselves together and act as a whole being in everything we do. Our thoughts and decisions must befit our place as the most evolved organisms on Earth. This is the ultimate aim of homeopathy as well: to integrate the human being, to make him whole. This is the only way nature intended the noble science of medicine to be. Everything else is either violent or dissociative in nature. Therefore it is time we really understood what Hahnemann meant when he said "aude sapere" – shed off your fears and dare to learn the truth.

References

[1] Kent, J.T (1996) reprint edition, *Lectures on materia medica*, New Delhi: B. Jain publishers (P) Ltd

[2] Murphy, Robin (1994) *Homeopathic medical repertory*, New Delhi: Indian books and periodicals syndicate

[3] Schroyens, Frederik (1998) *Homeopaths around the world*, in Synthesis Repertorium Homeopathicum Syntheticum edition 7.1, London: Homeopathic book publishers; New Delhi: B. Jain Publishers

[4] Vithoulkas, George (1988) *Essence of materia medica*. New Delhi: B. Jain Publishers (P) Ltd

[5] Vithoulkas, George (1997) *Materia Medica Viva*, 11 volumes. Alonissos (Greece): International Academy of Classical Homeopathy

Chapter 16

Using the Tools of Traditional Chinese Medicine Diagnosis to Prescribe Homeopathic Remedies in Psychological Cases

Dr. Joseph Rozencwajg, MD PhD NMD

Dr. Joseph Rozencwajg, MD PhD NMD
44 Karina Road
New Plymouth
4312, Taranaki
New Zealand
E-mail: jroz@ihug.co.nz

Abstract

The diagnostic methods of Traditional Chinese Medicine (TCM) are particularly useful to homeopaths in situations where very intimate problems might be very difficult if not impossible for the patient to relate to the practitioner. These methods allow the homeopath to pinpoint a group of remedies or a precise remedy without the need for the patient to perform a disturbing psychological "striptease".

1   Introduction

Why would we want to use the tools of Traditional Chinese Medicine diagnosis to prescribe homeopathic remedies in psychological cases? Homeopathic case taking is a well-established technique that goes into the deepest details possible, grilling the patient almost as if he were expected to reveal state secrets and coming back again and again to the same subject until the picture is clear. Anyone who has recently listened to Rajan Sankaran[17] can have no doubt about that.

And yet ... mental, emotional and spiritual issues are not the easiest to reveal. We have all been confronted with patients giving us only partial information, coming back time and again complaining that the treatments were not helpful, only to inadvertently reveal some crucial information when saying goodbye at the end of yet another difficult session, or during a fortuitous meeting in a shop, or during a social gathering. In contrast to purely physical situations that can be seen,

---

17 Rajan Sankaran is a leading homeopath from Mumbai who has developed a new method of case taking and case-analysis built on in-depth investigation into the main symptom until the level of so-called vital sensation is reached.

palpated, measured, quantified with tests or revealed through X-Rays, CT scans or MRIs, we depend on what the patients tell us or what we can sense or suspect through body language and the use of specific words during the consultation. Even the new methods of Sankaran and Scholten[18] depend on this type of information and are therefore subjective rather than objective (at least in my perception) - and are thus useful only inasmuch as the patient is open and honest and the practitioner alert and perceptive. These two writers are modern homeopaths who have created approaches very different from the usual classical methods; they themselves warn that their methods should not be used without a proper knowledge of and grounding in classical homeopathy.

Sankaran has created a system of interview that pushes the patient to reveal his deepest inner "disturbance" which is also expressed by gestures. The practitioner needs to be able to interpret these gestures, and this is not always easy, at least to me.

Scholten correlates the state in which the patient is, his evolution in life, with the rows and columns of the periodic table, whose elements are then used to prescribe the proper remedy; here too there is a lot of interpretation to be done; as hard as I tried, I have been unable to use these techniques successfully even though I have witnessed magnificent results by other, more skilled, practitioners. Fear, shame and self-loathing are often to blame for the states of secrecy patients may maintain in a consultation, but many situations are understandable: abuse and rape victims are still hiding their history, sexual orientations are not acknowledged, violence and anger are rationalized, controlled or uncontrolled pathologies like kleptomania, pyromania and paedophilia are rarely if ever admitted.

But the body does not lie. If one can read it, it will tell what state it is in and what remedy, or at least what type of remedy, it needs. There are windows of perception into the deepest mental situations even when the physical appearance seems to deny it: the bronzed athlete or the beautiful, sexually magnetic woman can be depressed, anxious or schizophrenic. They will just hide it better than the common human.

Traditional Chinese Medicine (TCM) does not differentiate between diseases of the body and diseases of the mind or the spirit, despite what can be read in recent publications. All signs and symptoms relate to patterns of energetic disturbances that can be understood by carefully listening to the patient, not only to the words but, even more importantly, to the way they are spoken, looking at him and especially focusing on the colours and their brightness, the eyes and the tongue, and palpating with special emphasis on that trademark of TCM, the pulses. Putting this information together leads to a specific pattern of imbalance independently of what actual or factual information the patient has agreed to reveal. Put differently, similar to homeopathic case taking it is not what the patient says, it is the way he says it that becomes relevant. With this approach the typical Western classification of mental diseases, the DSM, the labelling and pigeon-holing become irrelevant.

Homeopathic remedies can also be understood in terms of TCM classification and a basic repertory can be created. Early French homeopaths and acupuncturists like de la Fuye, the creator of

---

18 Jan Scholten, a Dutch homeopath who has done ground-breaking work on remedies derived from the table of the elements.

homeosiniatry, did correlate acupuncture points with specific homeopathic remedies; yet I have not been able to find consistent literature, either in English or French, describing remedies through the TCM vision. Acupuncture was my first introduction to the world of natural medicine and I suppose I have kept this perspective while learning other methods. The concepts about remedies and TCM exposed here and in future writings are therefore my own and entirely open to modifications. Comparing the TCM diagnosis and the remedies fitting that description narrows the choice, as with the system of repertorisation[19] used by homeopaths, but might also reveal unsuspected issues that can then be discussed with the patient. I often perceive Liver pulse disturbances in many patients; if there are no obvious liver organic pathologies; I then ask them about possible suppressed or repressed anger issues. This often opens the gates to a flood of information; often they tell me it is the first time they are talking about it. And I know, I am on the right track when the pattern of the pulse changes immediately after having asked that question. Not only is this an emotionally cleansing and a first step towards cure, it often changes the homeopathic repertorisation and the final prescription.

Homeopathy and TCM are both concerned with patterns. The energetic patterns of TCM lead to the energetic diagnosis of a perturbation, opening the way to an appropriate treatment, either with herbs or acupuncture, which resets the pattern to normal. The homeopath will selectively look at the pattern of behaviour that is typical of the individual patient and correlate this information with the pattern of a remedy. But in doing this, as already described, the practitioner depends almost exclusively on non-objective information as given by the patient, his family or friends, and the interpretation made by the homeopath, which can in turn vary according to his own situation. Both approaches are highly individualised; they explore the patient, not a label; they are in my opinion different instruments analysing the status of the patient and allowing a precise treatment. Both systems need to be studied individually, in the same way we study to interpret an ECG and an X-ray separately, with both tests giving more information together than each one on its own.

I will briefly cover the concepts of Yin and Yang, the Five Elements, the Seven Emotions, Tongue and Pulse diagnosis, introducing some homeopathic remedies that can be deducted while classifying the patients accordingly. This is not meant to be the ultimate information that will allow the reader to use it immediately in practice. Its purpose is to open a window, to offer yet another possibility to fine-tune the patient's evaluation and treatment.

---

19 A repertory contains symptoms on the mental, emotional, physical and general level and lists remedies for each which are relevant with respect to the symptom. Using several rubrics from a repertory a homeopath can thus select a remedy that qualitatively and quantitatively best covers these.

2   Yin and Yang

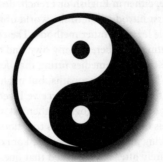

Yin and Yang are the two aspects of a totality. They represent the first basic division of a whole. Looking at the symbol, it is clear that there is no way to divide this figure into two equal parts containing one aspect exclusively; to reinforce this fact, right in the middle of the densest part of one aspect, there is a spot of the other. This represents clearly the notion that nothing is ever purely black or white, that each situation contains part of its opposite. Homeopathic remedies are no exception, as we know very well: the duality and the polarity of remedies is a clear fact. The cold *Sulphur* (usually warm), the angry, violent *Pulsatilla* (usually mild), the warm *Arsenicum album* (usually cold) (although we tend to see them as *Arsenicum iodatum*) are common patient types. What to expect in patients?

Yang is related to fire, heat, dryness, restlessness, hardening, excitement, speed, transformation, acute diseases of rapid onset with rapid changes, insomnia, red face, loud voice, talkative, craving for cold drinks and thirsty, scant urine of dark colour, constipation, a red tongue with yellow coating and a full pulse. Of course not all of those symptoms and signs will be or will have to be present at the same time to determine that we are dealing with a Yang situation.

Homeopathic remedies like *Aconite, Belladonna, Sulphur, Phosphorus, Iodum* and some aspects of *Pulsatilla* immediately come to mind.

Yin is related to water, cold, quiet, humidity, softness, slowness, chronic diseases of gradual onset and slow development, sleepiness, pale face, craving for warm drinks although not very thirsty, a weak voice and rather quiet and silent, profuse urine of a pale colour, loose stools, a pale tongue with an empty pulse.

Natrum muriaticum, Dulcamara, other aspects of *Pulsatilla* have many of those characteristics. Since Yin and Yang are interdependent and often evolving into each other, most if not all patients will have a mix of different proportions of each, especially in chronic cases. The ability to recognise either situation is therefore helpful but a rather basic and crude tool.

3   The five elements

The Five Elements are nothing more than a way to describe developments and interrelations of dynamic situations in relation to the TCM concept of organs and their functions. The use of Western words does not do justice to that concept; those words should be understood in a wider, broader sense and the reader should try to forget for a moment the English meaning of water, fire, liver, kidney etc. and "go with the flow". At first glance, the description and the terms seem archaic and unscientific. Nevertheless they are based on careful observation of nature, of the evolution of the seasons, weather, natural events, their interactions and the implications those interactions have. Without going into too much detail (otherwise this would become a full textbook of TCM), we all have observed that water is necessary for the growth of plants, hence the concept that Water is the Mother of Wood; plants and forest are often burned by fires that need wood as a combustible and are extinguished by water, bringing the concept that Fire is the Son of Wood and controlled by Water. Each organ/function is related to one of the elements; the relationships between organs and functions would be the same as those between the elements. Using the Five Elements notion helps to refine the clinical picture we are confronted with and correlate the appropriate remedies.

Wood is related to Liver and Gallbladder, the colour green (as in bile), Wind, Anger and is rather Yang. Wind is non-static, mobile, restless, changing: *Pulsatilla, Rhus toxicodendron*, come to mind. Anger can be sudden and develop rapidly; so does *Nux vomica* whose association with alcohol and drugs having a deleterious influence on the liver organ and its use as a remedy for the effects of excessive drinking (hangover) are well known.

Fire relates to the Heart and Small Intestine, the colour red, Heat and Warmth, the emotion of Joy and is the most Yang of all elements. Most of the hot remedies in homeopathy will relate to the element of Fire, like *Sulphur, Phosphorus, Iodum, Coffea*, etc ...

Earth relates to the Spleen and Stomach (digestive system at all levels, meaning also digesting ideas), the colour yellow, the emotion of Pensiveness (as in buried in thoughts, ruminating thoughts), dampness and is neither Yin nor Yang. *Sepia, Thuja, China, Ignatia, Plumbum* all relate to Earth.

Metal relates to the Lungs and Large Intestine, the colour white, Dryness, the emotion of Sadness and is rather Yin. *Calcarea carbonica, Bryonia, Natrum muriaticum* are but a few that correlate with Metal.

Water is related to Kidneys and Bladder, the colour black, the emotion of fear, cold (rather than wet, paradoxically) and is the most Yin of all. *Arsenicum album, Lycopodium, Silica, Mercury* belong mainly to the Water element.

As in homeopathy, the usefulness of this system is to collect objective findings from the patient, put them together and compare this to the remedy that covers best most if not all of the findings. Without going into the details of Chinese physiology, each and every organ, function or element has an influence on others and is influenced by others, as in conventional medicine: a heart pathology will give lung symptoms, congestive heart failure comes with dyspnoea and pulmonary oedema; the same will happen within the system of TCM but without being limited to material, organic functions.

A patient seems to be "depressed" but does not tell much more than that; he has digestive problems and claims that humidity makes his joints ache; his skin has a yellowy, ochre tinge; as we are going to see later, the centre of his tongue is covered with a heavy white-yellow coating and his Spleen pulse is weak, giving the sensation as if the artery is empty. All this information can be collected without a single word being said; it leads to the element Earth and the Organ Spleen: recurring thoughts, previous events not "digested", assimilated, leading to the conventional diagnosis of "depression" and the possible remedy Ignatia. And now, it is possible to ask in a tactful manner questions that will evoke the situation of "ailments from" and the remedy Ignatia, or at least lead to another remedy that has also the material characteristics determined by observation and examination. For some patients, it saves the need to dig deep into past events that are buried and not ready to be unearthed unless under the effect and control of the appropriate remedy.

In TCM, different emotions and mental pathologies are related to different "organs" or rather functional systems.

4   The seven emotions as causes of disease and their relations to organs/functions

Chinese Medicine includes seven emotions as causes of diseases: joy, anger, anxiety, contemplation, grief, fear and terror. They cause disorders of the Qi with disharmony of Yin, Yang, Qi and Blood, all leading to disease. Each emotion is regulated by an organ and, reciprocally, each emotion can influence its organ. Eventually, all the emotions are controlled by the Heart and all reactions to emotions are manifestations of the Heart-Spirit or Shen. Homeopaths would understand the concepts of Qi and Blood as the "Vital Force"[20], with Qi being the more energetic, immaterial aspect, whereas Blood would be the material aspect and support for the Qi. Once again we see that in TCM there is no real separation between what in western medicine is called body and mind.

The Organs-Emotions relations, and therefore pathologies, are as follows:

Heart	Joy
Liver	Anger
Spleen	Contemplation
Lung	Grief
Kidney	Fear

The emotions of Terror and Anxiety are related to the Qi in all five Zang (Organs). All emotions also have an effect on Qi in general:

• Excessive Joy relaxes the activity of Qi: deranged Mind, inability to concentrate, mania.
• Excessive Anger drives the Qi upwards: the Liver Qi and blood are driven upwards, associating the well-known physical symptoms to the expression of anger.
• Excess Contemplation creates stagnation of the Qi: it also consumes the Yin Blood of the Spleen, leading to less nourishment for the Heart-Spirit (Shen), bringing palpitations, amnesia, insomnia, dreaminess.

---

20 Samuel Hahnemann used the term "vital force" and described it as a "spirit-like" force that sustains and maintains life. It is the Vital Force that produces the symptoms in its effort to rid the body of disease.

- Excess Grief exhausts the Qi: essentially the Lung Qi, causing dizziness, lassitude, and dispiritedness.
- Excess Anxiety depresses the Qi: especially on the Liver and Lung Qi, with depression or stagnation of their respective Qi and the associated physical symptoms.
- Fear drives the Qi downwards: derangement of the mind, indecision, bewilderment.
- Terror disturbs the Qi: moves the Qi downwards, with incontinence of urine and faeces. Fear and Terror are of course related, Terror being a form of ultimate Fear, hence both act on the Kidney.

There are some other imbalances that are relevant to emotional and mental perturbations, like a superabundance of Liver Yang causing violent rage or overworking of the mind (the workaholic) consuming the Blood and impairing the Spleen, causing the symptoms of palpitations, amnesia, insomnia, dreaminess (Heart) and anorexia, abdominal distension and loose stool (Spleen).

This relates in homeopathy with the well-known rubrics "Ailments from...." and especially the emotional components like sexual abuse, rape, anger, etc,...as well as the rubrics contained in "Fear", "Anxiety", "Delusions" and often "Dreams". It must be remembered that notions like "Yin Blood of the Spleen" are specific to the philosophical concept of the human body's function in TCM; this does not mean that TCM practitioners believe there is a specific type of blood related to a specific organ; such are the pitfalls of literal translations; those concepts have to be understood but cannot be evoked properly by western languages without lengthy paraphrases.

All this does not mean that TCM does not recognise the Brain as being involved or at the origin of mental and emotional disturbances. The Brain is one of the Extraordinary Organs. Classical authors wrote that "The Brain is the seat of the Original Spirit" and that "A person's memory is in the Brain". They list the functions of the Brain as being the seat of mind, consciousness and thought; where mental activity takes place and where the primordial spirit is kept. What Western Medicine attributes to the nervous system is in typical holistic TCM manner distributed to the different functions of the different organs as well as Qi and Blood. Despite the recognition of the higher, integrative functions of the brain, the different mental activities are attributed to different organs:

Heart	Spirit, Shen
Lung	Superior Soul, Po/Pho
Liver	Inferior Soul, Hun
Spleen	Memory, Yi
Kidney	Conception, Zhi

As a general rule, all mental diseases will be clinically treated through the Heart, Liver and Kidney. The Heart governs the Mind and all mental activities, the Liver regulates the mental activities by smoothing the activity of the Qi and the Kidney nourishes the Brain by producing marrow through Yin Essence. Blood of course is the material basis for mental activity; its deficiency creates a lack of spirit whereas its disturbance creates mental disorder.

Now that we recognise the patient's problem as being an excess of Yin or Yang, originating through the effect of given emotion(s) and acting on given organ(s) or function(s) through history, we need the tools to confirm it in a positive, objective manner, independent of beliefs, attitudes, moral or religious concepts, which is also reproducible and teachable. We find those tools in the examination of the **Tongue** and of the **Pulses**. It is also necessary to know the influences of the pathogenetic factors alluded to previously (Fire, Wind, Humidity, Dryness and Cold) on the tongue and on the pulses. This requires in-depth study and experience, preferably by apprenticeship, but I will present the basic principles in what I hope will be an immediately useful manner.

5 Tongue diagnosis

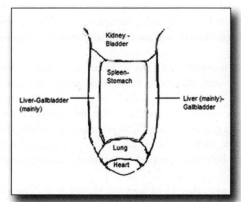

Fig. 1: Location of the organs on the tongue according to TCM. Drawing by Dr. J. Rozencwajg, NMD.

The tongue is divided into areas representing the different organs/functions. The base of the tongue represents the Kidney and Urinary Bladder, the extreme tip of the tongue represents the Heart, the area around it the Lungs, the sides of the tongue the Liver and Gallbladder with the right side more significant to the Liver and the left side more to the Gallbladder.

We first look at any general changes in the tongue, not forgetting that these might be caused by organic pathologies not to be missed: a dry parched tongue is seen in dehydration or mouth breathing, TCM relates it to Dryness or Heat/Fire; a pale tongue is the mark of clinical anaemia, with possible lack of brain oxygenation causing mental or emotional problems, which indeed should be investigated; TCM insufficiency of Blood correlates well here; a purple-violet tongue means cyanosis and a conventional differential diagnosis is indispensable; TCM has it as Blood Stagnation. A healthy tongue is pink with a slight clear coating. A thick coating (TCM calls it "fur", as in furry tongue) indicates Humidity; becoming yellow makes it Heat or Fire, so thick yellow makes it Humid Fire and thin yellow Dry Fire, and so on. The shape and form of the tongue has also some relevance: indentations, deformations ... all these notions are also found in the homeopathic repertories under Mouth, Discolouration, so this is nothing new for homeopaths - it just has to become another way of using information we are supposed to collect anyway during the interview.

Local changes are relevant of course. For example, the Red discolouration of the tip in TCM shows a situation of Fire in the Heart. The 2005 Complete Repertory mentions 58 remedies; 50

of them are also found in relation to Heart and Circulation problems. Combine this with Mind, Anxiety for example, and you are left with only 44 remedies, all of them having a red tongue tip, a cardiac action and anxiety, the more prominent being *Argentum nitricum, Arsenicum album, Phytolacca, Rhus toxicodendron, Rhus venenata, Sulphur, Apis, Fluoricum acidum, Lachesis, Lycopodium, Nitricum acidum*, all this using very general notions. Of course, the TCM Heart and our repertorial heart are different, but it has to be remembered that the TCM Heart includes the physical, anatomical heart that is mentioned in the repertories; therefore, although not strictly equivalent, an assumption of similarity can be made and this has been confirmed repeatedly in my clinical practice.

6   Pulse diagnosis

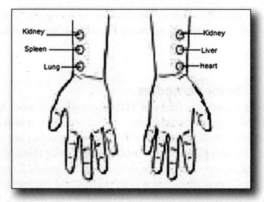

Fig. 2: Location of the organ's pulses according to TCM, hands are palm up, pulses felt on the radial arteries. Drawing by Dr. J. Rozencwajg, NMD.

Chinese Pulse Diagnosis is another trademark of TCM, although it is also well represented in Ayurvedic medicine. It is an art and a science that requires long period of practice and mentorship, if possible, to be useful in all its details and intricacies; after all, the most eminent practitioner and teacher of Pulse Diagnosis, Leon Hammer, wrote a book of no fewer than 812 pages about it! Even for a beginner it is not that difficult to use this tool in its basic form.

`On the right wrist, the Lung pulse is found closest to the radio-carpal articulation, on the radial artery; next to it, no more than a finger width as shown in the drawing for more clarity, is the Spleen pulse, then the Kidney pulse. On the left wrist, Heart, Liver and Kidney pulses are found in the same order. It is not very complicated to recognise a strong pulse, a weak pulse, a fast or a slow one. An empty pulse is the one you feel but which disappears on compression; a tense, taut or stringy pulse give the impression of a guitar string vibrating under the finger. Good descriptions can be found in articles and books available everywhere; it is then a question of habit to take the pulse in every patient (as old school doctors always did, as well as looking at the tongue), and to try to understand what is felt, then correlate it to the case.

For example, all pulses being weak and the Kidney pulse almost not perceptible at all conveys the notion of general weakness, lack of Qi and specifically of Kidney Qi, which correlates very well with the very widespread situation of adrenal exhaustion and burnout we tend to find in increasing numbers of our patients. It often indicates the prescription of an Acid remedy[21] but, as an aside, it is generally wise to repair the function of the adrenal and pituitary system before giving the homeopathic remedy, in order to allow the body to react to it; otherwise the remedy will fail, not because of a poor prescription but because the physiology cannot carry on the information provided by the remedy: this is another story altogether but it has been demonstrated time and again in my practice.

As stated earlier, an anomaly in the Liver pulse often shows an anger situation, either recent, in which case the pulse will be strong, taut, stringy, or ancient and repressed with a weak liver pulse. The beauty of pulse-taking is that it changes immediately when either the right treatment is given or the right question is asked, as I have seen repeatedly not only with an immediate change during acupuncture, but an immediate change during questioning while taking the pulses: often this has allowed me to ask direct questions, feel the reaction even before having an answer and reorient the anamnesis properly towards the roots of the problems. The patient is amazed, and relieved, by the accuracy of the questions, opens up and reveals the innermost workings of his mind.

7   Some remedies

Describing remedies in terms of TCM energetics is a work in progress, as is creating a repertory using TCM diagnosis to find homeopathic remedies. It will be published as soon as a decent working tool is created. For the time being, some remedies are obvious. These are very common remedies. As I mentioned earlier, I almost automatically think in terms of TCM diagnosis when seeing a patient and always examine the tongue and the pulses. I remember many years ago being amazed at how the Chinese diagnosis was so precise, and commenting that the remedy chosen had many of the same characteristics, especially in acute febrile diseases. It was from this time that I started looking carefully at the relationship between an energetic pattern as seen in TCM and the energetic pattern of the remedy prescribed. When they did not correspond, at least in general terms, my prescription was not the best that it could be. I am now in the process of refining that knowledge. The list below represents my personal opinion and experience with these remedies and is certainly far from being written in stone.

Yang remedies: *Aconite, Belladonna, Sulphur, Phosphorus, Iodum, some aspects of Pulsatilla.*

Yin remedies: *Natrum muriaticum, Dulcamara, other aspects of Pulsatilla.*

Wind remedies: will often be found in the rubric Generalities; contradictory and alternating states: *Ignatia, Pulsatilla, Tuberculinum, Abrotanum, Aloe, Berberis, Carcinosinum, Natrum muriaticum, Platina, Sepia, Staphysagria, Thuja* are the major ones.

Fire or Heat remedies are the expected ones like *Sulphur, Phosphorus, Iodum, Coffea.*

---

21 Homeopathic remedies made from acids are known to be indicated for states of mental, emotional or physical depletion.

Earth remedies: *Sepia, Thuja, China, Ignatia, Plumbum.*

Metal remedies: *Calcarea carbonica, Bryonia, Natrum muriaticum.*

Water remedies: *Arsenicum album, Lycopodium, Silica, Mercury.*

8   Conclusion

Of course, it can be said that most of the remedies mentioned here are polychrests[22], which will appear anyway in any usual repertorisation - so what is the point? Isn't this just a nice intellectual exercise but otherwise a complete waste of time? It certainly is when the patient is totally aware of what is going on with him, does not hide anything, either consciously or unconsciously, and tells his story in full with complete honesty. Many years of experience in both conventional and non-conventional medicine have made it clear to me that this is rarely the case. Finding shortcuts that allow the practitioner to understand the core problems while allowing the patient to maintain a certain level of discretion until he realises that it is possible to tell everything without problems, or ways to realise there are some deeply buried, hidden, forgotten but very active pockets of maintaining causes, seems worthwhile to me. Those shortcuts are the patterns of TCM diagnosis as revealed through listening to how the patient presents his problem, examining the pulses and the tongue, writing down an objective TCM diagnosis, albeit a lot less precise than what a TCM practitioner would do, then finding the remedy or remedies that best cover the case homeopathically (the usual repertorisation) and eventually selecting the ones to study more in detail before prescribing; the selection is made on the basis that the remedy fits the TCM pattern as well as the homeopathic pattern.

References

[1] Leon Hammer (2005) *Chinese Pulse Diagnosis: A contemporary approach*. Seattle, Washington: Eastland Press
[2] Giovanni Maccioccia (1989) *The Foundations of Chinese Medicine*. Edinburgh London Melbourne and New York: Churchill Livingstone
[3] Roger van Zandvoort (2005) *The Complete Repertory* edition 2005 in Mac Repertory Version 8.0.1.11. (2009), San Rafael CA: Kent Homeopathic Associates

---

22 A term used by homeopaths to indicate remedies that are very well-known and therefore regularly used, as opposed to so-called small remedies. Small here does not necessarily mean 'less' in terms of usefulness, but rather in terms of the knowledge built up about them.

Section 3: Research, Ethics, and Theory

Chapter 17
Is Homeopathy Useful in Psychotherapy?

Jane A. Ferris, PhD

Jane A. Ferris, PhD
5 Birdsnest Court
Mill Valley, CA 94941
USA
E-mail: drjaneferris@gmail.com

Abstract

This chapter summarizes the research findings of a clinical psychology dissertation on the interaction of homeopathy and depth psychotherapy. Psychotherapists were interviewed about their experience when homeopathic remedies were given to their psychotherapy patients. Thirty-nine descriptions of improvements in patients were identified. Details and complications to be considered by mental health therapists and homeopaths are discussed. The research finds that homeopathy can work synergistically with psychotherapy to move patients towards greater awareness and wholistic functioning.

1   Introduction

Wholistic psychotherapists see the importance of a new paradigm shift in consciousness that demands the release of old concepts of healing. They are searching for alternatives to modern psychopharmaceuticals and new ways to include the mind-body in their work. The philosophy and practice of homeopathy may have much to offer psychotherapy as we explore integrative methods to transform the human being. Jungian psychotherapy, particularly, shares a history with homeopathy that can be traced back to origins in alchemy and the Vitalist tradition [1] [2] [3].

The synergistic partnership of homeopathy and psychotherapy seems promising; however, we need to ask what actually occurs when homeopathic remedies are introduced into the psychotherapy field. Is the psychotherapeutic process enhanced or is it disturbed in any way? In what ways are homeopathy and psychotherapy similar and in what ways are they different and work in exclusive areas of the human experience?

Psychotherapists need to investigate the effectiveness and validity of homeopathy if they are going to refer their clients to homeopaths. Are homeopathic remedies useful for clinical depression, addictions, suicide, dying, borderline issues, psychosis, and other severe mental illnesses? Can they replace medications or be used in conjunction with them? Do remedies have adverse effects that must be understood? Can psychotherapy be shortened or deepened with homeopathy?

There are other questions within the psychotherapeutic frame. How are the transference, counter-transference, and the energetic field between therapist and client affected by homeopathic remedies? Are dreams and the body changed? When is it appropriate to refer for remedies? What factors determine when to refer for homeopathy rather than medications or other alternative practices?

Psychotherapists might also wonder how to introduce the subject of homeopathy to clients and how to work with clients when the proper remedy is not found or is antidoted, or when aggravations occur. There may be concern about the openness of homeopaths to consultation and what value therapists may find in this type of consultation. Therapists will want to know how to become better educated about homeopathy and how to find effective homeopaths.

This chapter is a review of introductory research into these questions where only some of the questions can be explored. It is therefore also an invitation to conduct more research on this topic.

2   The research

I was curious to discover how psychotherapists experience the introduction of homeopathic remedies into the therapy process with their patients. As a participant researcher in my dissertation [4] I was involved in my own experience of therapy and homeopathic treatment and many of my clients were seeing a homeopath during their depth psychotherapy. I was able to observe the movement of the psyche before and after homeopathic remedies were taken.

The research itself consisted of interviews with thirteen professionals. Seven are therapists and six are therapist-homeopaths. Common themes were identified that might give a more comprehensive insight into the world of psychotherapy and homeopathy.

The research participants indicated a special interest in a wholistic approach to therapy and healing that includes the body, and the importance of the spiritual and transcendent in their lives. Their trust in homeopathy came from their personal transformative experiences with remedies or from the experiences of their children or close associates. These were significant enough in their life stories to lead them to incorporate homeopathy into their practices. The intensity of their personal experiences with homeopathy is clear in the interviews.

One participant remembered her first reaction to a remedy: "It was like a storm had broken and the sun was out. I started to have flying dreams and dreams where I was doing daring things. I noticed an emotional shift at a very deep level." A psychoanalytically-oriented therapist observed: "I think the remedy made it possible for me to start differentiating myself from my therapist and get into a negative transference." One male participant noted: "About ten years earlier I had put a lid on my emotional life and this remedy essentially blew the lid right off." A woman recounted: "All the grief I had been unable to feel in the year preceding the breakup came tumbling out."

A homeopath-therapist described her experience when *triturating* (grinding the substance in milk sugar with a mortar and pestle) a remedy: "We resonate with the remedy and we really know that substance, how it can be used, and what it has to offer. Those remedies are vibrating with energy on a collective level, on an archetypal level, on a spiritual level." Another therapist reflected: "A new remedy had an enormous effect. I used to bite my nails to the quick and I have stopped. My energy is much higher, and I'm not depressed. I feel better than I have ever felt before in my whole life." Participants noted that when they observed a child getting significantly better after months of trying other methods of cure it was clear it was not a placebo effect.

2.1 Observations

Thirty-nine descriptions of improvements after the introduction of homeopathic remedies were noted in the interviews. I list the descriptions in groups:

- There is the very physical, yet emotional, subtle-body experience of the "opening of heart energy," "touching the life force," and "returning to essence." Therapists noted that clients had "greater distance from and disidentification with problems," were "more loving," and "more able to discuss new issues."
- More expressions that the participants used when describing their clients' experiences include: "opening to feelings," "feeling positive and safe," "stability, grounded, balanced, and centred," "more empathy," "world is friendly," "movement out of difficult relationships," "experience grief," "more decisive," "less obsessive," "opening and strengthening," "move to deeper work," "increased resiliency," "emotional shifts," and "more available and connected." All of these are signs of improvement in self-awareness that is the purpose of psychotherapy.
- "Decreased suicidality," "improvement of serious mental problems," "personality changes," "reduced medications," "less depression," "attachment issues improved," and "shorter therapy" are encouraging to see and warrant much more research. "Spiritual healing," and "easier dying" speak of spiritual subtle-body aspects of homeopathy.
- "Increased energy," "better sleep," "fertility improved," "weight loss" and "other physical symptoms improved or cured" are important indications that psychosomatic aspects frozen in the body are transformed into psychic manifestations.
- Dreams are an important barometer of the movement of psyche. Co-researchers observed "more movement in dreams," "increased dreaming," and "dreams as messengers of healing."

A homeopath-therapist mentioned the importance of the remedy metaphor for understanding clients in new ways and a new lens for understanding dreams.

As a homeopath I may think of a Bird remedy in relation to a flying dream. Could a fear of flying mean Bromine? Fear of inflation? Is this a mineral remedy or is this a gas? What does it mean? Cannabis, dreams of flying? Is it about the fall? This is what we do as therapists hearing dreams on two or three levels … Especially with animal remedies the client will stop being in victim-aggressor mode and the dreams will change. Mineral remedies are more about the emptiness. I had one fellow who had dreams of nuclear waste before I became a homeopath. I am sure he was a Plutonium and if I had given that remedy his dreams would have changed. When I give a remedy things change in dreams.

One therapist explained how remedies can help a patient in therapy by working on another energetic level.

> *Particularly when people feel shattered or fragmented, a remedy will help them hold together and be able to have whatever feelings are there. I am thinking of one person in particular who was taking a tree remedy, White cone pine. It would consolidate her and she was able to tolerate her feelings and her situation again. Homeopathic remedies can change a therapy. A clinic patient I worked with for years experienced a depression and a layer of being stuck that nothing was touching.*
>
> *When she took a remedy everything changed in unpredictable ways. I couldn't have guessed how it was going to be. It was like she touched her life-force. It was not therapy that did it. After the remedy she could use the therapy, but I don't believe that if we had worked for 10 more years it would have helped her that much. I feel sometimes you have to work on another level. There is something about the heart energy that increases. There is a layer of healing that is not touched if you don't do homeopathy.*

Many participants felt that therapy proceeds more quickly and deeply when used in conjunction with remedies.

> *I think that clients move through the psychotherapy process more quickly with homeopathy. The first thing I see is defensiveness and fear and attachment to the defences . . . People assume that their defences are themselves. "I am my defence. This is who I am. I'm not going to change." People become less identified with that defence when given a proper remedy. It gives that moment of reflection so they can pull back and be curious. It is easier to ask, "What am I doing." The remedy helps them to disidentify. It gives them a break. It addresses the fear factor. If you aren't as identified as a defence you aren't as attached. It's not who you are. It is easier to think of changing.*

One therapist said, homeopathy gives therapy a "jump-start" that takes it out of the pathological realm and deepens the client's essence.

> *After she began homeopathy it was much easier for her to express anger. She began to sleep better and arrive in therapy with many more dreams including dreams of the ocean. There was also a detoxing reaction. She was able to talk about suicide attempts from many years before for the first time. She expressed "Everything has opened up since I saw the homeopath." A year later she was given a feminine remedy, Sepia (Cuttlefish), that addresses the oppressed feminine, for one who is devoted but is distant from family, and for one who loves dancing but is sexually inhibited. After this remedy she felt great. She wasn't feeling anger in the same way and got off of Prozac.*

Some of the therapists were concerned that homeopaths often do not follow up clients or set a safe framework.

> *Sometimes homeopaths don't do enough follow-up to let people know what the process is going to mean for them. You can't just give someone a remedy and say, "I'll see you in a month." All of a sudden the client can get hit by a reaction. I think you need to let people have some framework to indicate what is about to happen to them.*

Participants discovered that clients often don't realize they have changed after taking remedies.

> People do tend to forget that homeopathy even worked at all ... There is a good story about this. One very depressed man was given Mustard, a flower remedy. The next time he came in he was much better. He had been depressed for years. He told me that he wasn't feeling better because of the remedy; it was because he had gone out and gotten a job. It didn't occur to him that he hadn't gotten a job earlier!

A homeopath-therapist emphasized that in homeopathy everything makes sense and nothing is discarded. "It is an incredible experience to sit in this field where everything is actually possible and can be heard. There is no judgment about it. It is such an expanded field." She sees homeopathy as an alchemical process. "They are not so stuck in problems anymore because something expands. The container becomes bigger and that also expands the container in the therapy as well."

A therapist expressed that remedies add something extremely valuable to the therapeutic relationship.

> When a client has taken a remedy it seems there is something extra working with the person's strengths, with the person's needs, but not against the person. There is something very positive about it. The whole frame of it is positive as opposed to "we'll cut off this piece; we'll get rid of it." There is also a dimension of hope. I know that a homeopathic remedy is part of the essence of the person. So that it deepens their essence. I have a sense of integrity about it.

Participants often talked about other modalities they use in their therapy that have an energetic feeling similar to homeopathy. Sandplay is an interesting example.

> Sandplay feels similar to homeopathy. It is energetic. It is working silently and we trust this process. The energies of the body and psyche will be constellated in the sand. You don't have to talk about it. This is a very different way to look at the movement of the psyche. Often sandplay allows the deep unconscious to be expressed in a way that is not conscious to the person. Their hands are doing it. There is a deep trusting of an energetic level that is below verbal, that is all symbolic, totally symbolic ... Images come alive because you are touching them and feeling them. In homeopathy you are taking something energetic that comes alive in you.

Suicide was addressed by several therapists. One told about a client who had a secret suicide plan despite presenting with a happy-go-lucky demeanour. The homeopath did not know about the secret suicide plan but prescribed the remedy *Hemlock*.

> Eventually she was given Hemlock (Conium maculatum – the very poison Socrates was forced to drink to end his life) which I thought was fascinating considering the homeopath didn't know about the suicide ideation. The cough stopped over a couple of months and she ended a destructive relationship that we had talked about for years and got nowhere with . . . She stopped seeing him right after the remedy. She was building new relationships, her life was expanding, and she was no longer obsessed with ending her life. I was impressed with the layers that the remedy was able to reach that talk therapy alone could not.

A homeopathic remedy improved the life of a psychotic patient who didn't want to be on medication.

> One patient in particular was too paranoid to do psychotropic medication. She was actively psychotic but some of her friends went to homeopaths before her psychotic break so she came to me for homeopathy. I was able to give her the remedy and she kept seeing me for psychotherapy. After about a month she shifted. A few weeks on antipsychotic medication pulled her enough out of the psychosis and for the rest of the time she was totally managed with Anacardium, a tree remedy. She came to me after her second psychotic break and hasn't had another hospitalization. She's married and doing fine after 5 years.

A woman in hospice was lifted from depression and was able to continue in depth psychotherapy for six years before she died.

> I gave her a combination of Aurum muriaticum natronatum (gold salt) and Ambra grisia (ambergris). Three days later her depression had lifted. She lived another six years and I continued to see her. We had to have a party when they kicked her out of hospice because she was going to live. She continued in long-term depth psychotherapy with me. It was extraordinary work to do at her age. She originally had a conflicted relationship with her son but it ended in a good and peaceful way. She didn't die and she had this opening. With the remedy she regained enough vitality and time to do the healing so that she died a more whole person, a less fearful person, and not a depressed person. She was at peace with who she was.

Many of the therapists value the mutually beneficial relationship they have with homeopaths who work with their patients.

> We usually have an initial consult with each other after my client's first session. I give some history, and the homeopath shares some initial impressions. I am always fascinated that she can get to basic information that I wasn't able to obtain as a therapist after 3 or 4 years. It is often about substance abuse or something pretty significant that didn't come out. Somehow something triggered it for the client in the homeopathic interview so they talked about it. She found out something important about almost every client. Often our consultation is while she is still searching for a remedy if she didn't find it during the initial interview. Whatever insight I offer must help her put some pieces together. She feels it fills out the case and helps her a great deal. It gives her a larger picture.

> I may call the homeopath later because I have seen some change, or I am so amazed, or to thank her for the help, or to say that the client is looking worse. I call freely as I would a psychiatrist. I like the collaborative feeling. Part of what I don't like about private practice recently is the solo-ness of it and how much it is done behind closed doors. It is important to sense if clients are open to being talked about before consultation. You have to be sensitive to that. My clients seem to feel safe with the process of being talked about with the homeopath and they seem to enjoy it.

All of the participants mentioned the importance of appropriate timing when considering referral to a homeopath or introduction of a remedy into therapy.

Sometimes it is important to wait to refer to a homeopath until you have a solid frame with someone.
Psychological work ahead of time may make it possible for people to tolerate more life energy that will
be released with homeopathy.

Another therapist says she refers to a homeopath when she sees that a client is stuck and circling
rather than spiralling.

The clients who are stuck or keep circling in their complexes are the ones I refer to a homeopath. I
see a complex as a point on a spiral. Every time we circle up the spiral we pass the point where the
complex touches, and every time the complex rears up again. "Here we are again." Each time you
reflect on it your relationship to a complex changes, the response changes. When I see people who are
not spiralling but are circling, I think that homeopathy is indicated. Homeopathy can help me work
with them to get them off of that circle and get them into the spiral. I think that every rung of the
spiral reflects more individuation, more self-awareness, more power over the complex, and more ability
to not be held by it.

Clients can be hesitant to participate in both therapy and homeopathy owing to the financial commitment.

Part of what impacts people is the cost of paying for a therapist and a homeopath. It is a lot to ask
people to do and I think that one of the referrals that I made really couldn't afford it. That will be
one of the deciding factors for the woman I just referred. Young women living in this urban area
don't have much disposable income and yet I remember hearing that some of the best candidates for
homeopathy are younger people.

Homeopathy is based on a deep empathy for the particular human being. If the therapist resonates
with the client and with the remedy, a profound healing environment can be created. Both the therapist and the client will gain a greater perspective on the client's life through the encounter with
homeopathy. The therapeutic field is affected by homeopathic remedies changing the experience of
therapist and client through an expansion of the field that includes changing dreams and transference / counter-transference issues.

I discovered that homeopathy affects the therapy and the therapeutic field. The interplay between two
people is always shifting and being impacted by any number of internal and external factors. When I
was given a remedy and I was no longer really depressed or really irritable, the therapy and the field
changed as well. There was more opening.

A therapist expressed how therapy went to a deeper place after a remedy was introduced.

We aren't spending nearly as much time on the negativity. She used to feel assaulted by negative thoughts
and be demoralized. That shifted almost immediately. The negativity isn't always there or right around
the corner. I feel our work deepened. I feel there is more connection to our work and we got to a very
deep place that we had skirted around. We were better able to get into it and it didn't destroy her to look
at some difficult things.

There are new developments in homeopathy that are making it more effective and more easily understood so that it can be more relevant to modern psychotherapy. Homeopathy can address the shamanic, energetic level of healing. Attachment issues that are central to therapy are being discussed in terms of homeopathic remedies including *Milks*, *Sugar*, and matridonal remedies connected with the birth process such as *Umbilical cord, Placenta, DNA* and *Amniotic fluid*.

Homeopaths understand the energetic factors that affect us from the past and from the collective. Therapists will benefit from exploration of the impact of these collective fields. Many of the participants take part in family constellation work, Genograms, and energy healing of various kinds.

2.2 Alchemical process: impact of research

Participants discovered that the interview process allowed them to consolidate ideas and experiences that had been waiting to arise in connection with homeopathy and therapy. They were given the space to review their own transformations with homeopathy as well as the journeys of their clients. In this review process the many tiny miracles that were witnessed in the therapeutic field, synergized by a potentised material, came to light. Invariably the co-researchers commented on their increased awareness of what has been occurring in their consulting rooms. There was the budding realization of the importance of this synergy.

This topic has acted upon every aspect of my own life. During these years I witnessed my clients opening either dramatically or more slowly with remedies. My trust in the process deepened and my increasing conviction that remedies contribute to therapy has strengthened. Several clients told me that they wished I had pressed them to try homeopathy sooner as they were discovering new ways of being in their lives that they had never thought possible. Therapy was more important for them as they began to realize how much more of life was now available to explore.

I discovered a dynamic interaction in the dreams of my clients and in my own dreams when homeopathic remedies are introduced. Even when I am not aware that a client has taken a remedy I can often see its action in the dreams.

Professionally, I am now more acutely aware of the necessity to involve all aspects of the client in the therapy: mind, emotions, spirit, and body. There is a significant loss when the body is ignored and a wholistic perspective is not maintained.

3   Conclusion

Psychology underwent profound changes after the development of psychotropic medications. Our culture increasingly depends on the use of medications and cognitive behavioural adjustments in order to condition people to a fast-paced lifestyle that demands immediate solutions that may be band-aid approaches to healing.

The therapists in this study are pioneering an alternative model of understanding the psyche from a wholistic, energetic point of view. They are candid about the successes and challenges in this new partnership of disciplines.

Homeopathy offers a treatment that can shift psychological states without suppressing and without side-effects. It can help clients become more available and connected to the therapist and more able to do the psychological work. The transference, counter-transference and therapeutic field are positively impacted. Clients have more distance from their problems, increased resiliency, decisiveness and stability, and are able to move out of difficult relationships and situations. The participants also observe increased energy, openness to feelings, empathy and love. There is evidence that remedies are useful for serious mental health conditions and for those who are dying. Therapy is described as being shorter and general health improved. Changes in dreams indicate psychological movement. Medications can often be reduced or eliminated. Homeopathy offers a cost-effective, less toxic, and more integral treatment that has immensely beneficial social and economic implications.

Homeopathy works synergistically with psychotherapy to move the client towards greater awareness and wholistic functioning. It is especially useful when therapy is stuck. Some clients have difficulty relating to the idea of homeopathy while others have problems staying with the process. Homeopaths can have challenges finding the proper remedy, adjusting for aggravations, and preventing antidoting. The therapist and client need to have the ability to wait for the process to unfold. Consultation with a homeopath, on the other hand, can give both therapists and homeopaths new perspectives on their clients.

Homeopathy is a wholistic medicine that provides healing on levels of being that may not be easily reached in psychotherapy and works well in partnership with it. Homeopathy also addresses the generational aspect of symptoms that may not be touched by the therapeutic exploration of individual life history.

Education of therapists and clients about homeopathy is imperative in this medically-oriented culture where we have been conditioned to assume that we are separate selves living on the earth. Homeopathy in concert with the containing function of psychotherapy awakens us to the realization that we are living, vital organisms woven into the pulsating web of life; moving us from alienation to intimate connection, from doing to being.

References

[1] Wood M (1992) *The Magical Staff: The Vitalist Tradition in Western Medicine*. Berkeley: North Atlantic Books
[2] Whitmont E (1980) *Psyche and Substance: Essays on Homeopathy in the Light of Jungian Psychology*. Berkeley: North Atlantic Books
[3] Whitmont E (1993) *The Alchemy of Healing: Psyche and Soma*. Berkeley: North Atlantic Books
[4] Ferris J (2008) *Homeopathy and Depth Psychotherapy: A Vital Partnership*. Ph.D. dissertation. Pacifica Graduate Institute, Dissertations & Theses: Full text. ProQuest. Web. 10 Sep 2009

Chapter 18
Research Issues in Homeopathy in Mental Health

Corina Güthlin, PhD[1] and Harald Walach PhD[2]

1) Corina Güthlin, PhD
Research Methodology & Project Management in General Practice/Institute for General Practice
Johann Wolfgang Goethe University
Theodor-Stern-Kai 7
D-60590 Frankfurt am Main
E-mail: guethlin@allgemeinmedizin.uni-frankfurt.de

2) Harald Walach, PhD
University of Northampton
School of Social Sciences & Samueli Institute for Information Biology
Boughton Green Rd
Northampton NN2 7AL, UK
E-mail: harald.walach@northampton.ac.uk

Abstract

This Chapter summarizes empirical studies looking at the importance of Complementary Medicine in Mental Health (Research). It highlights research issues in homeopathy and reviews existing studies on homeopathy in mental disorders and mental health symptoms.

1   Introduction

Homeopathy in mental health care: The first author of this chapter is for the most part a researcher in a setting (evaluation of complementary therapy and general practice in a university hospital) in which there are rather sceptical if not hostile views towards using homeopathy in mental health care. Some of the doubts stem from the view that mentally ill patients are too difficult a patient group to be treated without the utmost care (thus, assuming that only pharmacological treatment may be complemented by psychotherapy is a prerequisite for such care). The other preconception regularly found is that there is no valid research in homeopathy. We would like to discuss both in this chapter.

We are sure that not only in our academic institution it would not be considered as ethically appropriate to randomly assign patients with severe depression to homeopathic treatment or, say, a serotonin reuptake inhibitor (SSRI). Although it might work in some cases, there is not enough evidence to safely introduce homeopathy instead of SSRI to start a study assuming this (and therefore randomising patients). Does this sound like a vicious circle? Well, it is.

Although academic departments in some countries may not be as openly hostile and allow more homeopathic research, possibly even understanding that several different research approaches might be necessary when searching for evidence, it is the view of the authors that the only way to overcome this vicious circle is to be acutely aware of it.

In this chapter we will not only review features, results, and problems of research in homeopathy, but also point to some solutions. There are some well done studies and systematic reviews capturing the effects of homeopathic treatment in mental health issues, but before reviewing the evidence we would like to familiarize our readers with the patient's perspective and ask "what do patients expect from homeopathy and other complementary and alternative (CAM) therapies?"

One regularly stated reason for turning to CAM is the dissatisfaction with conventional therapy [1]. We found support for this in our own longitudinal observational study in a mixed patient sample with a large percentage of patients reporting emotional problems as a reason for seeking homeopathy or acupuncture. Seventy percent sought help from a homeopathic doctor because other treatments lacked efficacy; 60% of the respondents felt other treatments were effective but fraught with too many side effects [2]. In patients with mental health disorders this could mean two different things. First either they do not want to rely on psychoactive drugs [3], or do not view these drugs either as their preferred treatment or as contributing to their wellbeing [4]. Patients from an inpatient study of psychiatric care felt frustrated from being offered medication instead of human contact [5]. One patient cited in a qualitative study put the trade-off of CAM treatment vs. drug use like this: "There are no side effects [with CAM] and I feel in control; with the Prozac I felt it was in control of me." [3]. Secondly, mainly depressive patients find neither medication nor psychotherapy completely helpful and satisfying. Outcome data supports the common notion that less than 50% of all depressed patients seeking psychiatric help experience lasting relief through drugs or cognitive behaviour therapy [6,7].

In line with the idea of push and pull factors [8] which lead to CAM use, dissatisfaction would clearly push people away from conventional treatments whereas mental health specific pull factors could be the general notion that CAM is good for your wellbeing and recreation [9]. This is supported in the media [10] and becomes particularly important as research shows that patients with mental and behavioural disorders who suffer from low quality of life turn to CAM [11]. Apart from general wellbeing, calmness and emotional stability, patients with serious mental illness also mentioned improved sleep or improved cognitive functioning or improved clarity of consciousness as perceived benefits of CAM [9]. Another pull factor is the wish to physically support the body with another "natural option" besides psychotherapy or with an option that is in line with their own belief system [12]. Interestingly, when patients are asked about the helpfulness of CAM treatment for the treatment of their anxiety attacks and depressive symptoms, about the same proportion of patients who find conventional treatment helpful (between 60-70% depending on the underlying problem) finds CAM treatment beneficial (50-60%) [13]. With this large percentage of patients finding CAM favourable, we can assume a significant portion of these respondents will not only turn to CAM but stay on this treatment.

2   Research in homeopathy

A cursory search of the literature within the National Library of Medicine (http://www.ncbi.nlm.nih.gov/) gives us a very rough estimate of the research basis in CAM and mental health care: when doing a search with the keywords "Complementary Medicine" (as a Mesh heading) the library returns 130,098 references. Only 0.3% (N=362) of these references deal with the Mesh heading "Mental Health" whereas another 9.8% (N=12,700) cover the Mesh heading "mental disorder". When doing the same with "Homeopathy" as a keyword (not as a Mesh heading) we end up with 3,832 references in total. Of these 0.3% (N=1) have to do with "Mental Health" (Mesh Heading) and 2.8% (N=108) cover the topic of "Mental disorders" (Mesh heading). This shows us that mental disorders play only a marginal role in CAM and mental health is covered even less. It also shows us that the evidence base of homeopathy and mental health care is even more limited.

Some authors claim the right question to ask here would be "Are homeopathic dilutions any more than placebo?" [14] whereas others state that there are many more pertinent questions to answer when researching homeopathy. For example two authors who have more than 20 years of expertise behind them propose [15, p. 239]:

> Our suggestion would be that we should be asking different questions than whether homeopathy is different from placebo. These questions include: How effective is homeopathy compared with other treatments? What is the baseline chance of patients improving or being healed under homeopathic treatment? How stable are treatment effects? What are good prognostic indicators for success in homeopathic treatment? How much does success with homeopathy cost compared to conventional treatment? What are the risks of side effects in homeopathy weighed against the odds of improvement?

In terms of promising and useful research designs the authors continue [p. 240] to "*suggest that some of the following studies could be a main focus of any research agenda in homeopathy*":

- Observational and cohort studies to determine the general effects of homeopathy.
- Combined with an analysis of large sets of prognostic factors on doctors and patients, among them personality traits, measures of expectancy, hope, self-involvement, sympathy.
- Randomized comparison studies to determine effectiveness compared with alternative treatments.
- Quasi-experimental comparison studies in natural, self-selected groups to find out about the importance of self-selection.
- Combined with measures of cost and safety.
- Studies of biological activity of Serially Agitated High Solutions or the question of whether homeopathic dilutions are placebos should be delegated to stable, basic research models.
- Those who still believe in the superiority of homeopathy over placebo in clinical trials should try to replicate one of the promising positive results reported so far and book a therapist for the time after the trial.

After setting the agenda for homeopathy research and beginning to map results from homeopathy and mental health care to research designs and questions, we feel that a serious warning is in place.

The authors of the lists above correctly stated that until 2002 there was no research whatsoever which can answer the pertinent questions and there is a significant lack of trials and studies reporting results from the latter research designs. Bearing this in mind we have to expect a lot less research in mental health care. This is in fact what we found even today in 2009, and thus we cannot provide definite answers under the following subheadings.

2.1 Research in homeopathy and mental health care

In order to provide a comprehensive picture of research that links homeopathy with mental health issues, we would like to present results from basic research as well as from large and small quantitative and qualitative studies.

2.1.1 Basic research

Basic research in homeopathy is rather scarce compared to clinical studies. Thus, as we would expect, studies exploring homeopathy in cells, plants or animals which model situations applicable to the mental health context are even rarer.

Additionally, the general notion is that results are difficult to repeat, effects are seen then and again, but no generic rule exists about what test systems, which dilutions or what remedies yield consistently positive results [16]. One study from Brazil reports two experiments in Swiss mice and the application of *Chamomilla* (6 C). The data suggests that mice getting Chamomilla per os recover more quickly after stressful conditions compared to controls. Regarding the antidepressive effect of Chamomilla in mice, the results show that Chamomilla is less effective than amitryptilin, but definitely alters behaviour (swimming test) compared to baseline. The conclusion from this behaviour test model is that mice are less susceptible to depression after application of Chamomilla [17].

For all who would like to embark on basic research of homeopathy and mental health models we would like to share the advice this author had to give. He points out that, particularly in testing basic research models for mental health context, it is important to control for the effect of ethanol (mostly part of the manufacturing process of homeopathic remedies) as ethanol clearly has anxiolytic and antidepressive effects.

2.1.2 Systematic reviews and randomized controlled studies

Prominent research results from conventional depression treatment set the stage for what effect sizes could be expected in mental health research involving placebo controls, more specifically in depression research. A meta-analysis done by Kirsch et al. on published and unpublished data showed that people got better on medication, but they also got better on placebo, and the difference between the two was small, namely roughly a third of a standard deviation [18]. Clinical significance was only found in (a few relatively small) studies conducted on patients with very severe levels of depression. These results were based on data from all clinical trials conducted for marketing approval of the six most widely prescribed antidepressants approved in recent years in USA, which represent all but one of the selective serotonin reuptake inhibitors (SSRIs) approved during the study period. This result is virtually identical to one published in parallel pointing out the relative lack of effectiveness of SSRIs compared to placebo, mainly due to the strong placebo effect [19].

Apart from the small effect size which has to be expected in depression care, there is a significant lack of large and well-conducted randomized controlled studies (RCTs) in homeopathy and mental health problems. Thus, to date it is not possible to draw any definite conclusion with respect to the effectiveness of homeopathy over placebo or even over conventional care in the areas of psychiatric diseases [20]. Bearing in mind what was said at the beginning of this chapter that researchers and clinicians are often openly against the idea of applying homeopathy in psychiatric care, there is virtually no room (or money) for doing randomized controlled studies.

Moreover, with small effect sizes large numbers of study participants are needed, complicated by the fact that patients seeking CAM are often unwilling to be randomly assigned to treatments. A feasibility study of an RCT of homeopathy for depression in general practice showed tellingly: In this three-armed study (comparing individualized homeopathy vs. Prozac vs. placebo) the recruitment total over nine months was 31 patients who were potentially eligible out of 230 patients who were seen for depression. Of these, 23 met the inclusion criteria using DSM-IV and Hamilton Rating Scale for Depression (HAM-D), 11 could be randomized and 6 completed the study [21]. The major reason for not entering the study was the preference for homeopathic treatment. Thus, patients were not prepared to take the risk of getting either Prozac or placebo, but were prepared to embrace homeopathy.

Apart from the latter study which was too small to report results in terms of effects, there is one controlled study in the field of depression and anxiety [22]; see below. A study of individualized homeopathy versus placebo in fibromyalgia patients reported less depression in homeopathically treated patients [23]. Other RCTs studied the effectiveness of homeopathy in generalized Anxiety Disorder, in Chronic Fatigue Syndrome or in Attention Deficit Hyperactivity Disorder in a juvenile sample. These studies will be described in detail below. One two-armed pilot study comparing homeopathy with placebo in Pre-Menstrual Syndrome suffered also from recruitment problems [24], nonetheless results are available and will be presented below.

2.1.2.1 Randomized controlled trial in depression and anxiety

There is one published RCT comparing a homeopathic complex therapy (L 72) with the use of Diazepam in mixed states of anxiety and depression [22]. Although the initial report states that L 72 is as effective as Diazepam with a slight trend in favour of homeopathy, subsequent systematic reviews pointed out major flaws. These were: inappropriate use of Diazepam as this is an anxiolytic drug, but not useful in treating depressive symptoms. Also, missing information on the randomization process, as well as on blinding, compliance and co-interventions led to quality scores below the threshold for including trials in a systematic review [25].

Another RCT compared the results of a placebo group of 22 patients with the psychiatrically confirmed diagnosis of generalized anxiety disorder to a drug group of 22 patients which were treated with individually assigned homeopathic remedies [26]. Initially patients got one single dose of the homeopathic drug in 1M or 200C potency (or placebo), but were re-evaluated after six weeks and the remedy could be changed if necessary. Results were the score on the Hamilton Rating Scale for Anxiety (HAM-A) as primary outcome with the Hamilton Rating Scale for Depression (HAM-D) and other scales measuring depression, anxiety, wellbeing and subjective distress as secondary outcomes. In terms of effectiveness of homeopathy over placebo, no difference whatsoever could be detected, either at five weeks or at ten weeks after the initial dose. However, all measures except trait anxiety showed highly significant improvements in both groups over time.

The authors themselves point to the problem of small sample size and hence not enough power to detect small differences in this study. But the authors also conclude that as there was no difference between the groups, not even a large sample size would have yielded significant results. Apart from the fact that one might not be inclined to repeat such a study in the light of these results, there is some more information to infer from this study. 1) It might be a wiser choice to use anxiety disorders as a paradigm for testing homeopathy rather than depression. At least the publication does not give an indication that rescue medicine or concurrent psychiatric treatment had to be allowed, which does not seem feasible given the problem of possible suicides in depression. 2) The improvement over time might be due to the "placebo" effect of either homeopathic or placebo treatment. In fact, the size of improvement was in the range of differences seen in other studies when placebo was given to anxiety patients. But, as no waiting list control group was part of the study design, normal fluctuation or regression to the mean could also have contributed to the effects. Thus, if one is to go through the bother of a clinical study in anxiety disorders, including the necessity of convincing the ethics committee to consent to a study in psychiatric patients without offering them conventional treatment, one should consider a three-armed study in order to learn more about possible placebo effects in mental health care.

2.1.2.2 Randomized controlled trial in Chronic Fatigue Syndrome

A triple blind placebo-controlled study tested the efficacy of classical individual homeopathy in chronic-fatigue outpatients [27]. Patients were assigned to the study after thorough and standardized diagnostic procedures were performed in order to confirm diagnosis of Chronic Fatigue Syndrome (CFS). All 103 patients could be randomized; 50 were randomized to placebo and 53 to homeopathic medicine. This sample size was a little lower than the pre-calculated sample size of 60 per group that would be needed in order to detect a difference of 3 points on a standardized questionnaire measuring chronic fatigue (called MFI). Homeopathic remedies were prescribed after the usual homeopathic prescription process leading to different remedies for different patients. Patients were regularly seen at intervals of approximately four weeks over six months altogether, suggesting that homeopaths could switch to another remedy during this time if appropriate (although this was not clearly indicated in the publication). Although there was no significant effect of homeopathy over placebo on the pre-defined main outcome variable (MFI mental fatigue score), the authors conclude that there was an equivocal and weak effect of homeopathy as more patients improved in the homeopathy group compared to placebo.

A similar result was found in a study including 30 participants who were randomly allocated either to classical homeopathy or to placebo [28]. The treatment group showed a significant intra-group improvement from baseline to both the second (p = 0.001) and third consultations (p=0.002). The placebo group did not show any significant differences for these periods. However, inter-group analyses failed to reveal any statistical significance for both outcome measures (CFS questionnaire and visual analogue scale measuring energy level).

Thus, it might be worthwhile to further examine the possible effects of homeopathy in Chronic Fatigue Syndrome, but to date there is no definite result as to whether patients benefit from homeopathy in these symptoms beyond a placebo effect.

2.1.2.3 Randomized double-blind placebo-controlled crossover trial in Attention Deficit Hyperactivity Syndrome

This unique RCT adapted the usual RCT procedure by incorporating features to address two problems in homeopathy studies: one, that homeopaths cannot rely on the remedy picture in the placebo group if they have to change the homeopathic prescription; and, two, that randomly picked patients might not benefit as much from homeopathy as patients who consciously turn to homeopathy following positive experiences.

The study design was as follows:

1. Prior to the RCT the study group conducted an open-label study where they treated children with Attention Deficit Hyperactivity Syndrome (ADHS) with classical homeopathy and made the following observation: children respond to Q potencies in terms of having less ADHS symptoms. However, if treatment was stopped for four weeks symptoms reappeared (albeit not as intensely) and disappeared again if treatment was restarted.
2. Hence, in the screening phase of the study, the authors defined eligible patients for randomization as those for whom an adequate remedy had been found and whose symptoms deteriorated under no treatment by at least 50% compared to an open-label prior phase where classical homeopathy was applied.
3. 62 eligible patients in the age range of 7-15 with confirmed diagnoses of ADHS were then allocated to two groups with a random sequence of first homeopathy and then placebo treatment vs. first placebo and then homeopathy.
4. Statistical comparisons were made for homeopathy vs. placebo sequences and the assumption was also tested of whether symptoms ameliorated under placebo.

As the results showed that patients benefited from homeopathy significantly more than from placebo on a standardized scale measuring typical symptoms of ADHD (Conner's Global Index) during the first part of the trial, the study provided sound evidence that homeopathy is significantly more effective in ADHS than placebo. It also showed that it is highly likely that patients will benefit from homeopathy (provided they benefited once) as it could be repeatedly shown that symptoms returned when homeopathy was stopped and vanished when homeopathy was given. This study confirmed the results of a previous study that had also found benefits from homeopathic treatment in ADHD; the study design was contentious, however, as placebo was given to children without any information to their parents [29].

2.1.2.4 Randomized controlled double-blind pilot study on Pre-Menstrual Syndrome

Pre-Menstrual Syndrome (PMS) as a paradigm for testing the effects of homeopathic treatment was used by the authors [24] on the following grounds:

1. PMS symptoms could be grouped in clusters which make it easier to integrate the homeopathic approach of individually assigning remedies into a trial.
2. There is no satisfactory conventional treatment for PMS.
3. Psychological factors have an important role in PMS symptoms.

23 women were included in this trial and were allocated to either homeopathy or placebo. The prescription of a homeopathic remedy followed a simplified practice. Five clusters of symptoms were built beforehand mirroring the commonly used homeopathic remedies *Lachesis muta, Natrum muriaticum, Sepia officinalis, Nux vomica* and *Pulsatilla pratensis*. Women were then screened for typical symptoms by applying a score for these symptoms. According to the value on the score it was determined to which cluster they belong and hence which remedy out of the five they were given. The mean score of a menstrual distress questionnaire (MDQ) summarized over two months was given as the baseline value and this was compared to mean scores summarized over the following three months. The results showed significant improvement in the homeopathy group whereas no significant improvement was found in the placebo group.

Despite these encouraging results conclusions should be drawn with care. Whereas the appropriate statistical analysis would have been to compare the mean symptoms of both groups after three months, the approach taken here was to separately compare pre-post means. Hence, due to the pilot character of the study one could consider it a worthwhile basis for looking more deeply into the effects of homeopathy in PMS, but evidence for effectiveness is still to be determined.

It might be instructive at this point to glance aside to homeopathy's younger brother, *Bach flower remedies*. Although not strictly speaking homeopathic, such remedies have some commonalities with homeopathy, in that they are produced by a specific, "subtle" process, in this case by placing flowers in water and leaving them to soak in the sunlight. Afterwards they are also strongly diluted such that no molecule of the original substance is present. A combination of Bach flower remedies were tested that were picked especially for their anxiolytic effects by a specialist therapist. Students who suffered from test anxiety received either Bach flower combinations or placebo in a double-blind randomized study before an exam, and all received Bach flower remedies before the second exam, which occurred roughly a week later. Although there were strong anxiolytic effects and students reported great relief on the Spielberger anxiety measure, there was no difference between the flowers and placebo [37]. This study points to the huge potential for self-healing through appropriate mechanisms such as expectation and hope [31].

2.1.3 *Various other types of studies*
There are a number of case series reporting the results of homeopathic treatment in patients with various mental health problems, all of them dating back to the 1990s [32,33,34,35]. One of the case series explicitly looked at psychiatric problems [32] whereas the others described the treatment of other health problems but included symptoms like depression.

Davidson et al found in their study that homeopathic treatment of twelve patients with various mental health problems (Anxiety Disorders, Attention Deficit Hyperactivity Disorder, Depression, and Chronic Fatigue Syndrome) led to up to 50% reduction in symptoms on standardized questionnaires [32].

The most recent case series included 100 cancer patients with mood problems (mainly depression and anxiety) [33,36]. The results showed improvements in anxiety and depression measured with the Hospital Anxiety and Depression Score (HADS, [37]) and improved quality of life as measured by the EORTC-QLQ-30 [38].

Prospective outcome studies studying large unselected samples of patients treated with homeopathy in Germany show that mental health problems or psychological problems associated with other diseases play a significant role in homeopathic practice [39,40]. One study reports that about 6% of the treated complaints relate to mental health problems [39]. These studies show that patients overall (not only those with mental health problems) are very satisfied with homeopathy and report relevant effects.

Interesting single cases were presented at a homeopathic case conference [41] where interested readers will find detailed information. The cases with mental health problems included a boy with hyperactivity and clumsiness, a woman with breast cancer and panic attacks, a baby with eczema and behaviour problems, and "the case of the ultimate pessimist", a middle-aged male who presented with depressive symptoms.

A qualitative study not particularly concerned with mental disease but performing a secondary analysis of data sets from qualitative studies in cancer patients and patients with other chronic diseases can nevertheless cast light on concepts including mental health [42]. The study describes experiences with diseases followed by CAM treatment as states like *stuckness, unsticking* and *unstuckness*. These experiential states are clearly mental-health related. Stuckness was described by patients as repetitively responding in the same dysfunctional manner to a crisis owing to illness, work stress or family problems. The important feature of this state was that the dysfunctional part of it was only obvious to study participants after they had experienced some form of transformation after CAM treatment. Unsticking was the point where transformation started, e.g. referred to as "flipping a light switch" which caused pain to vanish for the first time after a long period. Unstuckness was experienced as the state after the unsticking transformation process was reliably detectable for patients. It was like being freed from long-standing patterns of stuckness. Apart from studying efficacy or effectiveness of homeopathy this study clearly indicates that the effects of homeopathy include not only improvement in somatic symptoms, but also some form of psychological transformation.

2.2 A practical guide to research

After reviewing the evidence base of homeopathy in mental health our readers might ask, "What is the best way to further contribute to this evidence?" We would therefore like to provide ideas for research designs that might be suitable to answer this question (see Table 1). This overview is by no means comprehensive for there is bountiful literature showing direct ways of performing research in homeopathy and CAM (see [43, 44]). Rather than providing cookbook research protocols, we offer examples of possible research questions (and the appropriate designs to evaluate them). In doing so, we hope to encourage our readers to embark on their own research in homeopathy.

Table 1: Examples of possible research designs and questions

Type of Research	Possible Designs	Aim	Possible Examples
Basic Research	In vitro, plant or animal models	To provide replicable models which could demonstrate biological effects and mechanisms	To compare effects of high diluted homeopathic remedy (HDR) to controls, e.g. succussed water, and/or standard medication
Remedy provings	Open remedy proving or blinded proving	To describe symptoms yielded by HDR	Extract mental health symptoms from overall symptoms and compare frequency of mental health symptoms over remedies or over a placebo-HDR comparison
Clinical Research	1) Randomized controlled trial	To show effects of HDR which are likely to be attributable to homeopathy	3-armed trial comparing SSRI vs. psychotherapy vs. psychotherapy plus HDR
	2) Pre-post-comparison	To study if HDR is likely to contribute to patient's symptoms	Monitor depressive symptoms over 12 months in patients who currently do adhere to anti-depressive medication but stop it due to being not comfortable with SSRI and take HDR instead. Compare symptoms with 12-months-period before taking homeopathy
	3) Outcome study	To study diagnoses, symptoms and improvement of symptoms in large sample of patients	Study frequency of mental health related problems in homeopathic practice and assess symptoms regularly over at least 1 year
Clinical Audit	1) Criteria-based audit	To study existing practice and compare it against standards set beforehand	Study frequency of hospital admissions due to mental health problems in homeopathic practice to ensure (and demonstrate) that it does exceed a certain threshold
	2) Patient surveys	To collect patients' views	Ask a sample of patients (e.g. patients with mental health complaints who turned to homeopathy recently) about their satisfaction with homeopathic care
Qualitative Research	1) Focus groups	To collect views and attitudes of groups of people	Run a series of group discussions with mental health patients who have experiences with standard treatment and homeopathic care and ask them what care they seek under what circumstances
	2) In-depth interviews	To gain in-sights into peoples' behaviour, attitudes, fears, etc.	Interview homeopaths asking them what whole person care involves for them in order to describe mental health issues in routine homeopathic care. Interview patients with treatment experience in homeopathy and conventional care about their experiences, the differences, the changes they observed, etc.

3   Conclusion

Reviewing psychological symptoms is a feature of the homeopathic interview and thus of homeopathic treatment itself. One might therefore think it should be easy to capture the effects on these symptoms in research studies. Although we are sure that discussing mental health and psychological symptoms has some effect on patients in everyday practice, it is much more complicated to extract the size of the effect in a sound scientific way. There are scientific approaches like grade of membership analysis which show some support for the homeopathic concept of constitutional types that include symptoms like sleep or anxiety [45], but capturing effects reliably is another matter altogether.

Randomized controlled studies are certainly at the forefront of well-conducted studies to extract effect sizes. However, one might debate whether comparing homeopathy to placebo treatment is the best way to discern relevant effects [46]. Nevertheless, most of the randomized controlled studies in the field of homeopathy and mental health care are studies comparing homeopathy to placebo, whether in general Anxiety Disorder, or Pre-Menstrual Syndrome, Chronic Fatigue Syndrome or Attention Deficit Hyperactivity Syndrome. The only study comparing homeopathy with a psychoactive drug (Diazepam) in mixed depressive and anxiety states shows that homeopathy is at least not inferior to Diazepam. This is a small study and there is only one report available which gives some results but lacks important features (e.g. statistical tests) in order to rely on the results. Even if one could convince the local ethical committee to repeat this study and design a non-inferiority trial (assuming and testing the hypothesis that homeopathy is not less effective than Diazepam), one would need even more patients to demonstrate this reliably than in ordinary randomized controlled trials (assuming and testing the hypothesis that homeopathy is superior to placebo).

In terms of clinical studies, one could design a study that compares homeopathy to a well-implemented and appropriate standard model of care. This might be easier in syndromes like Pre-Menstrual Syndrome (where no effective standard care is available) or in Attention Deficit Hyperactivity Syndrome (where homeopathy was shown to be effective over placebo). One might even venture to start out with a randomized wait-list controlled study in patients with a mental health problem who do not receive sufficient relief from standard treatments to study whether homeopathy might have anything to offer, leaving aside the question of whether it is placebo.

Apart from these concrete ideas, this chapter explicitly gives practical advice on different study designs and the interested researcher and/or novice also finds the appropriate questions which could be answered by the different designs.
In addition, we have to bear in mind that mental health care is certainly more than treating mental disorders. As one qualitative study showed that CAM (and homeopathy) can help patients to overcome their stuckness in illness symptoms and behaviour (something very much in line with results of case series, case reports and even large outcome studies) it seems that homeopathy can yield "mental *health*" effects, but this is not captured by the standard randomized trial comparing homeopathy to placebo.

Frankly, all types of studies are very welcome in this field, be it a thoroughly documented case study which helps to understand the improvement of clinical symptoms; be it a qualitative study which elicits important features of homeopathy in the field of mental health care; or be it the randomized or quasi-randomized study looking more closely at the real-world effects of homeopathy.

References

[1] Astin JA (1998) Why Patients Use Alternative Medicine. *JAMA* 1998; 279 (19): 1548-1553.

[2] Guethlin C, Lange O, Walach H (2004) Measuring the Effects of Acupuncture and Homoeopathy in General Practice: An Uncontrolled Prospective Documentation Approach. *BMC-Public Health* 2004; 4 (6): 1-33.

[3] Badger F, Nolan P (2007) Use of Self-Chosen Therapies by Depressed People in Primary Care. *J Clinical Nurs* 2007; 16 (7): 1343-1352.

[4] Lowe B, Schulz U, Grafe K, Wilke S (2006) Medical Patients' Attitudes toward Emotional Problems and their Treatment. What Do They Really Want? *J Gen Intern Med* 2006; 21 (1): 39-45.

[5] Lilja L,Hellzen O (2008) Former Patients' Experience of Psychiatric Care: a Qualitative Investigation. *Int J Ment. Health Nurs* 2008; 17 (4): 279-286.

[6] Fava GA, Tomba E, Grandi S (2007) The Road to Recovery from Depression - Don´t Drive Today With Yesterday´s Map. *Psychother Psychosom* 2007; 76 (260): 265.

[7] Rush JA, Trivedi MH, Wisniewski SR et al. (2006) Acute and Longer-Term Outcomes in Depressed Outpatients Requiring One or Several Treatment Steps: A STAR*D Report. *Am J Psychiatry* 2006; 163 (1905): 1917.

[8] Boon H, Brown JB, Gavin A, Kennard MA, Stewart M (1999) Breast Cancer Survivors' Perceptions of Complementary/Alternative Medicine (CAM): Making the Decision to Use or Not to Use. *Qual Health Research* 1999; 9 (5): 639-653.

[9] Russinova Z, Cash D, Wewiorski NJ (2009) Toward Understanding the Usefulness of Complementary and Alternative Medicine for Individuals with Serious Mental Illnesses: Classification of Perceived Benefits. *J Nerv Ment Dis* 2009; 197 (1): 69-73.

[10] Wu P, Fuller C, Liu X et al. (2007) Use of Complementary and Alternative Medicine among Women with Depression: Results of a National Survey. *Psychiatr Serv* 2007; 58 (3): 349-356.

[11] Yamada K (2007) Low Level of Quality of Life in Patients with Mental and Behavioral Disorders Wanting Complementary and Alternative (Kampo) Therapy. *Qual Life Res* 2007; 16 (5): 787-792.

[12] Rickhi B, Quan H, Moritz S, Stuart HL, Arboleda-Florez J (2003) Mental Disorders and Reasons for Using Complementary Therapy. *Can J Psychiatry* 2003; 48 (7): 475-479.

[13] Kessler RC, Soukup J, Davis RB et al. (2001) The Use of Complementary and Alternative Therapies to Treat Anxiety and Depression in the United States. *Am J Psychiatry* 2001; 158 (2): 289-294.

[14] Mamtani R,Cimino A (2002) A Primer of Complementary and Alternative Medicine and Its Relevance in the Treatment of Mental Health Problems. *Psychiatric Quarterly* 2002; 73 (4): 367-381.

[15] Walach H, Jonas W, Lewith GH (2002) *Homeopathy*. In: Lewith G, Jonas W and Walach H (eds): Clinical Research in Complementary Therapies: Principles, Problems, and Solutions. London: Churchill Livingston: pp229-246.

[16] Baumgartner S (2005) Reproductions and Reproducibility in Homeopathy: Dogma or Tool? *J Altern. Complement Med* 2005; 11 (5): 771-772.

[17] Pinto SA, Bohland E, Coelho CP, Morgulis MS, Bonamin LV (2008) An Animal Model for the Study of Chamomilla in Stress and Depression: Pilot Study. *Homeopathy* 2008; 97 (3): 141-144.

[18] Kirsch I, Deacon BJ, Huedo-Medina TB et al. (2008) Initial Severity and Antidepressant Benefits: a Meta-Analysis of Data Submitted to the Food and Drug Administration. *Plos Medicine* 2008; 5 (2).

[19] Turner EH, Matthews AM, Linardatos E, Tell RA, Rosenthal R (2008) Selective Publication of Antidepressant Trials and Its Influence on Apparent Efficacy. *N Engl J Med* 2008; 358 (252): 260.

[20] Pilkington K, Kirkwood G, Rampes H, Fisher P, Richardson J (2006) Homeopathy for Anxiety and Anxiety Disorders: a Systematic Review of the Research. *Homeopathy* 2006; 95 (3): 151-162.

[21] Katz T, Fisher P, Katz A, Davidson J, Feder G (2005) The Feasibility of a Randomised, Placebo-Controlled Clinical Trial of Homeopathic Treatment of Depression in General Practice. *Homeopathy* 2005; 94 145-152.

[22] Heulluy B. (1985) *Essai randomise ouvert de L 72 (spécialité homeopathique) contre diazipam 2 dans les etats anxiodepressifs*. Metz: Laboratoires Lehning 1985.

[23] Bell IR, Lewis DA, Brooks AJ et al. (2004) Improved Clinical Status in Fibromyalgia Patients Treated With Individualized Homeopathic Remedies versus Placebo. *Rheumatology* 2004; 43 577-582.

[24] Yakir M, Kreitler S, Brzezinski A et al. (2001) Effects of Homeopathic Treatment in Women with Premenstrual Syndrome: a Pilot Study. *Br Homoeopath J* 2001; 90 (3): 148-153.

[25] Kleijnen J, Knipschild P, ter Riet G (1991) Clinical Trials of Homoeopathy. *BMJ* 1991; 302 (6772): 316-323.

[26] Bonne O, Shemer Y, Hom RC et al. (2003) A Randomized Double-Blind Placebo-Controlled Study of Classical Homeopathy in Generalized Anxiety Disorder. *J Clin Psychiatry* 2003; 64 (3): 282-287.

[27] Weatherley-Jones E, Nicholl JP, Thomas KJ et al. (2004) A Randomised, Controlled, Triple-Blind Trial of the Efficacy of Homeopathic Treatment for Chronic Fatigue Syndrome. *J Psychosom Res* 2004; 56 (2): 189-197.

[28] Saul W (2009) *The effectiveness of homeopathic simillimum therapy in Chronic Fatigue Syndrome (CFS)* (Thesis, accessed 7th July 2009) 2005: http://ir.dut.ac.za:8080/jspui/bitstream/10321/44/16/Saul_2005.pdf

[29] Lamont J (1997) Homoeopathic Treatment of Attention Deficit Hyperactivity Disorder. *Br Homoeopath J* 1997; 86 (196): 200.

[30] Walach H, Rilling C, Engelke U (2001) Efficacy of Bach-Flower Remedies in Test-Anxiety: A Double-Blind, Placebo-Controlled, Randomized Trial with Partial Crossover. *J Anxiety Disord* 2001; 15 (359): 366.

[31] Walach H, Jonas WB (2004) Placebo Research: The Evidence Base for Harnessing Self-Healing Capacities. *J Alt Complement Med* 2004; 10 (Suppl. 1): S103-S112.

[32] Davidson JRT, Morrison RM, Shore J, Davidson RT, Bedayn G (1997) Homeopathic Treatment of Depression and Anxiety. *Alt Therapies Health Med* 1997; 3 (1): 46-49.

[33] Thompson EA, Reilly D (2003) The Homeopathic Approach to the Treatment of Symptoms of Oestrogen Withdrawal in Breast Cancer Patients. A Prospective Observational Study. *Homeopathy* 2003; 92 (3): 131-134.

[34] Clover A, Last P, Fisher P, Wright S, Boyle H (1995) Complementary Cancer Therapy: a Pilot Study of Patients, Therapies and Quality of Life. *Complement Ther Med* 1995; 3 (3): 129-133.

[35] Zenner S, Weiser M (1999) Homeopathic Treatment of Gynaecological Disorders: Results of a Prospective Study. *Biomed Ther* 1999; 17 (1): 31-35.

[36] Thompson EA, Reilly D (2002) The Homeopathic Approach to Symptom Control in the Cancer Patient: a Prospective Observational Study. *Palliat Med* 2002; 16 (3): 227-233.

[37] Zigmond A, Snaith R (19983) The Hospital Anxiety and Depression Scale. *Acta Psych Scand* 1983; 67 (6): 361-370.

[38] Bjordal K, Kaasa S (1992) Psychometric Validation of the EORTC Core Quality of Life Questionnaire, 30-Item Version and a Diagnosis-Specific Module for Head and Neck Cancer Patients. *Acta Oncol* 1992; 31 (3): 311-321.

[39] Witt C, Ludtke R, Baur R, Willich S (2005) Homeopathic Medical Practice: Long-Term Results of a Cohort Study with 3981 Patients. *BMC Public Health* 2005; 5 (1): 115.

[40] Güthlin C, Lange O, Walach H (2004) Measuring the Effects of Acupuncture and Homoeopathy in General Practice: An Uncontrolled Prospective Documentation Approach. *BMC-Public Health* 2004; 4 (6).

[41] Cannell M, Prunella M, Pettigrew A, Davies C (1999) Case Reports Presented at the Faculty of Homoeopathy Case Conference, Oxford, 13 March 1999. *Br Homoeopath J* 2000; 89 29-42.

[42] Koithan M, Verhoef M, Bell IR et al (2007) The Process of Whole Person Healing: Unstuckness and Beyond. *J Alt Complement Med* 2007; 13 (6): 659-668.

[43] Lewith G, Jonas W, Walach H (2002) *Clinical Research in Complementary Therapies*. Edinburgh: Churchill Livingstone.

[44] Kane M (2004) *Research Made Easy in Complementary & Alternative Medicine*. Edinburgh: Churchill Livingstone.

[45] Davidson J, Fisher P, van Haselen R, Woodbury M, Connor K (2001) Do Constitutional Types Really Exist? A Further Study Using Grade of Membership Analysis. *Br Homoeopath J* 2001; 90 138-147.

[46] Walach H, Falkenberg T, Fonnebo V, Lewith G, Jonas WB (2006) Circular instead of Hierarchical: Methodological Principles for the Evaluation of Complex Interventions. *BMC Medical Research Methodology* 2006; 6 (29).

Chapter 19
Ethical and Practical Implications for Homeopaths in Mental Health Care

Kate Chatfield, MSc RSHom[1] & Joy Duxbury PhD[2]

1) Kate Chatfield, MSc RSHom
School of Health and Caring Sciences
University of Central Lancashire
PR1 2HE Preston
United Kingdom
E-mail: kchatfield@uclan.ac.uk

2) Joy Duxbury, PhD
Divisional Leader for Mental Health
University of Central Lancashire

Abstract

In this chapter we explore some real-life practical issues that have arisen for homeopaths in the UK whilst working with people who have mental healthcare problems. These issues are considered in the light of ethical principles, discussing potential ethical dilemmas and how homeopaths might attempt to resolve them.

1   Introduction

This chapter was inspired by the results of a survey of UK homeopaths carried out in 2006/7. For this project we formed a multi-disciplinary team at the University of Central Lancashire comprised of homeopath and researcher Kate Chatfield, conventional mental healthcare worker and researcher Joy Duxbury and statistician Anna Hart. Together we designed a survey to seek information about the types and extent of mental health disorders people are presenting with for homeopathic treatment and to explore the views of homeopaths about their perceptions, experience and treatment of clients with these problems. Many potential practical and ethical issues emerged from the information that the homeopaths provided. Some of these may be peculiar to the treatment of people with mental health problems, others are more generalised. What became clear was the need for more explicit ethical guidance for practitioners and the profession as a whole.

In this chapter we draw upon findings of the survey to illustrate potential practical and ethical implications of working in this area. We are not ethicists and do not seek to offer definitive guidance but rather refer to general guiding principles that might be adopted in particular situations. We begin by outlining these guiding principles and the place of ethics in medicine.

2   Ethics in medicine

Whilst it can be argued that there are universal and overarching ethical principles, there are no ethical codes of conduct that carry in their entirety across cultures, across time, and across all professions. Codes of medical ethics are as old as the healing profession itself, dating back at least to the Hippocratic Oath 2,400 years ago. This oath served as the principle guiding force on issues such as patient confidentiality, refraining from causing harm and injustice, for most of the Western world until the 19th century when individual medical associations began to form codes of conduct for their own members. It was not until the 1960s, however, that ethical issues in medicine started to attract increased levels of attention from outside the medical profession and bioethics emerged as a distinct academic discipline. At this time advances in medicine such as organ transplants, contraceptive pills, life support machines and the like initiated widespread debate about the ethical implications of such interventions. This was also the prime era of the civil rights campaign in the United States, and revelations of abuse of human rights in the name of scientific or medical research directly challenged accountability within the medical profession.

There now exist a plethora of codes of ethics and many of them could be claimed to be directly relevant to the practice of homeopathy. No one code can cover all possible events but sound general principles can be applied in virtually any situation.

Current thinking in healthcare ethics tends to focus upon the four principles that are outlined by Beauchamp and Childress [1] as the foundation for ethical professional practice:

- Respect for autonomy
- Beneficence
- Non-maleficence
- Justice

2.1 Respect for autonomy

Respect for autonomy means respecting the capacity of an individual to be self-determining, to make decisions for themselves without undue pressure, coercion or other forms of persuasion. Paternalism occurs when actions of a healthcare practitioner override or do not seek the wishes of the patient, believing that they are better able to decide what is in the patient's best interests. Respect for autonomy implies that paternalism should be avoided as much as possible such that, whether or not the doctor knows best, s/he should not make important decisions on behalf of 'competent' patients. The word 'competent' here is crucial as there may be times when the personal judgment of the practitioner is required for assessment of competence. There may also be cultural and legal issues that influence the extent to which this principle is adhered to, some of which will be discussed later in this chapter, but the abiding message is that even where the practitioner acts in the patient's own interests, it is important that the patient's own choices and wishes be respected if possible.

2.2 Beneficence

The principle of beneficence describes an obligation to act for the benefit of others. Acting in this way might involve preventing or removing harm, or it might involve the active promotion of some good (health, for example). The aim of beneficent action will be to produce the best we can out of a range of possibilities. It can involve cost/benefit analysis such that the 'best' here will be the possible action in which the benefits produced maximally outweigh the costs or the risks. Put simply, it is to always act in the best interests of the patient.

2.3 Non-maleficence

Duties of non-maleficence require us to refrain from causing deliberate harm. Generally, obligations of non-maleficence are more stringent than obligations of beneficence, but again a cost/benefit analysis may need to be undertaken to identify the best possible action. In some situations harm may be unavoidable and then we must be sure that the benefits outweigh the harm.

2.4 Justice

It is possible to obey both the principles of non-maleficence and the principle of beneficence and still not behave in an ethical manner, for these two principles say nothing about how benefits should be apportioned. In a given case it may well be that we can only procure a major benefit for some people by slightly harming the interests of others. The principle of beneficence may say we should go ahead, but then the benefits and costs will be unfairly distributed. The principle of justice requires that we do what we can to ensure that costs and benefits are fairly distributed.

In this chapter we will be referring back to these four principles because they can form a useful working model for practitioners. It should be kept in mind however that there is philosophical debate about both the validity of basing ethical decision-making upon 'principles', and about the choice of these four principles in particular. Ethics evolves and changes with time and at any one point reflects what is considered to be ethically appropriate by that society. The principle of autonomy for example is generally more highly valued now than in previous times and perhaps more so in some countries and cultures than others. The increasing popularity of some forms of complementary and alternative medicine (CAM), including homeopathy, has in part been attributed to 'dissatisfaction with medical paternalism' [2]. Patients appreciate both that they can choose their own treatment modality and that their wishes and opinions are valued in the therapeutic relationship.

Health professionals invariably have more knowledge about their subject than the patients who consult them and hence a power differential often exists that is unavoidable. Consequently health professionals must be even more cognisant of ethical practice and seek to behave in an ethical manner at all times. They are normally governed by Codes of Ethics for their profession but these inevitably fall short of telling us what to do in every conceivable situation. For the health professional to behave in an ethical manner involves far more than simply adhering to a code of ethics. Julie Stone [3] wrote specifically about ethics in CAM practice outlining major aspects of ethical practice for the practitioner. In addition to adhering to a professional code of ethics they also included things such as:

- The competence of the practitioner
- Boundaries between the practitioner and patient
- The patient's right to make decisions based on informed choices
- Respect for the patient's culture and values
- A responsibility to consider their options in the light of existing ethical theories
- Awareness of any particular laws governing his or her sphere of practice
- Awareness of professional developments and research underpinning their therapy to ensure competence

3   Ethics in treatment of people with mental health problems

The treatment of people with mental health disorders can bring with it a whole host of additional ethical challenges. For conventional medics who wholly adopt a biomedical model of disease, treatment involves an attempt to identify and treat an underlying physical pathology even if patients themselves do not acknowledge that they are sick. In this case the autonomy of the patient is completely overruled in favour of medical paternalism. The debate about how to achieve balance between respect for autonomy on the one side and medical paternalism with public protection on the other continues to baffle policy-makers in the mental health field [4].

The current policy in the UK of increased care in the community, where people are treated in their own homes, can lead to situation where autonomy is actually reduced rather than increased. Assertive Community Treatment (ACT) aims to ensure that engagement is maintained even when the patient expresses a desire to reduce treatment [5].

It has been argued that there is a moral hierarchy of mental disorders, each provoking value judgements and some carrying a high level of social stigmatisation. Personality disorder, for example, is considered so stigmatising a diagnosis that patients can ask to be reclassified as schizophrenic [4]. Homeopathic philosophy would have us believe that disease labels are unimportant to the homeopathic diagnosis. Whilst this may be the case for finding a suitable remedy, it is not unimportant for responsible case management and it is not unimportant for the patient. Homeopaths are required to straddle medical paradigms and this can generate its own challenges. Moral distress is a common phenomenon in healthcare workers [6] and they are often caught between what they think might be best for their patients and the institutional constraints or overriding decisions of other healthcare professionals [7]. It could be reasonably argued that for health professionals who straddle medical paradigms the potential for moral distress is even greater.

Homeopaths have a moral duty to work out how they can best treat patients in an ethical and responsible manner. It may be that they are already doing so but little research has been undertaken to find out what is actually happening in practice. The survey presented here helps to shed some light on what is happening in practice in the UK by asking the homeopaths themselves.

4   The survey

The Society of Homeopaths (SoH) is the largest professional organisation for homeopaths in the UK with approximately 2,000 practising members. One tenth of these members (200) were randomly selected from the register to participate in the survey. A questionnaire that included both open and closed questions was developed. Definitions of nine individual mental health disorders, drawn from the mental health charity MIND [8], were embedded within the questionnaire for reference. The open questions focused upon the views of homeopaths about their experience of treating people with mental health problems. They asked specifically for homeopaths' experiences and opinions on a number of issues such as what helped and hindered treatment and any challenges encountered. Questionnaires were posted out in September 2006 and responses to the questionnaire were anonymous.

Results from the quantitative part of the questionnaire provided us with some information about the homeopaths and a picture of what kinds of mental health problems patients present with. Of the 200 surveyed homeopaths 96 (48%) responded. Of these 72/96 (75%) were aged 45-64; 78/96 (81%) were female and most, 67/96 (70%) had spent 5-19 years in practice. Most of those surveyed, 49/96, (61%) saw no more than 9 patients per week with 62% (60/96) stating that they see patients at home, 51/96 (53%) in clinic, some at both home and clinic and 9/96 (9%) in neither place.

The most commonly treated conditions fall into the categories of anxiety and mood disorders, reflecting the known prevalence of these disorders [9]. Results also indicate, however, that homeopaths are treating people with a full spectrum of mental health disorders. For example, a substantial proportion (57%) state they have treated patients with schizophrenia and 78% state that they would.

The sample of homeopaths spans years of experience and no clear association was found between time in practice and either willingness to treat each condition or level of confidence felt about doing so. Over 90% of respondents would be willing to treat all disorders mentioned except schizophrenia regardless of length of experience. Those who have treated schizophrenia in the past were more likely to say they would treat it in the future, suggesting that experience of treatment is not acting as a deterrent.

The qualitative part of this survey contained open questions that invited homeopaths to write about their opinions and experience. Amongst other things, we asked about what factors they felt helped and hindered treatment and about any challenging situations that had occurred. Despite some differences in views expressed by the homeopaths, a number of generic concerns were raised and these are outlined below within the context of the questions that were asked on the questionnaire. Direct quotes from the completed questionnaires are used to illustrate the most typical responses.

4.1 Question: Please tell us about factors that you believe can help or hinder treatment of patients with mental health problems

By far the two largest factors mentioned by the homeopaths in response to this question were those of being able to work collaboratively and not feeling as if they are on their own with the patient, and the influence that allopathic medication is having upon the patient. Two lesser factors were to do with patient compliance and patient use of recreational drugs.

4.1.1 Collaborative working and support

This was mentioned by 60 homeopaths. Homeopaths in the UK often work alone, seeing patients for appointments every 4-6 weeks. Many concerns were raised about the need for support of the patient by other healthcare workers, friends and family. Working in an environment of collaboration was the most commonly expressed helpful factor. This collaboration may be with mental health care workers but also a positive relationship with the patient's GP and family was viewed as essential. It was evident that a number of patients enlist the support of 'non-conventional' practitioners in part of a treatment package. Generally homeopaths recognised this as a positive influence. Social support for clients, largely from family members, was highly valued by homeopaths and seen to be indicative of a client's progress when consulting a homeopath.

"Working in conjunction with conventional medications and those who administer them is much more successful." (#62)

"Patients with severe mental health problems often need 24-hour support which is not practical within my practice." (#9)

"Several patients also use the counsellors and psychotherapists at the clinic where I work. We frequently have case conferences, which we all feel helps us to do the best we can for our patients. Patients comment that they feel supported and are happy to know that we can provide more than one route to health." (#48)

Many reported positive experiences of integrated care, such as:

"Worked as part of ward rounds on acute mental health team for three years. ...Gradually became accepted as a team member with something to contribute." (#57)

"I work on wards for acute mental health problems; they are very open-minded and holistic." (#35)

Broadly speaking, the support sought by most homeopaths in their work was from other professionals. However, this was not always straightforward and poor liaison and partnership working was reported as problematic for many. If the support and collaboration is not available then this is viewed as an impactful hindrance.

"If the patient doesn't have other support then I have to think twice about whether I can take them on. Just seeing me every four weeks often isn't enough." (#39)

"Medical profession advising against homeopathic treatment has definite negative issues for the patient to address and vice versa." (#94)

There are few examples of SoH members working within an integrated team of healthcare professionals for the treatment of people with mental health problems. Consequently it is likely that the majority of homeopaths are practising outside of the conventional healthcare system and therefore without access to standard support networks available to mental healthcare professionals. According to Stone [3] it is rarely ethical for practitioners to work in isolation from professional colleagues, a situation that we in the UK often find ourselves in. Perhaps the profession as a whole should be asking how integrated healthcare and/or collaborative working might best be promoted. In the meantime, individual homeopaths might consider whether it is ethical to take on those patients who are in obvious need of a network of care that cannot be provided.

4.1.2 Allopathic medication

52 respondents mentioned allopathic medication as something that can hinder treatment. Various reasons were identified:

1. That it slows down the patient's reaction to remedies.

"Antidepressants slow down treatment, particularly Seroxat and Effexor." (#52)

2. That suppressive effects of the drugs can mask the true symptoms of the patient.

"They are usually on very heavy chemical drugs which hinder establishing symptoms of the disease rather than side-effects of the drugs." (#14)

"Major tranquillisers like Chlorpromazine make it impossible to see the case." (#56)

"The most difficult thing is that the medication masks the true picture and I rarely see a person before they are given medication for OCD, schizophrenia, or Bi-Polar Disorder." (#30)

3. Of those who mentioned the issue most believe that remedies can work in spite of allopathic treatment.

"To my surprise I do not find that medication hinders treatment if LMs are used. I have successfully treated people on antidepressants, antipsychotics and mood stabilisers." (#27)

"Although I find it difficult to treat through long-term medication I have seen homeopathy succeed in such cases." (#34)

"Drugs can make treatment more difficult but I would always be prepared to treat in spite of this and have sometimes been surprised by how well remedies can act in spite of drugs." (#44)

Some disagree:

"Allopathic drugs make people with schizophrenia incurable homeopathically." (#47)

4. There is awareness that reduction of allopathic drugs is a complicated issue ...

"The standard 'chemical' approach to mental illness makes symptom recognition quite difficult ... and it is always tricky and ethically dangerous to suggest any changes to prescribed drugs." (#79)

... but can sometimes be done in co-operation:

"Their current medication can hinder their treatment. Although I still find patients improve and generally I aim to gradually reduce their medication with the full cooperation of their doctor." (#3)

The issue of how to deal with allopathic medication use raises many ethical principles. The ability to take a homeopathic case might be affected by the mental health drugs that the person is taking but this can be true for any type of pathology. Homeopaths must respect the autonomy of the patient and this can at times be in conflict with they might believe to be best for the patient. Current ethical guidance in the UK would have us place autonomy of the patient as paramount in cases where the patient is capable of positive self-determination. As with any case that is taken, the right of patients to self-select the treatment(s) that they believe are right for them must be accepted even if it makes the job more difficult. This holds true for any treatments or therapies that the person chooses, not just allopathic medications.

Also important for homeopaths here is the principle of non-maleficence. Homeopaths must make sure they do no harm, such that advice to patients about their use of other medications or treatments will not cause any harm. It has been known for patients to inadvertently develop the idea that they can cease all other medication when they begin homeopathic treatment.

"One bipolar patient on daily homeopathic prescription took himself off lithium overnight without informing anyone." (#94)

It is part of a practitioner's ethical responsibility to ensure that patients understand how homeopathy works and to explain to them the possible consequences of changing treatment regimes.

On a more controversial note, it might be asked where the responsibility of the homeopath lies if they believe there is good evidence to demonstrate that harm is being caused by the conventional medication the patient is taking. There may appear to be compelling ethical reasons for discussing such concerns with the patient, but this is an extremely delicate issue. In trying to avoid harm of one kind there is a danger that another might be caused if the patient should become confused or distressed. Professional homeopaths in the UK can be considered experts in the field of homeopathic interventions and as such qualified to give advice on this matter. Matters of conventional medication use will normally fall outside their expertise and hence they may be in contravention of professional codes of conduct if they advise against its use.

Tension of this kind might arise more commonly for professional homeopaths who work outside a conventional healthcare system, but can also exist as a result of conflicting beliefs or differing health paradigms. As previously stated, moral distress is a common phenomenon in healthcare workers [6] and perhaps a constant challenge for homeopaths who adopt a medical philosophy that is contrary to the dominant one in most countries. This issue is not exclusive to the area of mental health and one that will no doubt continue to be debated for some time to come.
On a positive note most who responded to the survey believed that homeopathic remedies can work well even when the patient is taking allopathic medication; the treatment may just take longer.

4.1.3 Compliance

Patient compliance was mentioned as an important factor by 32 respondents. Many different factors were mentioned as having an impact upon compliance but essentially they all entail an understanding of what homeopathic treatment involves and having commitment to the process. There was recognition that this is not always easy and perhaps very different from the nature of the treatments that have already been experienced.
Whether individuals were able to successfully follow and comply with homeopathic treatment appears to be dependent upon three additional sub-themes: cost, personal motivation and the long-term nature of the problem, and subsequent treatment.

"Many people expect 'quick fixes' even for deep-seated conditions." (#38)
"Successful treatment is likely to take 1-2 years for severe cases with 3-4 weekly appointments." (#10)
"The patient has to be committed to the treatment. They have to want to go through the process." (#12)
"It is often very difficult to maintain a proper process of follow-up treatment due to financial constraints." (#22)

When people consult a homeopath for the first time, they may not know what the therapy involves or what outcomes to realistically expect. In these situations, and from an ethical standpoint, it is even more important for the practitioner to openly discuss the form of treatment being offered, what it entails, and what could be achieved, as well as to discuss alternative treatment strategies. If the patient is to engage fully with the process then informed consent is essential. The fact that outcomes cannot be precisely predicted should not deter us from explaining as best we can what the patient might reasonably expect to happen during the consultation and treatment.

4.1.4 Recreational drugs
Eight responders mentioned the use of recreation drugs as a potentially hindering factor to treatment.

> *"One patient also took cannabis, which made case more difficult as it was a major factor in depression and did impede effectiveness of remedies." (#28)*

But as is the case with allopathic medication these are thought to obscure the picture and perhaps slow down the treatment but not to present a major obstacle to cure.

4.2 Question: Please tell us about any challenging situations that have resulted from treating patients with mental health problems
Experience of challenging situations was not described by all homeopaths, but of those who did respond to this question their responses fall into three categories: safety issues, reactions to treatment and boundary issues.

4.2.1 Safety
Concerns about safety for both patient and homeopath were frequently expressed and many specific examples of challenging situations described. These concerns were commonly intensified by frustrations regarding poor follow-up and obstacles to effective inter-professional working. 15 homeopaths described situations where the patient posed an actual or potential danger to themselves or others:

> *"I broke confidentiality with a young borderline schizophrenic and explained to him that I would do this. In my judgement he was a potential danger to himself and was exhibiting behaviour close to stalking a female neighbour." (#72)*

Nine of the fifteen mentioned patients with suicidal thoughts and tendencies. There appears to be a lack of clarity around assessment of actual threat ...

> *"Not being sure about the severity of patient's illness, e.g. suicidal thoughts – are they actively suicidal? At what point should others be alerted re confidentiality." (#37)*
>
> *"I think the most difficult situation I have found myself in was when one of my patients telephoned me to say she couldn't carry on and was going to commit suicide. Luckily I persuaded her to contact other services who were very supportive and she was able to move onwards without ending her life." (#9)*

... some of whom subsequently committed suicide:

> *"Following the disturbing suicide of one patient with manic depression I would not want to treat this condition again*

a) For my own state of mind's sake

b) For the patient's sake" (#80)

Eleven homeopaths described events that have arisen during consultations resulting in them having concerns for their own personal safety. This appears to be especially the case for those who work from home often on their own. When personal safety is compromised this is largely due to fears over violence from clients, threatened, implied or more subtle forms such as a heightened demand for time and attention. This can then lead homeopaths to question the level and suitability of arrangements needed to ensure greater security and safety.

"A patient suffering from schizophrenia (sent by a member of his family) displayed aggressive behaviour in response to being asked questions during case taking. This could have been dangerous but was thankfully diffused. I would – if ever again- only treat such a case in a clinic with a support system / security in place" (#5)

"I have felt very uncomfortable with a male patient who was telling me about his violent dreams – I was still practising from home then." (#67)

Five homeopaths described situations which they felt were outside the bounds of their competence:

"A man with a history of violence and domestic violence was outside my competence to treat without the involvement of a psychotherapist. He refused to go to any therapist or NHS mental health care practitioners and I chose not to treat him." (#72)

"Young single man, diagnosed schizophrenic, treated for 18 months. Very anxious mother demanded support and information I could not provide. Client also had florid delusions which were extremely disturbing, especially as I did not have adequate mentoring." (#23)

Issues of safety for both patient and homeopath may raise worrying concerns but they are rare and not experienced by all. In comparison to the number of patients that would have been treated by these 96 homeopaths during their careers, the number of worrying incidents is probably quite small. Fears may be exaggerated by feelings of isolation or vulnerability in the workplace. It is clear from both our findings and professional body registers that homeopathy in the UK is currently numerically speaking a female-dominated profession, a significant proportion of whom state that they work from home. However, even if practise is currently safe, in the vast majority of cases this should not deter us from asking if anything could be done to further enhance safety for all concerned.

Mental health care practitioners are required to carry out a risk assessment exercise for patients. This is used to predict whether patients are a danger to themselves or others but the practice is widely challenged for its lack of accuracy and inherent discrimination [10]. The main problem with the existing risk assessment instruments is that they are not reliable and often greatly overestimate the risk of serious acts of violence. Subsequently, many persons are detained in order to prevent one seriously violent act. In fact, serious acts of violence by persons with mental health problems are rare. Studies examining whether individuals with mental illness are more violent than the non-mentally ill have yielded mixed results [11, 12, 13]. In a study of psychiatric patients released into the community, most were not violent [14]. A weak relationship between mental illness and violence was found but violent behaviour was greater only during periods in which the person was experiencing acute psychiatric symptoms. Contrary to popular belief, a diagnosis of schizophrenia was associated with lower rates of violence than was a diagnosis of depression or of Bi-Polar Disorder.

In spite of this apparently rather confusing picture painted by research, the official stance is that mental health service users are vulnerable to a number of potential risks often related to their own behaviour such as self-harm, aggression and violence, and sexually disinhibited behaviour [15]. Issues of safety may rarely arise but when working with patients we accept an obligation to notify appropriate authorities if there is a serious risk of harm to others. However, how we determine what is 'serious' as well as whom and how we notify is a matter that has yet to be resolved for homeopaths in the UK.

Just as with risk assessment for violent behaviour, suicide risk assessment is difficult, as some homeopaths have found. Suicide risk assessment inherently involves an assessment of human emotions, thinking and behaviours, which vary considerably with individuals depending on their age, culture, and personal circumstance [16]. The diversity of human behaviour and experience precludes accurate, foolproof suicide risk assessment techniques. However, developing a greater awareness of the risk factors and potential antecedents for suicide increases the likelihood that significant risk factors will be spotted during treatment [17].

Some homeopaths described situations that they felt were outside the bounds of their competence. The principle of non-maleficence requires us to be able to recognise such situations and act accordingly. It is not a bad thing to feel that some situations are outside our competence but it would be unethical to continue to treat the patient regardless. A challenge for homeopaths is how to effectively assess bounds of competence whilst continually working with different kinds of patients, different kinds of illness, different approaches to treatment and new remedies.

4.2.2 Reactions to case taking and treatment
Eighteen homeopaths described reactions to the case taking or treatment that were challenging for themselves and the patients. For example during case taking:

> "Two patients having to leave half way through the first consultation because talking was creating intense anxiety." (#27)

Aggravations, return of old symptoms and stirred memories/emotions were all mentioned as possible reactions to the treatment:

> "Dealing with painful issues as they emerge as part of the healing process." (#33)
> "Severe aggravations or exacerbations of part of the condition – sometimes associated with underlying trauma." (#56)
> "Conditions getting worse not better because remedies, although apparently well-indicated, stirred the unconscious even more than it already was in schizophrenia. The danger is that we attempt to cure when what is needed is appropriate care." (#4)
> "Return of old symptoms in constitutional treatment which can be alarming for the patient and relatives." (30)

Bearing in mind our ethical principles, these experiences raise several questions:

- How is it possible to take a case in such a way that trauma and anxiety is avoided?
- Given that we are obliged to cause no harm, is aggravation inevitable?
  - o If no then how can we be sure to avoid it?
  - o If yes then how can we weigh up the costs and benefits to the patient?
- Should it be explained to all patients that aggravations/unpleasant reactions/return of old symptoms are a possibility so that they can make an informed decision about whether to undergo treatment?
- Is it always in the best interests of patients to treat them with homeopathy?

It is likely that opinions amongst homeopaths will differ on these matters and further research might be necessary to find solutions. However, they are important ethical questions that need to be addressed by the profession.

4.2.3 Boundary issues

Another major cause of significant concern to thirteen of the surveyed homeopaths is the problem of establishing and maintaining therapeutic boundaries between themselves and patients which can result in professional conflict for the homeopath. Specific and somewhat worrying examples were given, such as:

> "Young single woman with schizoid symptoms, no formal diagnosis, socially isolated, with unsupportive family and GP became unhealthily dependent upon myself and her psychotherapist." (#23)
> "Patient who fell in love with me and stalked me for years." (#11)

Phone calls appeared to be particularly problematic:

> "Patients with anxiety can be very demanding. One patient kept ringing me through the night about 10 times." (#5)
> "Frequent telephone calls between appointments." (#22)
> "Late-night phone calls from patients in a depressed state." (#42)

Homeopaths are not the only healthcare professionals who can have problems in maintaining clear therapeutic boundaries. Problems for all CAM professionals might be exacerbated when working outside of conventional healthcare settings, particularly if they work from their own homes. In addition, the psychotherapeutic nature of some interventions (such as homeopathy) can produce a significant power imbalance that facilitates transference and counter-transference [18]. These factors make it even more important for the homeopath that great care be taken in the setting and maintaining of clear therapeutic boundaries. It is the responsibility of the homeopath to provide a safe space for patients. When boundaries become blurred, the potential for harm to the patient increases. [19]

4.3 Implications

Two major recommendations for ethical practice in the treatment of people with mental health problems emerge from consideration of the results of this study:

1. That education and training programmes should incorporate sufficient training in the treatment of people with mental health problems and ethical practice.
2. That greater collaboration and integrated practice might avoid many potential problems and may be safer and more effective for the patient.

4.3.1 Education and training

Homeopaths in the UK come from a wide variety of backgrounds and homeopathy is often not their first career choice. A study involving 223 members of SoH found that 53% had qualifications at degree level and above in addition to their homeopathic qualifications [20]. 26% of those questioned had qualifications in some form of conventional healthcare (doctor, nurse, midwife etc) but most professional homeopaths in the UK do not have specialist qualifications in the treatment of people with mental health disorders. Whilst there is much in homeopathic literature that describes treatment of people who have mental health problems, this is primarily reported in the form of case studies. There is no specialised training available in homeopathic psychiatry in the UK and the amount of time devoted to this area during training varies considerably between colleges. An extensive and in-depth book such as this is long overdue and provides a welcome addition to the homeopathic literature.

In addition, it is widely recognised that ethical issues are ubiquitous in healthcare but how many homeopaths have received ethics education in their professional training programmes? Ethics education and training can help healthcare practitioners develop confidence in their decisions and know-how to take appropriate action and tap into available resources when needed [21]. CAM students require explicit training to understand the boundaries which exist and why they are important; their education and training must include clear advice on what actions are and are not acceptable [18].

Homeopaths registered with SoH are bound by a Code of Ethics and Practice [22] to ensure professional conduct in practice. The National Occupation Standards in Homeopathy identify elements of competence and good practice. In order to achieve competency in the provision of homeopathic treatment for people with mental health problems homeopaths need to assess their own knowledge, skills and experience to ensure that they are practising safely and effectively. However there are no specific guidelines at present for what constitutes safe and effective practice. Homeopathic philosophy teaches that the person is an integrated whole of mind and body and as such no part should be treated in isolation. Consequently most homeopaths will view themselves as being providers of healthcare for persons rather than particular types of ailments and speciality training has to date been rare. However, it is becoming more widely acknowledged that certain groups of patients require practitioners to have more specialised knowledge and competence, particularly with respect to case management.

4.3.2 Collaboration and integrated practice

It is clear from this survey and many other studies [23, 24] that many people are choosing homeopathy either as an alternative or an adjunct to conventional treatment for mental health care problems. Homeopaths in the UK often work alone in private practice but it is evident that collaborative working is highly valued when treating people with mental health care problems. Homeopathy is not a statutorily regulated profession in the UK, so there is no legal definition of who can call themselves homeopaths and there is no established infrastructure that allows for a widespread integrated approach to treatment. A significant challenge for the profession in the UK is how to establish a safe, supportive, collaborative environment for effective treatment and case management of people with severe and enduring mental health problems.

Collaboration might include an integrated working approach in which homeopaths work as part of a healthcare team. In 1993 The Prince of Wales founded The Prince's Foundation for Integrated Health to promote integrated healthcare for all in the UK. The foundation is currently writing guidelines to encourage the development of integrated health in National Health Service mental health services by setting out the governance infrastructure and providing a guide to service development. How widely the guidelines will be adopted and whether they can be practically implemented remains to be seen.

Collaborative working is not simply about integrated healthcare. Indeed many homeopaths choose to work 'outside' of the system. One broad interpretation of the results of this survey is that many homeopaths in the UK believe that being the only person who is treating or supporting the patient can lead to an unsustainable position that challenges treatment. Collaboration in this sense can include the patient's social network as well as GPs, mental health care workers and other CAM practitioners. In addition to the obvious benefit to patients, collaborative working can also support the homeopath, essential if the homeopath is to function in a healthy and effective manner.

4.3.3 Study limitations and recommendations

This study has various limitations that should be taken into consideration when interpreting the results. The main limitations are as follows:

- No formal diagnoses of patients were requested for the survey and hence we only have homeopaths' opinions about what they were treating.
- The questionnaire was only sent to members of the Society of Homeopaths in the UK. Whilst this is the largest sole professional organisation in UK there are more than ten other organisations with smaller numbers of registered members.
- Medically qualified homeopaths in the UK may have different experience as they have access to a support network not available to those outside the National Health Service.
- The UK homeopaths that were surveyed provide only a UK perspective. They work alongside the NHS framework in the UK and this may be different in other countries where homeopathy is either more or less widely accepted and there are different systems of public healthcare.

Primary recommendations from this study are that:

- Similar studies be carried out in a range of different countries with different healthcare systems
- Ethical principles be more widely considered and debated in relation to homeopathic practice around issues such as informed consent of the patient and ethical tension for the practitioner.
- Educational programmes for homeopaths incorporate sufficient training in the treatment of people with mental health problems and ethical practice.
- The homeopathy profession consider how to work towards greater collaboration and/or integrated practice for the treatment of people with mental health care problems.

5   Summary

In this chapter we have attempted to describe some of the practical and ethical implications of working with patients with mental health problems. Whilst ethical challenges might be rare, they do appear to exist, and this survey has highlighted some that have actually occurred for homeopaths working in the UK. Issues around allopathic medication use, lack of collaborative working, safety, reactions to treatment, boundaries and compliance raised the most concerns.

Homeopaths have a well-documented history of success in treating people with mental health problems and current trends indicate that by 2020 mental health problems will contribute to 15% of the global disease burden [25]. If homeopathy is to be accepted as a viable treatment option then clear guidance on what constitutes safe and ethical practice is crucial.

References

[1] Beauchamp T & Childress J. (1994) *Principles of Biomedical Ethics* (4th edition). Oxford, Oxford University Press

[2] Balneaves LG, Kristjanson LJ, Tataryn D. (1999) Beyond convention: describing complementary therapy use by women living with breast cancer. *Patient Educ Couns*. 38: 143–53

[3] Stone J. (2002) An *Ethical Framework for Complementary and Alternative Therapists*, London, Routledge

[4] Eastman N, Starling B. (2006) Mental disorder ethics: theory and empirical investigation. *J Med Ethics*, 32: 94-99

[5] Szmukler G, Appelbaum PS. (2008) Treatment pressures, leverage, and compulsion in mental health care. *J Mental Health*, 17: 233-244

[6] Kalvemark S, Hoglund A, Hansson M, Westerholm P, Arnetz B. (2004) Living with conflicts - ethical dilemmas and moral distress in the health care system. *Soc Sci & Med*, 58: 1075-1084

[7] Jameton A. (1984) *Nursing Practice: The Ethical Issues*. Englewood Cliffs, NJ: Prentice Hall

[8] Stewart G. (2007) *Understanding mental illness*. London: Mind publications;

[9] WHO World Mental Health Survey Consortium. (2004) Prevalence, severity, and unmet need for treatment of mental disorders in the World Health Organization World Mental Health Surveys. *J Am med Assoc*. 291(21): 2581-90

[10] Scott CL, Resnick PJ. (2006) Violence risk assessment in persons with mental illness. *Aggression and Violent Behavior*. 11: 598–611

[11] Link BG, Andrews H, Cullen F T. (1992) The violent and illegal behavior of mental patients reconsidered. *Am Sociol Review*. 57: 275–292

[12] Steadman HJ, Mulvey EP, Monahan JR, et al. (1998) Violence by people discharged from acute psychiatric inpatient facilities and by others in the same neighborhoods. *Archives Gen Psy*. 55: 393–401

[13] Torrey E F. (1994) Violent behavior by individuals with serious mental illness. *Hosp & Community Psy*. 45: 653–662

[14] Monahan J. (1997) Actuarial support for the clinical assessment of violence risk. *Intl Review of Psy*. 9: 167–170

[15] National Patient Safety Agency (2006) *With safety in mind: mental health services and patient safety.* Patient safety observatory Report. NHS

[16] New Zealand Guidelines Group and New Zealand Ministry of Health. (2003) *Best practice evidence-based guideline: the assessment and management of people at risk of suicide.* For Emergency Departments and Mental Health Service Acute Assessment Settings. Wellington

[17] Boyce P, Carter G, Penrose-Wall J, Wilhelm K, Goldney R. (2003) Summary Australian and New Zealand clinical practice guideline for the management of adult deliberate self-harm. *Australasian Psychiatry*, 11(2):150—155

[18] Stone, J. (2008) Respecting professional boundaries: What CAM practitioners need to know. *Comp Ther in Clin Prac*. 14:2–7

[19] Pepper RS. (2008) Boundaries, ethics and chaos theory in psychotherapy. *J.Eurpsy* 1:1353

[20] Chatfield K, Partington H. (2004) Professional homeopaths in the UK: *Who are they? Conference presentation.* Alternative and Complementary Health Research Network: Nottingham

[21]Grady C, Danis M, Soeken KL et al. (2008) Does education influence the moral action of practicing nurses and social workers? *Am J Bioeth*. 8(4): 4-11

[22] Society of Homeopaths. (2004) *Code of Ethics and Practice*. Milton Keynes: SoH publications

[23] Relton C, Chatfield K, Partington H, Foulkes L. (2007) Patients treated by homeopaths registered with the Society of Homeopaths: a pilot study. *Homeopathy*, 96:87-89

[24] Spence DS, Thompson EA, Barron SJ. (2005) Homeopathic treatment for chronic disease: a 6-year, university-hospital outpatient observational study. *J Alt Comp Med*, 11: 793-798

[25] Murray CJL, Lopez AD, editors. (1996) *Global burden of disease: a comprehensive assessment of mortality and disability from diseases, injuries, and risk factors in 1990 and projected to 2020*. Cambridge, MA: Harvard University Press

Chapter 20
Neuro-Psychic (Dis)Orders and Homeopathy: Biophotonic Connections

Prof. Dr. Traian D. Stănciulescu

Prof. Dr. Traian D. Stănciulescu, Romania
Str. Oancea nr. 1. bl. D12, et. 4, ap. 19
700351 Iassy
Romania
E-mail: tdstan@uaic.ro

Abstract

The present chapter makes the connection between homeopathy and mental health care from the emergent perspective of *biophotonics*, the new science of biology and laser technology. This connection is able to clarify some phenomena and processes which have previously been obscure and/or unknown such as: the *"ultraweak bioluminescence"* (emission of biophotons) generated by all living systems, identified with the "vital force" or "life force" of homeopathy; the "biological laser" mechanism of remedies, involving the "nothingness" of super-high homeopathic dilutions or the vibratory information of the "living light" (aura); the exogenous and/or endogenous "holographic resonance" able to deliver the "energy-information traps" (sources of electrons and biophotons) inside the human body, for stimulating the self-healing phenomenon of *similia similibus curentur*; the holographic functioning of the brain; and the mnesic[23] role of membranous "liquid crystal" structures and of the human aura (as a "memory field") in explaining the unrecognized causes of mental illness.

Through clarification of these issues, the therapist – homeopath and/or psychiatrist – could better understand the wholeness of the illness semiosis[24], being able to combine the rationality of science and the intuition of the therapy for generating its main desirable effect: human health (re)harmonization.

*(The field of science represented by the author in this article is highly specialized. Although for many this article may still be a tough read, the author has nevertheless succeeded in making the content accessible to homeopaths and other health professionals. The beginning of the final section of this article, **Summary and implication of the healing process**, explains*

---

23 Mnesic: relating to memory (mneme in Greek).

24 Semiosis: the activity or process (symbolic or mental) involved when something acts as a sign* to an organism, producing meaning. *Sign: anything which stands for something else, to someone, in some capacity.

in a nutshell the practical relevance of the subject, and reading that first may help to keep an overview while reading the full article – The Editors).

1   Instead of an introduction: towards a (meta)physical synergy

To help understand the subtle mechanisms of human becoming, the cognitive resources of many sciences that refer to man – from Philosophy (Metaphysics) and Psychology to (Bio)Physics and Anthropology, Medicine and Semiology[25] – are to be correlated in an inter- and trans-disciplinary way. This is the only way that HUMAN SYSTEMS SYNERGY can be described and relevantly explained, meaning: the functional power of the whole is greater than the sum of its constituent elements.

This is why, in the forthcoming paragraphs, I will synthesize the explanatory principles of an emergent discipline – BIOPHOTONICS – so as to fruitfully combine it with NEUROPSYCHOLOGY and HOMEOPATHY. These correlations define the title of the scientific approach symbolically described through the meanings of the triangle presented below (See Fig. 1).

Figure 1. An essential connection for human health: "mens sana →←in corpore sano" (from neuro-psychic disorders → via homeopathic therapies → to integral health).

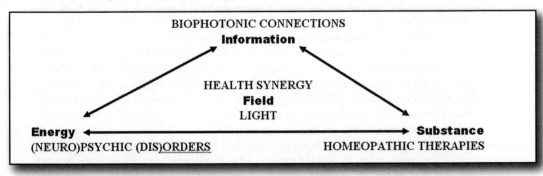

A number of further general and specific considerations are to be mentioned in order to illustrate the meanings of this B(N)PH triangle [*Biophotonics → (Neuro)Psychology / Psychiatry → Homeopathy*], which synthesizes the Protagoras saying: "*Man is the measure of all things…*". As general metaphysical premises, necessary for the "physical" (therapeutic) applications of the present study, we can state that:

- "*Everything is vibration*" (Rig-Veda) / "*Everything is wave*" (Max Planck). Or, in Albert Einstein's terms: "*Everything is light in different concentration degrees*": from the not-created light to the light created on the first day and being present both in the wave of particle-photon, in the Sun and Moon, in the bio(psycho)luminescence of living organisms and also in the "vital force" of the homeopathic remedy.

---

25 Semiology/Semiotics: the study of signs & communication (including how meaning is constructed and understood).

- *Knowledge of created realities implies the following inverted direction*: from the visible effect to the invisible cause or in the case of a disease from studying semio-logical symptoms to decoding the causes of getting ill.
- When disorders appear (chaos) at the level of a random whole (such as the human organism), *reinstating the order (cosmos / health) implies the regulation of the disorder appearing in the informational field waves of the whole and only then of that manifested at the level of the "particle" or (bio)physical subsystem.*
- If *"Complex Light"* [26] is responsible for all that is, it means that *both health and disease will be correlated with light involvement*; the theoretical and practical synergy between Biophotonics, Psychiatry and Homeopathy will be used in this *transdisciplinary* sense, with LIGHT as a common denominator / basis.[27]

Through the analysis of the BPH triangle, two categories of *specific interpretations* can be grasped:

a) *Separately analyzed*, and from the perspective of a standardized scientific approach, the above-mentioned disciplines in the three corners of the triangle seem to offer only vague and limited insights (insufficiently elaborated, justified and generalized) into a small number of aspects of a reality as complex as the Universe itself: HUMAN LIFE. This is because:

1. it is hard to consistently appreciate from the perspective of academic knowledge what *biophotonics* means – a science as old as life itself but only recently rediscovered in the lab as a discipline of the "living light";
2. very little is clear about the "black box" of cerebral functioning, about *neuro-psychism*[28] in other words, because it is unclear whether madness, for example, is a malfunction of cerebral substance or of the whole body, whether it is the result of an energetic (electromagnetic) imbalance, or simply, from an informational point of view, an effect of "karmic accumulations" or the "punishment of the gods";

---

26 Through the concept of "complex light" we have named all the possible manifestation of the (bio)electromagnetic spectrum in its many facets from the metaphysically non-created light to the light physically created through the Big Bang (Fiat lux!), to the biological light of plants, animals and man respectively and to cyclical or spiritual (noesic) light.

27 It is amazing to note that all these (meta)physical premises of creation have already been assumed and intuitively introduced in the practice of homeopathy itself. This starts with the choice and usage of a substantial source with specific information; as a remedy it becomes a source of sanogenous* "spiritual light", is diluted in water and then impregnates the neutral substance (lactose). The process ends with its transfer by "holographic resonance" to the living body already prepared to receive it through the BPL (Bio-Psycho-Logical) attributes of the personality. (*Sanogenesis: the processes involved in creating or maintaining health; the opposite of pathogenesis.)

28 It is necessary to consider the semiological link between the "neuro" and "psychic" dimensions of brain activity, in order to encompass both aspects of the "vital signs" of health, namely a) neuro-cerebral activity, representing the signifier - hardware, the support / base of any activity of b) the signified-software, which is defined by the human subject's emotional affective mental states. As each of these dimensions manifests itself through the other (and since Biophotonics makes novel links between the hardware's structure and its effects on health condition and mental disease) this conjunction should perhaps have been explicitly mentioned in the title of this study.

3. little can be said either about the therapeutic power of *homeopathy* (starting from the symbolic story of the patient's life) to heal the layers of the human body through therapeutic effects manifested beyond the limit of the Avogadro number, signifying substantial "nothingness".

The conclusion that certain ignorance seems to hover over the elements of the symbolic triad defining the field itself of our scientific approach normally brings up the following question: When uncertainty seems to dominate, would it not be normal for the combination of a triple "obscurity" to lead only to total cognitive "darkness"? A positive answer to this question would put paid to such an approach before it even gets started. Fortunately in order to proceed, the existing experience of *synergy effects*[29] comes to our aid.

b) *Initially followed in a correlated way* in their dynamics, then taken in pairs, and finally judged as a coherent ensemble, the elements of BPH acquire a hitherto undiscovered explanatory force, offering a new understanding for the whole that defines HUMAN HEALTH. Taking into account these correlations, we can state that:

1. *The Logical Sequence* implied by the present study is as follows: *Biophotonics*, a novel explanatory premise about the working mechanisms of the human body and the contextual conditions that could generate a certain disease → *Neuro-Psychology (Psychiatry)*, which describes the mental disease situations that are to be overcome → *Homeopathy* which creates biophotonic healing strategies for neuro-psychic malfunctions. In other words: premise / context → disease / disorder → therapy / healing is a very natural sequence.

2. *Dualistic, interdisciplinary pairings* that could be separated out from the BPH trianglular structure are as follows:
   - *Biophotonics* →← *Neuro-Psychology*: the conjunction is fruitful because, on the one hand Biophotonics offers neuro-psychology new explanations for a number of little-known mechanisms of the brain's holographic activity, of memory, of language, etc.; and on the other, psychiatry offers biophotonics the case-book records necessary to validate its assumptions, namely a series of neuro-psychic malfunctional categories that reflect the explanatory contents of biophotonics.
   - *Biophotonics* →← *Homeopathy*: the relationship is fruitful, as it has been demonstrated that biophotonics can offer a questioning explanation to all of the mechanisms posited in homeopathy; while homeopathy offers a practical field of application for the achievements of biophotonics.
   - *Neuro-Psychology* →← *Homeopathy*: a conjunction in which the former is a "language-object" for homeopathic therapeutic interventions, where a psycho-behaviouristic method of knowledge, a "meta-language" in turn, is necessary in order to establish the patient's framing as a certain human type, in a certain homeopathic treatment chart, in a case of neuro-psychic dysfunction; homeopathy contributes to the wealth of semantic content in neuro-psychology by defining new healthy behaviour, in which psycho-physiological manifestations are matched by symbolic, temperamental and character-based ones.

---

29 Let us remember, for example, that the combination of two "poisons" for human health – for instance, sodium and chlorine – does not always generate a stronger poison, but in this case a *sine qua non* food ingredient: our daily salt. A similar situation is defined by the integration of the three corners of the triangle in a functional whole.

3. *The Synergetic Triad* of elements integrating with each other suggests that: healing a patient with psychic malfunctions by implying human symbolism (in choosing homeopathic informational remedies) unconditionally supposes the activation of mechanisms and (bio)electromagnetic realities implied and explained in homeopathy.

In conclusion, through the above-mentioned connections, the following circuit:

explanatory theory (Biophotonics assumptions and clarifying patterning) → *practical malfunction* (crisis / neuro-psychology) → *effective resolution* (through homeopathic therapy)

... becomes an efficient framework for checking biophotonic theory, and for transforming it into a strategy which can be applied practically. To sum up, this is the declared intention and the theoretical-practical purpose of this study: *implementation of original synergetic effects for the benefit of human harmony and health*. Or, in other words: **Something new under the Sun ...**

2   Fundamentals of biophotonics: a necessary synthesis

First some defining aspects of the connection between biophotonics and homeopathy, (namely a series of clarifications associated by biophotonics with certain lesser-known aspects of homeopathic therapy) must be presented.

1. Generally speaking, BIOPHOTONICS was defined as early as the 1970-1980s by German specialists under the supervision of Professor Fritz-Albert Popp who – in the etymological sense – meant through Biophotonics: *Biology + photons / light = science of "living light"*. Detailed lab research of certain *"ultraweak luminescence"* or "delayed luminescence" at the level of any living system (vegetal, animal, human) has been highlighted by the observation – hard to accept at that time – *that this emission has properties similar to those of laser emission*. The coherent explanation of this finding realized by Romanian researchers in the last fifteen years has permitted a new definition of BIOPHOTONICS, understood as: *Biology + Photonics = theory / technology of "biological lasers"*. Completed with this new meaning, INTEGRAL BIOPHOTONICS could be defined as: *the science studying the processes of generating, storing, releasing and interaction of emissions of biophotons / biolumines-cence at the level of all living beings, in their quality of "biological laser" systems*.
2. Taking into account these contributions, HOMEOPATHY appears as a science of "therapy by light" [Stǎnciulescu, 2003a], based on the transfer of the waves / information complex of the extremely diluted remedy giving substantial support to the living body in order to trigger the self-healing process through a "holographic resonance" mechanism.

Understood as such, homeopathy represents perhaps the most direct application of biophotonics in the field of human health, implying processes such as: bio-electromagnetic mechanisms activated in preparing and administering the remedies (mostly of biological origin), triggering at the human organism level certain specific resonance processes with healing energo-informational effects, etc. The innovative consideration of these biophotonic aspects – awaited for more than two centuries – offers scientific explanations for homeopathy, capable of increasing its prestige.

2.1 Theoretical roots of healing by light

Two emergent theories – the *(bio)Photonic Theory of Energy-Information* (bPTEI) [Constantinescu & Stănciulescu 1993; 1995] and the *"Biological Lasers" Theory* (BLT) [Stănciulescu & Manu, 1995; 2002] – have correlated their efforts in order to explain the creative mechanisms that made the following possible:

1. light genesis of all hierarchic systems of the world (physical / cosmic in general and bio-psychological in particular)and their mutual interaction / influence through holographic resonance mechanisms, installed at the level of the (bio)photonic fields (cf. **bPTEI**);
2. the structure and function of biophysical systems under the impact of light radiation, the genesis of energo-informational (**EI**) resources of biophysical systems and homeostasis / health maintaining and their mechanisms (cf. **BLT**). In very general terms, in the framework of the present study[30] we should mention and describe: *a) The (bio)Photonic Theory of Energy-Information* and *b) The "Biological Lasers" Theory*.

a) The (bio)Photonic Theory of Energy-Information. This theory supposes that, according to Schrödinger's duality of particle-wave, any two substantial systems can interact with each other under certain conditions, taking into consideration that:

1. the equality of the wave phases and of the substantial vibrator's receptor / receiver, and therefore their resonance / coherence, is a necessary and sufficient condition for guiding the substantial vibrator by the coherent wave on an electric (geodesic) and mutual line;
2. the (elementary) *energy quantums* ($E = \hbar\omega$) intuitively associated with the electromagnetic wave's electric component, and the *information quantum* ($I = ik\omega$) associated with the magnetic component, may be considered as generating (through resonance) the electromagnetic field's quantums (photons), having the speed of light;
3. the super-luminous speeds ($v \geq c$) specific to the information quantums can be correlated to virtual photons (tachyonic type) which leads to a hypothesis of a universe built on frequency-ranked levels.

This universal model of the "holographic resonant universe", based on the physical phenomena of *modulation, interference and coherent interaction*, of a *"pars pro toto"* reproductive memory,[31] is also manifested between the two structural components upon which the existence of the human being builds its activity:

---

30 For a better understanding, my studies: Homeopathy and biophotonics: a (meta)physical approach to the «life principle», Homœopathic Links, volume 17 / 04, Winter 2004b, and: Two centuries of expectancy. From endogenous to exogenous homeopathy: biophotonic explanations will be quite profitable for the interested reader [http://www.hpathy.com/research/stanciulescu-biophotonic-explanations.asp].

31 A hologram is characterized by two attributes: a) it is a virtual coherent complex of waves, generated only by the action of a laser system; b) it supposes an informational connection between the parts and the wholeness, each part / element reproducing the attributes of the system. Such an understanding was possible only by using the postulates of biophotonics, involving the presence of physical or biological "natural lasers".

1. The *Fourier code* provides a mathematical description of the "auric biofield" ("matrix of light" / "vital force") – namely a fundamental wave and many subordinated harmonics – as a complex of invisible *bio-electromagnetic holograms*, able to conserve quasi-actively the "abyssal memory" of the (human) system. This energo-informational "organizing pattern", as an "individual consciousness", etc., has a central role in determining by resonance the individual's bio-psychic health, overlooked by traditional science.

2. The *informational codes* (holograms) generated by the "substantial vibrators" of the biological structures are explained by (b)TPEI through the role played by the organism's liquids (blood, lymph, linked water) and by the organic "liquid crystals" everywhere present in the human body (cells, organs, interstitial tissues, etc.). These represent an active support of the "biological memory", able to receive messages from the "auric biofield" memory of the body and to assume them as commands (resonant holograms) for an adequate *(re)organization of the substantial biological structures*. This is exactly what the "VITAL FORCE" of homeopathy does therapeutically (See Fig. 2).

Figure 2. The general mechanisms of "holographic resonance" (of homeopathic healing implicitly): the waves of the emitting source (a remedy, for example), namely the "informational hologram" of the emitter, specifically interacts with the waves of the receptor (cell, organ, etc.), by modulating its own vibratory state and by remodelling / normalizing the receptor's form, if necessary.

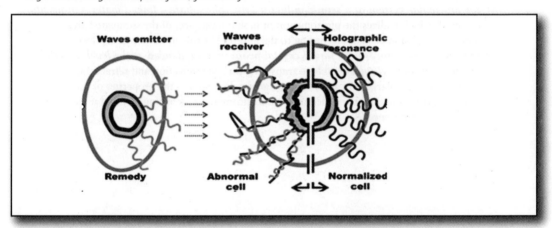

Relevant arguments for sustaining such a mechanism were formulated by Christopher Johannes, who developed the hypothesis that: "Interaction between the non-energetic information process and the energetic fields is proposed to be an essential feature of homeopathic potentization and therapeutic action" [2006]. This hypothesis – able to clarify the nature and genesis of the "Light Matrix" holographically comprising all the world's systems [Stănciulescu, 2007]– can at the same time implicitly clarify the functional principles of homeopathy.[32]

---

32 This paper represents a synthesis of some ideas already presented by the author in previous studies, with the addition of new aspects, in particular the innovative idea of the synergy between the triad: Biophotonics, Neuro-Psychism, Homeopathy.

Particularly, we could conclude that even homeopathic remedies are working in this way, by transmitting holographically the optimizing information-wave of the curative source (homeopathic remedies) to the body resonators (blood, water, membranous liquid crystal structures, etc.), within the human body systems, either directly – in the case of "endogenous homeopathy" - or indirectly, "exogenous homeopathy. (See section 3.2 of this article and my previous work [Stănciulescu, 2006a] for further explanations.)

b) The "Biological Lasers" Theory. Starting from the laboratory studies of light's interference with living matter realized by F.A. Popp et al. [1989], the two premises of the "Biological Lasers" Theory (**BLT**) [cf. Stănciulescu & Manu, 2002] have been formulated:

1. by its double quality – energetic and informational – light (electromagnetic field) plays an essential role in the structural and functional organization of living matter;
2. the mechanism which could explain this essential involvement is that of light amplification by stimulated emission of radiation, namely of a laser-type process.

According to BLT, two structural-functional systems are responsible for the *optical activity of the living organism* that generates bioluminescence – namely the homeopathic "VITAL FORCE" of the organism – as a "biological laser" phenomenon:

1. *the molecular system of a semi-conductor type (phosphate – linked water – molecular oxygen)*, which realizes the phenomenon of bioluminescence, of the stimulated and amplified emission of light (according to the anti-Stokes rule in non-linear optics);
2. *the organic structures with liquid crystal properties, evidenced at the level of cellular membranes and cytoplasm*, able to transmit – through reflection and refraction, birefringence[33], polarization and rotary magnetic dispersion – the properties of the (bio)laser-type emission: the coherence, monochromaticity, directionality and intensity of the light / bioluminescence (See Fig. 3).

---

33 The splitting of a light ray, generally by a crystal, into two components that travel at different velocities and are polarized at right angles to each other; also known as double refraction.

*Figure 3. The essential premises of the "biological laser" mechanism, the metamorphosis / modulation in fre-
quency of the incident* / external light namely:*

*a) the molecular structure of the bio-laser's "active substance" (symbolically speaking, the synergy of the four
cosmogonic** elements: earth / phosphate → water / organic linked water → air / molecular oxygen → fire /
light), able to unify living systems (plants, animals, humans); this mechanism explains how the external light
(EM visible and infrared waves) is absorbed, for generating the quantum phenomenon of "biolaser" emission.*

*b) the structure of membranous liquid crystals (phospholipids), able to generate the optic activity of the cells /
organs / organism, the transparency against light (EM waves)-- in other words, the piezoelectric*** energo-informational effects and diamagnetic memory genesis, the increase / modulation in frequency of bioluminescent
fluxes at the level of linked and intricate "biolaser" systems, etc.*

*(*Incident light is the ray or particles of light arriving at or striking a surface. ** Cosmogony: the study of the ori-
gin and development of the whole universe or a particular part of it. *** Piezoelectricity: the electricity generated
by crystals subjected to mechanical stress or electrical voltage.)*

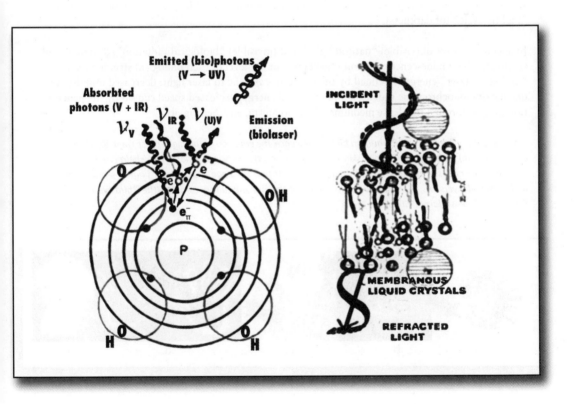

The premises presented above – already validated experimentally by the authors[34] – represent the basis of the major conclusions of BLT, namely:

1. The correlated action of the molecular semiconductor "biological-laser" and of the organic structures with liquid crystal properties allow to argue that the molecules, membranes, cell nuclei, cells, organs and the whole organism are functioning just like some "biological-laser" systems, both "linked" and "included". On the one hand, all these systems present evident structural analogies with technical lasers: optic resonator, active substance, etc. On the other hand, the functionality of these biological complexes generates a bioluminescent phenomenon, having all the above-mentioned properties of "natural laser" emission.

2. The structural-functional particularities of the six types of "biological-lasers" existing in the living complex body allow evidence to be provided for the correlated effects of four types of phenomena: Biochemical, Electrical, Magnetic and Photonic (BEMPh effects). These phenomena are characteristic of all the biological processes of the living body.

Through the energetic accumulation permitted by the presence of light, and through the energetic discharges which happen in light's absence respectively, it is possible to define two essential cycles which maintain the vital processes on a dynamic equilibrium: the "daily cycle" (of light) and the "nightly cycle" (of darkness).

By metamorphosis of (visible) "natural light" into (invisible) "biological radiation", deviated to ultraviolet, a bioluminescence emission is generated at the level of each biological structure. This "biological-laser" energy is defined by the properties specific to laser light: decreased impulse frequency of monochromatic radiation and increased energy; decreased speed caused by the penetration of light through the dense mediums of the organism, etc. (See Fig. 4).

Figure 4. Bio-psycho-logical (BPL) human bioluminescence, the emission of (bio)light of [cf. Guja, 1993]: (a) pelargonium leaf; (b) dragon fly; (c) human skin; d) human hand; (d) elderly individual with Alzheimer's disease (dementia): higher density and intensity of streamers, specific to the old age, together with right / left asymmetry and extended inversions; (e) electronographic image of the pineal-pituitary complex (the "third eye"), responsible for the super-sensorial activity of the brain.

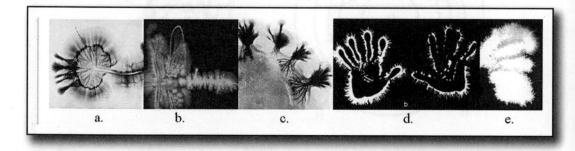

a.   b.   c.   d.   e.

The amazing analogy / correspondence between all biological systems, (starting from the molecular and membranous level up to the nuclear, cellular, organic and organismic one) represents the main contribution of BLT, which is able to clarify many of the therapeutic principles and practices of homeopathy.[35]

2.2 The model of hierarchical energy-information traps: on the genesis of the profound resources of human health

As BLT explains, after the process of light radiation in the human organism, at the cellular level (first and foremost in the nerve pathways, but not only here) and at the level of tissues and organs (the organs' complexes), comes the appearance of the *deep reserves of energy and information in the organism*. Thus, the living organism appears as a hierarchical system with "energy-information (EI) traps" having different levels of complexity, namely:

a) The cellular reserves of energy are made, first of all, at the level of "mitochondrial traps" (by means of the stock of electrons and protons deposited as a consequence of macroergical[36] processes, involving the synthesis of ATP and steroids respectively). *The reserves of information* are accomplished predominantly at the level of the "nuclear DNA trap", within which a large quantity of bio-photons is deposited, as demonstrated in the research lab under the guidance of F.A. Popp et al. [1989]. The circulation of energy-information (E-I) of this kind is made:

1. At the level of the nervous network system. On the one hand, this mainly transmits electrical impulses (as a membrane potential of action and repose, predominantly energetic); on the other hand, the interior also transmits biophotonic information (through a system of "optical fibers" within the cellular chain).
2. At the level of the "nadi"[37] network, as Indian thinkers call the subtle network through which vital information is received and transmitted in the entire body. This corresponds to the network theoretically postulated by the bio-structural model conceived by the Romanian Academy member Eugen Macovschi [1969] and recently validated empirically by electron microscopy; the two major E-I "nadi channels" (complementary "paths" of bioluminescence fluxes, one ascending and the other descending), run along the backbone.

b) At the organ level, the energy traps are predominantly represented by the nutritive reserves, (those of treacle polymer type or of the macroergical type). The informational resources are predominantly deposited at the level of the seven shiny vortex / chakra fields and they are interrelated with as many organic complexes as the organism itself has. Thus, the energetic-informational (E-I) circuit is conceived:

1. At the level of the major meridians (preponderantly energetic circuits), already mentioned by traditional Oriental medicine (eg. acupuncture) and evidenced by electrodermal measurements, correlating the physiological functions of all the major organs;

---

35 Details about these aspects are presented in my study [Stănciulescu, 2006b]: Homeopathy and Biophotonics (II) The "vital force": explanatory contributions of the "biological lasers" theory will be quite profitable for the interested reader [http://www.hpathy.com/research/stanciulescu-biophotonic-explanations3.asp].

36 Macroergic – Energy-providing, for example substances such as ATP.

37 Nadis: the body's subtle energy channels in traditional Indian thought, from the Sanskrit word for "tube, pipe", equivalent to the meridians in Chinese thought.

2. At the level of the complex informational circuits, defined by the bio-field fluxes around the nerves, the "nadi" micro-circuits and the meridians.

According to BLT, all these micro- and macro- E-I traps are embryo-genetically interrelated meaning that:

1. Every "informational trap" (bio-photonic / radiant) precisely placed at the cellular or organic level has as a necessary correspondent the energetic support of an "energy trap" (electronic-protonic or bio-chemical); everywhere in the organism we will find "pair-traps" diffused in this way, characterized by the relationship between a substantial substratum and/or energetic *shape*, belonging to a specific informational complex *content*. The number of these traps is variable; it depends on the maturity state of the organism, on its state of health, etc.
2. Every trap-complex, well placed at the cellular or organic level, is in a relationship of resonance / informational coherence (through identical frequencies) with other E-I traps, situated in other areas of the organism. The connection / coherence of these traps is accomplished by means of the actual process of embryo-genesis, taking into account that: (a) they belong to the same original embryological foil (endoderm, mesoderm, ectoderm); (b) they are subordinated / correlated to a major organic complex; (c) their connection is maintained by means of the E-I channels (meridian system, nervous system, "nadi" system) built during the process of embryo-genesis, as part of the structural effects of bioluminescence.

This is how we can explain the way in which – in the light of the organism's holographic structure – every zone in the organism (tissue, organ, etc.) always has, as an E-I reserve, one or more deposits hidden in some other location elsewhere in the organism. These deposits are in a coherence / resonance relationship (by means of identical frequencies) with other pair-deposits, embryologically or metabolically defined in the process of the organism's morphogenesis[38]. This E-I redundancy mechanism explains all the energetic and informational substitution phenomena specific to the human organism (the malfunction of one organ / zone is partially supplanted by the activity of another), the protective and regenerative mechanisms of the organism, etc., stimulated by appropriate frequencies such as those of homeopathic remedies.

Understanding the releasing mechanisms of E-I resources represents the key to any balancing / optimizing process of the human organism, and thus implicitly of homeopathic procedures. This is because what a remedy does, once inside the human body, is to stimulate by resonance / super-radiance the release of an E-I trap. This can occur directly, due to a "resonant tropism", or indirectly, by coherent commands addressed by the brain to the affected organs. In this framework, we could consider that each remedy is a type of computational "disk-system" able to remember the right functional and structural patterns – *frequency and amplitude (form)* – of a certain biological structure (cell, organ, organism) when it loses its "functional memory", becoming ill.

Consequently, the homeopathic "life principle" is present here as the holographic pattern that both governs the appearance of living systems (the DNA pattern) and that controls – as a

---

38 Morphogenesis: the biological process in developmental biology that causes an organism to develop its shape.

"morphogenetic field" [Sheldrake, 1981] – the similarity of different biological forms. It follows from this general condition that taking the main unique remedy, in a given homeopathic treatment situation, is often enough to optimize / restructure the hierarchical systems of the human body. The interdependent duality between "waves" and "particles" is quite clear: the waves are generated by the "substantial" (biochemical) activity of the body, and the (bio-photonic) activity of the waves determines the state of the substantial system, by assuring the homeostasis of the "vital body", in other words the health state of the bio-psycho-logical system.

Such a correspondence is well sustained in an exciting article by Alexandra N. Delinick: *"The organism's natural frequency / field is equal to the simillimum in homeopathy*. We give back to it, as a biofeedback mechanism, the same information, so as to achieve this kind of effect ... So, the remedy too has a certain natural frequency (electromagnetic wave frequency / field), and this means it has certain qualitative and quantitative information that it gives back to the cell and to the whole organism ... It comes in at the quantum level" [1995: 46-47]. It is possible to understand in this way how "order" (the pattern of health) emerges from "chaos" (the disorganization of illness), stimulated by the hierarchical types of information that the remedy contains.

Finally, in connection with biophotonics, homeopathy could be considered:

1. *biologically*: the science of healing with "potential light" which uses artificial "traps of light" (remedies) to stimulate the delivery of the "traps of light" (energetic-informational reserves) of the natural organism that can balance the states of that organism;
2. *psychologically*: as the science of helping the individual to evolve on their path in life.

3   Neuro-psychical (dis)orders: a biophotonic approach

Starting with a few general definitions accepted by biophotonics [Stănciulescu, 2003a],[39] in the following section I intend to analyze two problem categories relating to the subject of neuro-psychic / mental diseases:

1. Neuro-physiological principles implied in the brain's normal activity / functioning as mental health-sustaining hardware, representing the holographic mechanisms of human memory as a mediating programme (software) responsible for mental health;

---

39 From the explanations of biophotonics given previously, the following apply: ● LIFE means the capacity of any biophysical system (vegetal, animal, human) to generate, store and release biophotons , i.e. bioluminescence. A system/body that does not have this attribute/function (the aura or vital force) is by definition not alive. ● HEALTH describes a system's capacity to metamorphose natural light into "living light" (of the "bio-laser" type). This transfer requires transparency and occurs step by step at the level of the cellular liquid crystals (membranous and cytoplasmic) throughout the whole body; this process ensures its functional coherence. ● DISEASE supposes the living system's loss of capacity to correctly activate the biophotonic mechanisms. This occurs as a side-effect of an "oblivion / loss" phenomenon in terms of the essential properties of the "light matrix" (at the aura / software level) and/or at the level of the organism's support or hardware (for example the nervous system's complex of "biological lasers"), which ensures the correct processing of "living light". ● THERAPY (implicitly homeopathic) represents a combination of actions through which the organism's "forgotten" biophotonic functions are recovered (frequencies, amplitudes, intensities, etc.); or whereby the affected biological support structure is repaired, at each level of the organism (for example the Central Nervous System or the Vegetative Nervous System).

2 Defining the main situational aspects that characterize neuro-psychic clutter, with a view to establishing some possible healing strategies (primarily homeopathic ones).

3.1 Neuro-mental mechanisms of human health

For the present study a new understanding of the neuro-physiological mechanisms / principles facilitating brain functioning is necessary, with neuro-mental disease being generated by the malfunction of one of these mechanisms.

We will therefore discuss: *a) The main principles of brain functioning* and *b) The memory, as a basis of neuro-psychic health states.*

a) The main principles of brain functioning. From the perspective of biophotonics and psycho-neurology, I developed in another context [Stănciulescu, 2003b] a semiotic model of the principles which govern neurological activity, a model offering an original explanation of the brain's performance and its healthy functioning.

1. *The principle of energy-information unity*: any impulse received by the (nerve) cell will be homeomorphically[40] transformed into electrons and biophotons, due to the piezoelectric properties of the membranous liquid crystals. This mechanism suggests that the significative connection between the referent's[41] energetic-information properties (mechanical, visual, caloric, etc.) and its corresponding cerebral sign (as representation, information / the signified) is always mediated by one and the same electric and electromagnetic energy (as support / signifier).

2. *The principle of redundant propagation of information*: the same received information is transmitted "step by step" to the brain, by the complementary methods of BEMPh phenomena: by biochemical transmitters at the synaptic level; by membranous electric potentials and by magnetic cellular fields; and by biophotonic fluxes (which penetrate the interior of the cells, due to the membranous liquid crystals' transparency). All these methods transfer the specific information of the referent to the brain support, both chemical (liquid crystals, neuro-transmitters, etc.) and bio-physical (electric and magnetic fields, photonic flux).

3. *The principle of information simplification*: the complex of exterior information is decomposed into types of elementary information (such as frequency, intensity, phase, form, distance, etc.) at the level of the different sections of the neuro-analyzers, and these are received / registered in such form at the level of the posterior cortex. Consequently, each complex of stimuli belonging to a certain referent is first represented as an assembly of simple components (primary signs) at the level of the cortex, and after that as an integrative sign (visual, auditory, tactile, etc.).

4. *The principle of cerebral hierarchical functionality*: due to the holographic organization of the brain, biophotonics could explain why the major functions of the brain (such as

---

40 In chemistry, having a similar shape, but not necessarily the same composition, for example in the similar crystal form of different chemical compounds; in mathematics, two shapes are homeomorphic if they can be continuously stretched or bent into each other (eg. a square and a circle, but not a sphere and a doughnut).

41 Referent: something which is referred to; the specific entity in the world that a word or phrase identifies or denotes.

memory, for example) are both "localized" (at the level of the cortex, where simple information is received) and "not localized", because of the distribution of the memorized / signified
information at the level of the entire cerebral mass, having as signifier a substantial sup
port (the membranous liquid crystals), or an energetic one (bioelectromagnetic waves).

5. *The principle of holographic reception and information processing*: this mechanism is
   specifically activated in two circumstances: (a) at the level of the peripheral analyzers, where
   some signals are registered as "holographic points - objects" (optic, acoustic, etc.), and some
   as "iconic reproductions" of the referent; (b) at the level of the central nervous systems: the
   holograms are realized in the whole mass of the brain, being generated at the various deep
   levels of the brain, by the interference of the different (simple) information (coherent
   bioelectromagnetic waves, "biolaser" type ones) which describes the referent.

6. *The principle of the holographic memory's functionality*: the membranous liquid
   crystals could be considered as the substantial support (signifier) for the information
   (signified) carried by the stimuli (referent). Due to their diamagnetic properties, activated by
   the incident light (as a "sign" of the incident stimuli), the membranous liquid crystals are
   able to change specifically their position, configuration, etc., and to keep / memorize in this
   way (morphologically), for a certain time, a specific form (to inform = to put in form).

7. *The principle of holographic representation, by two categories of stimuli*: a) (in)direct
   excitation of the brain, by a *physical signal* (electromagnetic, for example), able to generate
   at the level of the signifier some resonant phenomena (predominantly energetic predominantly); b) stimulation by a *sign* (word, gesture etc), able to involve a certain resonance,
   predominantly informational, at the level of the signified.

8. *The principle of binary processing of data*: the "cerebral computer" operates with a
   system of information based on the presence or absence of the stimuli (light, sound,
   pressure, etc.), by an "On-Off", + / B, 1 / 0 mechanism. This mechanism permits the use of
   the formal rules of logic, through some basic operators: conjunction, disjunction, negation,
   implication. With the help of these "technical" operators, the brain represents the necessary
   "hard" information (the signifier) for the "soft" mind (the signified), able to generate the
   signs used by human thinking (inferences) to construct all its creative products.

Using all these biophotonic principles, we could rationally justify Karl Pribram's essential hypothesis [1971: 35-52] that the brain's activity (memory) is of a holographic type. Schematically, this
process is defined by the following succession of phases:

the transfer of objectual information to the brain through visual channels → registration of the
complex information at the cortex level as simpler information (volumes, shapes, colours,
positions, tastes, etc.) in specific areas → their redistribution and memorizing in the whole
cerebral mass → cerebral (synergetic) hologram constitution, having the liquid crystal structures
as physical support → the genesis of the complex signs / holograms describing the reality →
memory activation.

Taking all this into account and in order to understand the mechanisms of neuro-mental health, it
is both possible and necessary to study memory in different terms than previously.

b) *The memory as a basis of neuro-psychic health states.* Memory – the capacity to store and reflect or reproduce information preserved in a certain layer – represents the defining attribute of the correct functionality of any system generally, and of the human system in particular. Even though many theories have tried to elucidate the sometimes exceptional manner in which memory works, only partial evidence has been obtained, which has not totally clarified all the so-called implied aspects. In this case biophotonics can effectively contribute to explaining the two complementary memory types: *structural and functional.*

1. **The structural memory** supposes in its turn two complementary components, substantial-energetic and informational-undulatory[42], namely:

- *The substratum memory* is assured – according to the explanations of BLT – by the capacity of liquid crystals to orient diamagnetically in the membranous / cytoplasmatic field, in accordance with the nature and the attributes of the incidental stimuli: intensity, direction, shape, etc. This highlights the (hard) substantial support of the cerebral "mnesic[43] routes" of any object, phenomenon or process received by the brain through sensory stimuli (seeing, hearing, touching, etc.). The ensemble of the information received by the brain generates *bio-electro-magnetic interference fringes,* located in the liquid cellular crystals, at the level of the cortex and of the whole cerebral mass.[44]
These fringes compose the object-holograms that sustain the active memory and practical experience of the individual / person. In order to activate an object-hologram it is enough for a stimulus with similar properties to the initial one to appear, for the already existing cerebral hologram to resonate and thereby trigger awareness.

- *The field memory* is assured – according to bPTEI – by the property shared by biological systems of all sizes (whether nucleus, cell, organ or organism) of generating a certain biofield / vital force around them; this is able to conserve through the afferent[45] Fourier spectra a certain kind of information. The "auric memory" of the whole body is responsible for keeping / receiving a certain type of abyssal memory, transpersonal, having as extremes: the memory obtained at birth, by resonance with the cosmic electromagnetic ensemble, and the memory transferred from the cerebral or mental supports to the whole body's biofield (soul / aura), which has a certain autonomy, even after the subject's death (See Fig. 5).

---

42 Undulatory: wave related; wave like appearance or form.

43 Mnesic: relating to memory (mneme in Greek).

44 The complementarity of two theories that have been opposite until now is thus explained: a) the localizing theory (Gall, Nielssen, Penfield et al.), which postulates with factual arguments that the cerebral memory is located in specific centres of the cortex; b) the diffusing theory (Goltz, Lashley et al.), which considers that the whole holographic memory is distributed at the level of the whole cerebral mass.

45 Bringing inward towards a central part (eg: a nerve which transmits impulses to the brain).

Figure 5. Correlations between cerebral waves and bioresonant technology: a) holographic mouldings of the cerebral field that highlight the presence of circular waves extended in space [http://www.qhbiocybernetics.com]; b) the whole body aura image in a permanent oscillation (realized by the author with a BIOPULSAR REFLEXOGRAPH) presenting three hypostases* of a person's BPL (bio-psycho-logical) state: (1) normal state; (2) cerebrally stimulated state, from strong EM cerebral stimuli; (3) optimized state through the use of a Biophotonic Resonator to protect against EM smog. (*Hypostasis: in philosophy, the substance, essence, or underlying reality.)

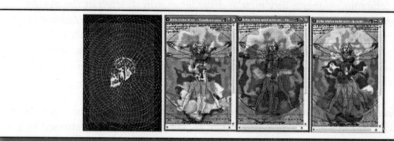

The pairing of "field memory" and "substratum memory" is similar to those of information-wave, particle-energy or sofware-hardware. Thus we can consider that any type of hierarchical *energo-informational trap*, as previously defined, that is constituted at the body's micro- and macrophysical level (from the level of atomic and macro - molecular traps up to cellular, organ or body levels) will suppose a specific type of memory.

2. **The functional memory** (which is processual) depends on the nature and quality of the stimuli that – tracing the path/track of neural cells – generate "vibratory echoes", mnesic processes that are susceptible to updating after a certain time from their generation / building. So, depending on the BEMPh triggering stimuli, the following types of memory can be defined:

- *bio/(psycho)photonic (F) memory*, (holographic and long-lasting) from the cellular and organic memory (of the brain or of the chakras), to the "auric memory" that is transferred beyond death, the field being infinite in both its storing and informational transfer possibilities;
- *electric (E) and magnetic (M) memory* (short-lasting) that lasts only as long as the time it takes to send the signal to the brain, through the cellular electric potential and the afferent magnetic field;
- *biochemical (B) memory* (medium-lasting) determined by the presence of chemical mediators (such as acetylcholine) at a higher synapse level, activating the "synaptic memory", that eases the signals passing from one neuron to another, using the linked "biological lasers" system.

In conclusion, we could say that the (in)correct functioning of memory is the first sign of neuro-mental health or disease. The formulated biophotonic explanations concerning the structure and functionality of different types of memory are in the position to clarify the greatest part of phenomena implied in the genesis of mental diseases (from the known ones to the parapsychical ones, most often mistaken for neuro-mental malfunctions). The correlation of these phenomena with homeopathy represents the practical contribution of my research.

3.2 Neuro-mental illness: biophotonic connotations

The pairing of neurology and psychology, interposed by biophotonics, that the present study is tracing, supposes the following postulate: *any mental disorder manifests itself at the psycho-emotional and affective level (software)*, but necessarily implies the presence of a neuro-mental support (hardware). In general the state of disease is generated by the appearance of a malfunction at one of these levels which gradually installs itself at the other level of manifestation. Within this context a display of the illness / neuro-mental disorder situation supposes the answer to some defining questions such as:

a) WHO can be affected by a random neuro-mental disorder? Neurological illness can affect anybody, no matter what age or social environment, when the subject is sufficiently stressed by a generating cause. Therefore beyond certain predispositions that mark its VITAL FORCE (such as the genetic heritage, the birth-established holographic resonance between the "cosmic light" matrix and the newborn's body, the psycho-social environment, etc.), the mental disorder can be considered a psycho-emotional answer through which the human being tries to get out of a certain crisis state. Neuro-mentally affected subjects undergo slight changes of shape and "vital field" parameters, contortions that – marked out by clairvoyance or by adequate bioresonant devices – could generate a "biophotonic semiology" of the health state in general, and one of the neuro-mental illnesses in particular (See Fig. 6).

Figure 6. Aura contortions of subjects with mental disorders of [cf. Brennan, 1996: 105]: a) informational (psycho-emotional field) type and: b) energetic type (of the sick body that affects the psyche).

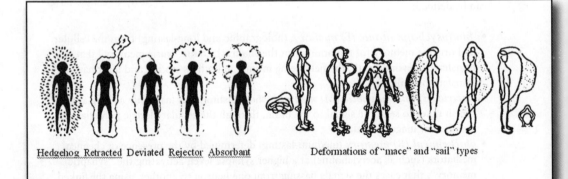

Hedgehog Retracted Deviated Rejector Absorbant   Deformations of "mace" and "sail" types

b) WHAT is (neuro)mental disorder / illness, HOW does it manifest itself and WHAT does it imply? A dictionary definition would describe "mental illness" or "mental disorder" as a group of anxieties that cause a more or less severe disturbance in thought, affectivity and social relationships. According to the severity of the malfunction we can distinguish:

1. *neuroses, undifferentiated* (neurasthenia, depression, anxiety, etc.) and *differentiated* (phobia, obsession, hysteria, schizophrenia, etc.) that manifest themselves particularly through irritability, functional and somatic disturbances, thinking and speaking disorders, etc. of a neuro-physiological nature;
2. *psychoses,* such as depressions, paranoid and delirious states, anxiety, etc., endorsing the main consciousness / personality disorders, manifested as asthenia, weariness, gloominess, hyper-sensibility, distraction, etc. generating malformations of the vital field and the physical decay of the neurological-membranous support (such as demyelinization in Alzheimer's).

c) WHY do neuro-mental disorders appear? Among the causes more or less known / admitted by the specialists, we must acknowledge:

1. *Individual reasons,* specific to the human subject's inner becoming, endorsing:
   - *objective reasons,* such as organic / neurological determinations related to birth trauma, hormonal and biochemical changes within the body / brain, the imbalance of trace elements, excessive alcohol or drug abuse, etc. All these affect the structure of the "biological lasers", with contortion of the cellular resonators and decay of the cooling system (generating opacity of the liquid crystals, which becomes lethal at 43-44 C);
   - *subjective reasons* related to psycho-social and cultural life parameters, to stress and depressing events, and also to virtually unrecognized childhood traumas[46] (which can affect the quality of holograms / mental liquid crystals and memory too).[47]

---

46 In this context we find an original explanation of the psychoanalytic mechanism of psychic pressing / depressing which is first and foremost a stress generator mechanism and then a psychosis generator. Thus, naturally, any order addressed to one processor of the brain through a wave / hologram, having the information of the operation which has to be executed, must be stopped by means of a feedback of the processing organ (by means of a counter-wave cut short by 180°). If this feed-back does not appear, the order has not been accomplished (correctly or at all) by the processing system and that unaccomplished order will remain a source of tension and of permanent oscillation between the brain and the processing zone. The order will be active even after it has been completely forgotten. Therefore, a tensioned event that took place during childhood, for example, and was unsolved at the proper time, can break through as a malfunction – after many years – in different forms of psycho-physiological disequilibrium (through neuro-mental disease); this is just how Sigmund Freud has explained the genesis of psychosis. In this situation, the cure implies stopping the order still present at the subliminal level (subconsciously). This operation requires awareness of the existence of a potential stimulus generated long ago, and the deliberate (mental) annihilation of its effects by understanding that the stimulus has become irrelevant for the present life of the involved human being.

47 The correlated ensemble of these aspects implicitly comprises the so-called spiritual causes of neuro-mental diseases, which take into account the human subject's BPL (bio-psycho-logical) personality. For example, the triggering of depression is often correlated with the lack of desire to live. When you continuously feel unhappy and discontented, when you blame yourself, you are already predisposed to depression through constant aggression against yourself. This has negative consequences for your nervous system and triggers diseases that are correlated with the vegetative nervous system and mental disharmony involving sight, hearing or perception; stress, tension, and worry cause insomnia, headaches, allergies, chronic diseases, ulcers, arterial tension, infections, etc. Mental background diseases derive from spitefulness, anger, negative thought and anxiety feeding. People that do not believe in God are predisposed to disease because of the decrease in immunity coefficient, through the lack of a positive tonus generated by the belief that "somebody up there loves you".

2. *Trans-individual reasons*, developed at the (bio)energo-informational field level supposing (un)conventional subjective-objective influences which are often overlooked by standard science; these are correlated to the presence of different field categories:
   - *noesic reasons* carrying the information of some presumptive "karmic determinations", the influence of events in other "past lives", and the imperatives of the "Akashic Records[48] destiny" in humanity's collective memory, etc.;
   - *psycho-social reasons* generated by perturbing bio-energo-informational actions, from the typical / plain "evil eye" to "black magic", etc.
   - *technological reasons* endorsing the harmful effects on the brain of electromagnetic waves generated by antennas and mobile phone devices, TV or excessive PC use;
   - *telluric / earthly and cosmic reasons* determined by the EI hyper- or hypo-stimulating effects of Hartmann and Curry[49] networks or knots, etc. or by solar / lunar / stellar field effects.

The exceptional significance – no matter the determined nature of the cause – of the brain in mediating health states and mental illness has led to the recent medical research view that *any disease including cancer has neuro-mental roots.*[50] Such a hypothesis – neurologically and psychologically justifying disease genesis – is essential to allow possible correlation with biophotonic hypotheses on the one hand, and with homeopathy therapeutic implications on the other hand.

Thus, from a biophotonic point of view, we can state that all these neuro-mental causes gradually (or precipitously) generating diseases affect the correct manifestation of those functional principles through which we have characterized the activity of the human body, in particular the brain's activity, that is:

1. *diminishing "vital force", the intensity of bioluminescence emissions*, by affecting absorption and the capacity for emission of stimulated light, due to insufficient natural light and its visual or epidermis-based reception, etc., depreciation of the semi-conducting mole-

---

48 The individual records of a soul's journey, also described as the Soul Records, Cosmic Mind, etc.

49 Global grids of two types of earth energy lines described by Dr. Manfred Curry and Dr. Ernst Hartmann; intersections of these have been linked to geopathic stress, with detrimental health effects.

50 It would suffice to recall in this context the slightly marginalized contributions of the German doctor Ryke Geerd Hamer, who detailed the "heresy" of German New Medicine [http://germannewmedicine.ca]. The nucleus of this theory is represented by the "Dirk Hamer Syndrome" hypothesis postulating that every disease has a neuro-psycho-emotional origin: the shock that surprises the individual affects a specified area, predetermined by the brain, causing a visible tomographic injury – like a clear set of concentric rings/circles. After the impact, cerebral cells transmit the shock to the corresponding organ (through a "holographic resonance" mechanism, already established since the embryo-genetic phase, as the BLT also explains), which pathologically modifies its shape and functionality. The disappearance of mental commands leads to the disappearance of the cause/disease thus leading to a healing process. There has been increased scientific interest in a new (un)conventional synthesis – theoretical and therapeutic too – in the field of human neuro-mental health. This is also demonstrated by the contribution of Dr. Dietrich Klinghardt [http://www.neuraltherapy.com]. His "neural therapy" supposes that each of the five fields (implicitly biophotonic) of human body systems – physical, energetic (electric) and mental, dream (intuitive) and spiritual – needs a particular therapy, starting from Homeopathy and ending with spiritual (auto)therapy.

cular complex phosphate / tied water / molecular oxygen state through an imbalance in trace elements (deficient food, with bioluminescence inhibitor "R's"), insufficient natural water consumption or incorrect breathing (in a populated environment);

2. *degradation of the quality of liquid crystals*, which affects: cellular and organic memory (cerebral memory, substratum first and then field), the correct bioluminescence transfer at the level of the whole living organism (a sign of organic disease and premature ageing), energy and piezoelectric transformation of exogenous information (followed by metabolism decay and weakening of the vital energy and immune system), efficient / redundant brain information transfer (followed by the loss of representing and recognizing capacity, generative visual and auditory language holograms, redundant information memorising), affecting the brain's "binary logic" default thinking.

Nature, the biophotonic causes and effects of neuro-mental diseases allow us to define them in a certain way, as "luminous diseases". Understanding them from this perspective, a series of therapeutic and prophylactic measures are to be formulated, by both allopathic and alternative medicine, and homeopathy in particular.

4   Homeopathic therapy for neuro-psychic disorders: the integrative assumption of biophotonics

The conception of Samuel Hahnemann is based on seven principles or functional laws, amply studied by homeopaths [Jayasuryia, 1997: 23-31]: the law of similars, the law of testing (proving), the law of the individualized remedy, the law of the minimal (homeopathic) dose, the law of the direction of healing (Hering's law), the doctrine of miasms, and the integrative principle of the "Vital Force" (life principle). Among these laws – already explained in terms of biophotonics (BLT) [Stanciulescu, 2003b] – the most relevant is the first one: *"Similia similibus curentur"*.

4.1 On the mechanism of resonance by light: *"similia similibus curentur"*

The basic homeopathic law – "what is alike must be cured by similar procedures" – involves the mechanisms of universal cybernetic feed-back. The reason this law is so general is because it corresponds to the first principle of genesis itself: RESONANCE / COHERENCE / LOVE, or the capacity of two or more systems to pull together. Similarly, if the disappearance of resonance/love generates illness or chaos in the body or cerebellum, emotionally or affectively, its (re)appearance restores the state of harmony of the whole. There is no simpler way to define the homeopathic healing mechanism.

Such a relationship is convergent with the hypotheses formulated by Hahnemann:

1. The symptoms / syndromes do not represent the illness itself, but the action of the protective mechanisms mobilized by the organism for counteracting the causal factors of the illness: physical (atmospheric condition, pollution, etc.), biological (viruses, bacteria, etc.) or psycho-social (different types of stress). According to BLT, such a defence reaction (the organism's struggle to regain homeostasis) is equally determined by:
   • *informational modifications* (generated by interference, resonance or modulation mechanisms) stimulated by different physical / biological undulatory factors (characterized by frequencies, intensities, amplitudes, etc.). First, such modifications happen at the

invisible level of the human organism's bio-fields; after that, the modifications will be transferred to the level of the appropriate receptor-organ (at the level of the membranous "liquid crystal" support, in fact) where they will determine the appearance of some specific symptoms;

- *energetic modifications*, evidence being found at the deep substantial level of the organism. (Affliction of the lung, for example, due to intoxication, will be followed by some specific symptoms: coughing, green / yellow expectoration, etc., which will affect the general (energetic) state of the organism.

2. In certain conditions, the elimination of the symptoms (by "antipathy" / "counter-pathy" / dissonance) represents one of the greatest dangers that classical / allopathic medicine can generate. From the homeopathic point of view, such suppression "cures" only locally (symptoms), but not systemically (causes). A semiotic distinction could be established between allopathic and homeopathic interventions, taking into consideration that:

- generally speaking, allopathic medicine supposes that the symptoms belong to illness itself; consequently, sometimes their elimination is considered to be the eradication of the illness itself;
- homeopathic medicine considers that symptoms are exterior signs of the organism's reaction against illness; consequently, since they belong to the healing process, the manifested symptoms must not be eliminated but amplified, in order to establish the true causes of the sickness and their eradication; by the elimination of the deep causes, at the level of the body – soul – spirit complex, the effects will implicitly disappear.

In conclusion, we could say that the appearance of symptoms signifies the beginning of the natural process of an organism's defence against illness. This process is stimulated / amplified by homeopathic intervention, when it is necessary, taking into consideration that:

1. *The sickness must be defeated with its proper instruments*, used differentially, from case to case. For example, it is known that the same information transmitted by a certain emitter (wave phase, for example) could generate different "magic effects" (white / black) at the level of the receptor: a) by the growth of wave amplitude (when the implicated waves / information are "in phase"), further generating a super-radiance / super-energizing mechanism; b) by cancelling the receptor's own waves, if these are not "in-phase" with the emitter's waves.

2. *A similar mechanism is activated in the situation of bio-energetic practices*, when the bio-energy of the therapist generates in the patient a benefic effect, if the ill person is under-energized, or a malefic effect, if the ill person is super-energized. We could discover in this context an explanation for the practical fact that the same homeopathic remedy could be benefic or malefic, depending on the deep cause of disease, the degree of dilution, the timing of the application, etc. Corresponding to its degree of dilution, for example, the remedy could act complementarily, to activate liberation of deep E-I resources, by different BEMPh reactions:

- *Bio-chemical reactions*, by molecular combinations, in the case of *low dilutions*, obtained especially from organic sources (plants, animal tissues, etc.), determining different reactions for: a) increasing the density of the cellular / nuclear masses, necessary for liberating the DNA / mitochondrial "traps" of biophotons and electrons; b) generating strong biochemical reactions involved in the modification of biological tissues. Due to these properties, low dilutions are used especially in cases of acute disease, which requires rapid and strong (biochemical / substantial) reactions.

- *Electric and magnetic reactions*, in the case of *medium dilutions*, obtained predominantly from mineral / crystalline or biological sources (such as clay and salt, or various different plant-powders), generating the increased presence of "biological (liquid) crystals" which will essentially influence the cellular electric and magnetic activity. This produces perceptible effects both at the level of the affected zone and/or of the deep E-I traps. Such dilutions are used in the case of sub-acute (functionally / energetically predominant) diseases.
- *Photonic (bio-electromagnetic) reactions* are generated by certain field-resonance mechanisms, in the case of high dilutions (which no longer keep the substantial properties of the remedies). The bio-field waves of the remedy will generate informational effects at the level of the cellular E-I traps. These remedies are used in chronic diseases, mental instability (in emotional / informational states), etc.

We could associate the above-mentioned effects – substantial, energetic, informational – with the three types of effects characterizing a homeopathic remedy: chemical, mechanical and dynamic. From the BLT perspective, all these effects could act differently, both by:

1. *stimulatory action*, in order to: a) increase cell membrane transparency to light, to generate better informational activity in the whole organism; b) generate a compensatory liberation of "energy", in the case of "yin-type illnesses" (supposing a lack of energy / light);
2. *inhibitory action*, in order to: a) decrease the membranous permeability to light (by generating opacity of cell membranes) of microbes, bacteria, etc., in order to destroy them; b) liberate adequate quantities of "information" (biophotons) necessary to decrease the excess of energy, in the case of "yang-type illnesses" (supposing an excess of energy / light).

Taking into consideration all these types of complementary BEMPh processes, we can understand now why homeopathic therapy is still considered to be "obscure" [Jayasuria, 1997: 116]. In this context, we express our conviction that such "obscurity" will be essentially clarified by the explanatory contributions of biophotonics.

The final conclusion is quite clear now: by its conceptual and methodological contributions, biophotonics represents the scientific framework for an integrative medicine of the future, with homeopathy as a hard nucleus, as the "medicine of energetic-informational fields", the "medicine of the soul-body connection", of psycho-mental and bio-physiological human states. Such a medicine will valorize *ab initio* the human quality of being the "face and likeness" of the Creator, being able to connect the two essential types of therapy / healing mentioned by Mekilta: "*Humans heal by contraries, God heals by similarity*" [cf. Vithoulkas, 2002: 24]. Or, as an integrative (meta)physical / therapeutic principle, both homeopathic and allopathic: *Similarity creates the necessary conditions that the opposition manifests.*

4.2 The homeopathic mechanism of neuro-psychic therapy: the release by resonance of energy-information traps

Understanding the releasing mechanisms of energy-information (E-I) resources represents the key to any recovering / balancing process of the human organism, and homeopathic healing implicitly.[51] Because what a remedy does, once inside the human body, is stimulate by resonance / super-radiance the release of E-I traps: directly, due to a "resonant tropism", or indirectly, by coherent commands from the brain addressed to the sick organs.

Usually, the E-I reserves of the organism are kept intact as long as the organism is in a state of equilibrium, that is, as long as something from outside does not forcibly intervene in their releasing / parting.[52] This kind of parting involves two complementary energetic and informational processes:

1. The breaking up of the energy traps determines an increase in the tension / potential of the assimilated electrical charges by means of a *super-energizing process*, a necessary process in exceeding the energetic limit of the trap (which unconditionally implies a physical limitation, such as the membrane). As far as the cell is concerned, for example, the size of this threshold is directly proportional to the thickness of the (substantial) mitochondrial membrane, differentiated in its turn according to the zone to which it belongs in the organism.
2. Escape from the interior of the information traps implies a *super-radiance* phenomenon, which is an increase in the amplitude of the traps' deposited waves / bio-photons, which can thus escape the resonance zone that keeps them in an energetic membrane / pellicle (of the "auric ovoid" type, surrounding not only the nucleus / the nuclear DNA, but also the cell, the organ and the entire organism) having a specific diameter. By means of super-radiance there appears exactly the energetic increase necessary for radiant flux, that is for the bio-photonic / bio-electromagnetic oscillations needed to overcome the power of attraction in the substantial nucleus / support to which they are connected.

Taking into account all of the above, one can conclude that, on the one hand, each of the two types of traps can function relatively independently, their release being determined by stimuli specific to each of them which can be energetic and/or informational. On the other hand, taking into account their functioning as a dual complex, beyond their relative autonomy the two processes mentioned above can be reciprocally initiated. Thus, in terms of homeopathic therapies (differentiated according to the dilution degree of the substances used for the remedy preparation) we could talk about:

---

51 In homeopathic language, the term "disease" refers to physical, mental and emotional pains as a totality; for any physical pain generates a psycho-mental one and vice versa. Therefore homeopathic remedies do not just treat a single organ but the whole body, in order to remove the cause that generated the disease. Homeopathy follows the principle that simply treating symptoms and organs can only offer temporary help, the real solution being the stimulation of the healing capacity of the whole body.

52 The previously mentioned research of the German specialists [Popp et al. 1989] denotes that deposits of bio-photons at the DNA level can be kept for hours, days or even years, being released only under certain conditions, as a kind of "delayed bioluminescence". The way in which bio-photons enter or escape from the DNA trap is not entirely explained by the specialists. This explanatory gap is filled by BLT.

- super-energizing by means of bio-electromagnetic fields (biophotons / bioluminescence), by a super-radiance phenomenon;[53]
- super-radiance as biochemical, electrical and magnetic (field) phenomena, by means of super-energizing mechanisms.[54]

No matter how it is accomplished, the super-energizing / super-radiance mechanism is absolutely necessary for the releasing process of energy and information from the hierarchical traps in the human organism and especially the bio-physiological optimizing process of the human being. This kind of process unconditionally implies the release and active presence of some of the E-I reserves, which are usually passive in the organism. Release of these reserves can occur in two stimulus situations: a) *natural* or b) *artificial*.

a) Release of E-I reserves during natural stimulus situations: Here, release of passive resources is accomplished through two categories of bio-psycho-logical (BPL) mechanisms, namely:

1. The *bio-physiological mechanisms* activated during some natural recovery processes, (such as the ones occurring during sleep) determine – through the extreme diminishing of exterior, especially photonic, stimuli – a decrease of pH, that is the modification of hydrogen ion concentration in the intercellular environment. Such modification can be the result of switching the polarity by means of the created *pile phenomenon* between the brain and peripheral organs. Precisely this difference of potential will contribute, by super-energizing / super-radiance, to the spontaneous (natural) release of some of the energy and information deposits required during the nocturnal activity of the organism. For, according to BLT, in the absence of generating light (night), all the vital functions are entertained by bioluminescent flux made and deposited during the day / light stimulation of the organism.
2. *The psycho-logical mechanisms* which are active in situations characterizing "life stress", determine, in their turn, the immediate or step-by-step releasing of energy and information under psychic tension, such as:
   - situations of *negative stress* ("distress"), such as strong negative shocks produced by danger, fright, accident, sleep deficiency, exhaustion, etc.;
   - situations of *positive stress* ("eustress"[55]), determined by activities which are pleasant, creative and successful for the human being.

---

53 A process of activating an energy trap (electrons) as the consequence of the nuclear biophotonic flux release. Under these circumstances, the field generated by the flux of the bio-photons released from DNA interferes with all the coherent mitochondrial micro-fields it encounters on its way to the central nervous system and to the decompensation zone it has to equalize. The increase phenomenon of the amplitude within the interfering waves is followed by an increase of the kinetic energy in the field. This increase is transmitted by means of the liquid membrane crystals at the level of the energy traps from which the electrons' reserves are released as a result of the super-energizing process.

54 It is a process determined by the presence around the cellular nucleus of electron flux already released from the mitochondrial traps, as a result of an energizing process. Such flux will implicitly activate the nuclear (magnetic) bio-field whose modified valorized parameters will be received by the inter-nuclear bio-photons (from DNA implicitly) as a super-radiant stimulus.

55 Positive, manageable stress.

In both cases, negative and positive stress, two categories of processes specifically activate: energetic and informational.

- *Energetic* processes are accomplished through releasing biological substances (secretions, hormones, neurotransmitters, etc.) in different zones of the organism, such as endorphins and adrenaline.
- *Informational* processes provoke the release of bio-photonic fluxes at the micro-biological level (cellular, from the nuclear DNA) or on the macro-biological level (the 7 chakras belonging to the organic complexes) which maintain in a radiant-matrix form (in the vibratory structures of the bioluminescent fields) the holographic image of the whole or of a certain zone of the organism. The specific action of these emanations mostly manifests itself at the level of zones that are coherent with the source from which the emanations have been released.

The qualitative distinction between positive and negative psychic states has to be interrelated in this context with the personality (psyche) of the individual, to which homeopathic medicine pays a great deal of attention. On the whole, and with respect to the psyche, we can discern two major types of personality: a) predominantly "constructive" (characterized by positive, optimistic, negentropic[56] thinking); b) predominantly "deconstructive" (characterized by negative, pessimistic, nihilistic, entropic thinking).

How do these two types of personality manifest on the energetic-informational ground? There is no doubt that both imply energy and information consumption, at least at the debut of the actionable state. The difference consists in the fact that:

1. *The positive personality*, by the nature of its activities, generates "benefic tensions" (of short duration and stimulating) which transform the initial energy / information consumption into a source productive of new energy, possibly to be deposited. This process takes place because the initial tension ("stressing") is maintained only as long as it is necessary in order to begin the constructive action, which – during its accomplishment – does not constitute itself as an unnatural energy consumer but begins to be self-sustaining. Thus positive psychic states generate, by means of their benefic effects (including the optimal stopping of the implementing commands), a situation of energetic-informational equilibrium. According to BLT, the risk of becoming ill for these positive personalities is correlated especially with illnesses of the "excess of light" type, such as gastritis, allergies, asthma, immune system weakness, etc.
2. *The negative personality* generates, by means of the dominant type of thinking itself, actions that do not stop implicitly and cannot be solved by means of self-control, maintaining an interior conflict, which becomes a supraliminal energy consumer. In other words, they are energo-phagous actions that consume a great part of the E-I resources of the organism. Unable to be compensated, these E-I reserves are eventually used up, generating a state of tiredness and exhaustion, which at length produces the physical / psychic disease of the individual. The risk of falling ill for the negative personality type is correlated predominantly with illnesses of the "lack of energy / light" type, such as anaemia, muscular hypotrophism, hepatic malfunctions, etc.

---

56 Negentropy: or 'negative entropy' is reverse entropy, meaning that things becoming more ordered (rather than less ordered, as in entropy).

This dichotomaic-reductionist distinction between human personality types (made with the intention of stressing the effects of benefic or malefic thinking) can also be found in, and fills in the nuances of, homeopathic propositions with regard to human categories. According to homeopathic theory, personality type is determinative for *susceptibility to certain illnesses*.

b) Release of E-I reserves in situations of artificial stimulation: We can use the following types of therapeutic methods or strategies – conventional, unconventional or mixed [Stănciulescu, 2005: 203-209]:

1. *Conventional therapies* are achieved through pharmaceutical (bio-chemical)action including natural types, or through procedures of artificial stimulation: electric (through various procedures of induction of types of electric power), magnetic (through the introduction of the patient to a variable magnetic field) or photonic (through laser-therapy, polarized light therapy, colour therapy, crystal therapy, etc.), as is done in recuperative spa treatments. By means of these practices, all the BEMPh effects (bio-chemical, electric, magnetic, photonic) that are highlighted by BLT can be used by the human body with a therapeutic-optimizing value. The effects of these practices are mainly of an energetic type.

2. *Unconventional therapies* suppose psycho-therapeutic practices, such as suggestion, hypnosis, meditation, prayer, etc., which are mainly informational and have as a goal the optimization of the human being by generating in the mind the status of optimum functioning, through conscious and unconscious regeneration of the informational-radiant matrix that configures each structure of the biological organism.

3. *Mixed therapies* suppose practices of the biological type (direct or distal) or technological energizing type (crystal therapy, sound therapy, etc.), and of the homeopathic therapy type, such as acupuncture, acupressure and reflex therapy. In all mixed therapies, the effects are implicitly dual because they aim at generating energetic effects by means of informational procedures or vice-versa.

We have to mention the fact that among the insufficiently-known processes involved in the procedures of the complementary therapies mentioned above, there are two mechanisms – clarified, in principle, by BLT – that have a fundamental role, namely:

1. The idea of information transfer from the biological field (of the aura of the organism, organ or cell) in the substantial support (of the physical body, of the organs, of the cells, etc.) has been developed within the framework of (b)PTEI.

2. The piezoelectric effect of organic liquid crystals (with their membrane) allows us to understand – according to BLT – the way in which a type of energy (and implicitly information) is turned into another type of energy (and implicitly information). It is known that when exposed to a certain pressure, liquid crystals release electrons and photons that reproduce in other ways the properties / values / characteristics of the incident stimulus. On the one hand, this phenomenon explains the fact that, regardless of the nature of the received stimuli, the language of the brain is unitary because it operates with electricity (electrons) and light (bio-photons). On the other hand, some processes of complementary therapy (such as acupuncture, massage, acupressure, reflex therapy, sound therapy, etc.) become explicit; these imply a process of transformation of the physical stimulus (pressure) into a neuro-

psychical one: a super-radiance / super-energizing mechanism necessary to change the energy and information traps upon which they act. It is exactly this mechanism which a homeopathic remedy stimulates, by acting objectively inside the human body, and not in a "magic" way, as many still believe.

In order to demonstrate that "magic therapy" is a practice quite rationally possible, let us remember, in this context, the practice of traditional native Americans, among others, who permanently wore around their neck a "magic medicine pouch" full of plants, crystals, etc. If this "talisman" was lost, the owner could become ill or even die, because they had lost the power of the substances to objectively stimulate the health of the body and mind by the resonance of the active substance of the "pouch" activated by light, by human palms and prayer, by love, etc.

PLACEBO, the sceptics would say from the very beginning. But such practices have been reconsidered by many as alternative homeopathic techniques, able to stimulate by resonance the human "life field". Among them, special attention should be paid to an innovative recent Romanian type of biotechnology [Stănciulescu et al., OSIM 2006], which uses a "bio-resonator complex" (a "biological laser" active substance) of several natural ingredients (vegetable and proteic), specifically selected and measured, placed on the human body as a pendant, button, etc., having a specific state of aggregation, a particular volume, form and colour, etc. (See Fig. 7).

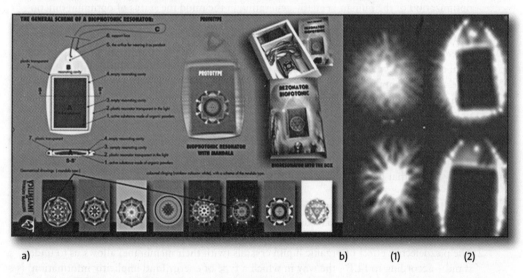

a)   b)   (1)   (2)

Figure 7. The main elements of the Biophotonic Resonator (BR): a) the active substance inside the transparent pandantive + coloured filter and mandalas; b) the electrographs of the active substance of a general stimulating BR (up) & a specific stimulating BR (down), as: (1) simple powder; (2) the powder inside the transparent pandantive, demonstrating a clear difference between samples.

Such an *exogenous source of homeopathic effects* is able to stimulate the Energy-Information of the living system's resources and to eliminate the causes of different illness states, including those that are neuro-psychic. The therapeutic power of these effects – biophotonically connected in the synergy of **homeopathy + chromotherapy + form-therapy** – could influence the health state of the human being, in two complementary ways:

1. *by using a powerful mixture of an active substance, emitting just a few general frequencies*, usually equipped with the white-violet or indigo filter and mandala, acting for the optimization of the general BPL (bio-psycho-logical) energy-information field, and implicitly for increasing the resistance of the organism's immune system. From a homeopathic point of view, the biological laser's active substance of the general stimulating Biophotonic Resonator (BR) could be considered to be a technological *polychrest remedy*, acting from the exterior of the human body; the very large spectrum of action (frequencies) possessed by the selected active substances (a homeopathic solid complex) offers a high probability that the normal "fundamental wave" of a certain unhealthy biological system (a person or, in certain conditions, even a group of persons) is present and, by its beneficent bioresonance, the harmony of the system can be (re)established.

2. *by using a harmonizing specific stimulating BR*, its active substance having a large spectrum of frequencies, able to stimulate / normalize specific types of hypo- and hyper-malfunctions specific to different levels (chakras) and organs of the human body. The action of this BR could be compared with that of *complex remedies*, used by some homeopaths.

As already explained [Stănciulescu, 2004: 105-150], from a biophotonic point of view homeopathic bioresonators have: (1) *an energetic function*: to deliver by a resonance mechanism the internal energy of the receptor system and to activate its growth / healing processes; (2) *an informational function*: to play the role of a "disk-system", able to remind the sick organism (which has lost its "matrix field memory") of its original "software" (the normal functionality of the brain, for example, determined by bio-electromagnetic frequencies and intensities, holographic forms, etc.).

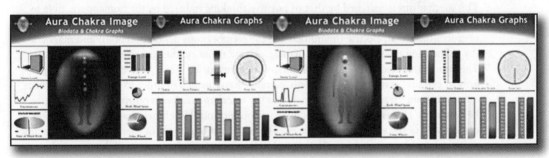

Figure 8. "Aura Vision System": the evident E-I change of a human "aura chakras image" (frequency / colour): from green-blue (a) to violet (b) and of the "aura chakras graphs" intensity from 70 % to 100%, after using a biophotonic resonator of type BR.

In conclusion, this practical application of "exogenous homeopathy" could fundamentally enrich homeopathic practice by concretizing the possibility of using the remedies as a (quasi)permanent external source (converter) of radiation. At the same time, such a healing alternative could represent the necessary step for accomplishing the amazing idea of Harry van der Zee [2004]: to conceive a "*transpersonal homeopathy*" able to cure / harmonize a whole human collective and, finally, the whole of humankind.

5   Summary and implications of the healing process

Briefly, remaining in the realm of neuro-mental disorders, let us imagine – as the framework of an integrative strategy – the simplified scenario of the next therapeutic situation:

1. A patient with a migraine, for example, supposing an energo-informational decompensation and headaches in the frontal area, being generated by a certain cause, a brain super-stimulation determined by a very intense look, an ocular reflection of biophotons;
2. By studying the case history, the therapist identifies a neuro-psychic type of personality (emotional, artistic temperament), and recommends swallowing an individualized homeopathic remedy, *Belladonna*, diluted to C100, by applying the homeopathic strategy: "*stress is converted to eustresses by using the similar stress*";
3. The remedy's information / frequency, dilutes itself under the tongue and quasi-instantaneously transfers to the level of the whole organism, in two ways: a) through the organic liquid system (water, blood, plasma) which adequately structures itself to the received information; b) through the nadi system of the organism (the EM pathway network);
4. With distribution at the level of the whole organism, the remedy's specific frequency operates through supra-radiance over the traps from a number of embryogenetically correlated points, resonating with them: on the sole and in the palm (between the index and forefinger), in the coccyx and cervical vertebral area, on the earlobe, etc.;
5. The supra-radiance effect releases the energetic and informational reserves, electron and biophoton fluxes afferent to all the above mentioned coherent areas;
6. This mechanism is matched by that of positive thinking induced by the homeopath, able to generate coherent effects of a BEMPh type, biochemical (by delivering different types of neurotransmitters), electric (by influencing the membranous action potential) and magnetic (by influencing the state of cellular diamagnetism / memory, the auric field intensity, etc.);
7. The cumulative electron / biophoton fluxes are transported – as a "wave train" that stops only at certain "stations", to take only certain "passengers", in order to discharge / let them off at a certain "train station" – directly to the *uncompensated cerebral area*, which is to be balanced. This is achieved through (bio)photonic and (bio)electro-magnetic stimulation respectively of the substantial trap area. The release of hormones in chemical mediator traps – through an electro-magnetic "holographic resonance" mechanism – will determine the same balancing effect.

What homeopathy does in this case is quite similar to what any other remedy type does or would do: a) *remind the body* (uncompensated area) *of essential information necessary for its correct functioning* (frequencies, intensities, amplitudes, etc.); b) *ensure the body's hidden E-I resources release*, in order to thus trigger the auto-healing process.[57]

In conclusion, if illness equalizes the entry of a human system into "chaos", it means that re-establishing health supposes the same generative mechanism as the "outer space" state, that only

RESONANCE / LOVE can determine [Stănciulescu, 2006a]. This is exactly what happens through *"similia similibus curentur"* in the case of homeopathic practice: it acts at the level of the energetic-substantial body systems (of their objective healthy processes) through the mediation of some unsubstantial principles, namely by the *"ultraweak (bio)luminescence"* / informational attributes of homeopathic remedies (having similar / resonant properties with the objective symptoms of the illness: colours / frequencies, extension / wave length, intensities / forms / amplitudes, etc.). By such a resonance, the appropriate deep resources of the body are delivered, having as an effect – after an initial amplification of the symptoms of the illness (meaning that the organism is strongly fighting against the illness) – the restoration of health. To find remedies with appropriate properties – able to stimulate by a super-radiance / resonance mechanism the delivery of energy-information resources and their circulation through the meridian systems exactly to the affected organs – represents the real medical art of a homeopath.

Acknowledgements

For stimulating my entry into the framework of homeopathy, I wish to express my deep gratitude to Professor *Fritz Albert Popp*, who credited my contribution in the field of biophotonics – and implicitly of homeopathy – by doing me the honour of writing the foreword to my book *"Signs of Light"* and to Sir *Anton Jayasuryia*, who personally credited my biophotonic interpretation of homeopathy. Very special thanks are due to my very special friends: Dr. *Harry van der Zee*, who first reviewed the above-mentioned book and previously published some of its ideas in *Homoeopathic Links*; Dr. *Manish Bhatia*, who supported the entry of my work into the public domain via the prestigious net review *www.hpathy.com*; Dr. *Christopher Kent Johannes*, who opened so many important doors for me to the international "dialogue on health"; and, finally, Dr. *David Cornberg*, who permanently stimulated my mind by pertinent questions and suggestions and made possible the best English editing of my texts. *In Love and Light*: THANK YOU.

---

57 At the same time, we must specify that an essential proportion of the therapeutic effect is represented – no matter what the nature of the remedy used – by the subject's correct mental training through: positive thoughts, faith in the remedy's beneficial outcome and anticipated "thanks" for the awaited result (health), mentally visualised. A PLACEBO effect, would the sceptics say once again. But, to claim that homeopathic remedies have "only" PLACEBO effects means to ignore that, from a biophotonic perspective: (1) a PLACEBO could be considered the strongest therapeutic effect which the brain / mind of a patient can generate, because – by activating the brain waves / cerebral holograms specific to positive thinking – two effective processes are determined: a) initiation of the proper BEMPh effects (biochemical, electric and magnetic, photonic), objectively, coherently and integrally initiated; b) mental (informational) preparation of the human body substratum (namely the more than 70% of the body found as water, blood, lymph fluid, etc. (as Masaru Emoto has already proven), to organize the liquid crystal structure of the cellular membranes and of the cyto-plasm, etc.; (2) a PLACEBO does not at all signify "NOTHINGNESS", as is sometimes claimed, but the objective force of the mind (the complex energetic-informational effects of bio-electromagnetic waves which coordinate the whole activity of the body), the objective result of a cerebral hologram complex, of the vibrations meant to prepare/structure the body's liquid substance or of membranous liquid crystals, and to free hormones and chemical mediators (such as endorphin, serotonin or melatonin) as a means of bio-chemically determining the auto-healing process which homeopathic remedies implicitly sustain.

References

[1] Brennan, Barbara Ann (1996) *Maini de lumină* (hands of light). Oradea, Hungary: Editura Hungalibris

[2] Constantinescu, Paul, Stănciulescu, Traian D. (1993) Resonance as a Principle of Universal Creativity. Photonic (Quantical) Hypothesis of Information-Energy. *Revista de Inventică*, 1993 nr. 12

[3] Delinick, Alexandra N. (1995), *On what primary level of the organism does the homeopathic remedy act upon? ...* A hypothesis, "Alonissos Teacher's Meeting", on Research, August 1995

[4] Guja, Cornelia, et al (1993), *Materi si spituralitate (Matter and spirituality)*, in Guja C (editor), Aurele corpurilor, interfete cu cosmusol (Body's auro, cosmic interfaces). Bucharest, Bulgaria: Editura Enciclopedica

[5] Jayasuriya, Anton (1997) *Homeopatia clinica (Clinical Homeopathy)*. Bucharest, Bulgaria: Editura Apimondia

[6] Johannes, Christopher (1996) Beyond the Avogadro limit: Homeopathy's quatum leap into a new era of medicine. *Journal of American Institue of Homeopathy*, Vol 89; 3

[7] Macovschi, Eugen (1969), *Biostructura (The Biostructure)*. Bucharest, Bulgaria: Editura Academiei

[8] Popp, F.A., Li, K. H., Gu, Q. (1989) *Recent Advances in Biophoton Research and its Applications*. World scientific, Singapore, New Jersey, London, Munich: Urban Schwarzenberg

[9] Pribram, Karl (1971) *Language of the brain. Experimental paradoxes and principles in neuropsychology*. Monterray, CA: Brookes/Cole

[10] Sheldrake, Rupert (1985) *A New Science of Life*. New York: Terrytown

[11] Stănciulescu, Traian D. (2003a) *Therapia prin lumina. Fundamente biofotonice ale medicinei complementare (Therapy by light. Biophotonic fundamentals of complementary medicine)*. Iasi, Hungary: Editure Christal Concept

[12] Stănciulescu, Traian D. (2003b), *Signs of light. A biophotonic approach to human (meta)physical fundamentals*. Iasi & Geneva: Editura Cristal-Concept & World Development Organization

[13] Stănciulescu, Traian D. (2004), Biophotonics and homeopathy: a (meta)physical approach to the life principle. *Homoeopathic Links*, volume 17; 4, Winter 2004

[14] Stănciulescu, Traian D. (editor.), Botez Mihai, Anastasiu, Gabriela (2005), *Homeopatie integrala. O (ne)conventionala sinteza (Integral homeopathy: an unconventional synthesis)*. Iasi, Hungary: Editura Performantica

[15] Stănciulescu, Traian D. (2006a,b) Two Centuries of Expectancy. From Endogenous to Exogenous Homeopathy: Biophotonic Explanations. *Hpathy4Everyone*, November Issue (2006a), www.hpathy.com/research/Stănciulescu-biophotonic-explanations.asp

Homeopathy & Biophotonics (II): The Vital Force. Explanatory contributions of the "biological lasers" theory. *Hpathy4Everyone*, December issue (2006b)   , http://www.hpathy.com/research/Stănciulescu-biophotonic-explanations3.asp

[16] Stănciulescu, Traian D., Constantinescu, Paul (1995), *Fundamente bio-fizice ale gîndirii creative (Bio-physical and psycho-logical fundamentals of creative thinking)*. research project nr. 76 A, National Inventics Institute & Research and Technology Ministry, Hungary

[17] Stănciulescu, Traian D., Manu, Daniela M. (2002), *Fundamente biofotonicii (Fundamentals of biophotonics)*. Iasi, Hungary: Editura Performantica

[18] Stănciulescu, T.D., Apopei, M., Poenaru, A., Brasoveanu, M. (2006) *Rezonator biofotonic (Biophotonic resonator)*, Bucharest, Romania: invention brevet, OSIM

[19] Stănciulescu, Traian D. (2007), *The Living Light Matrix: a biophtonic approach to human harmony design*, Papers of the First Global Conference of the Professional Lighting Design Convention (PLOC) and International Light Association (ILA), London, UK, Oct 24 -28

[20] Vithoulkas, George (2002), Homeopatia. *Medicina noului mileniu (Homeopathy. The medicine of the new Millenium)*. Iasi, Hungary: Editura Pan Europe

[21] Zee, Harry van der (2004) Transpersonal realms of homeopathy: treating beyond space-time limitations. *Homoeopathic Links*, Vol. 17; 3

About the Authors

Dr Hannah Albert, ND received her doctorate of naturopathy from the National College of Natural Medicine in Portland, Oregon. Also a visual artist, Dr. Albert felt an early resonance with homeopathy and was drawn to study with Louis Klein due to his visual teaching style, sense of humour, and Buddhist-influenced approach. In addition to completing Klein's Homeopathic Master Clinician Course, she has also studied with homeopaths Dr. Massimo Mangialavori and Dr. Jan Scholten. She has been in private practice since 2000 and sees patients in Seattle and Minneapolis.

Philip Bailey, MbBs MFHom DipHyp graduated in Medicine from the University of London in 1984. After completing his hospital internship he studied Homeopathy at the Royal London Homeopathic Hospital, graduating with the MFHom qualification in 1987. Philip went on to practise as a homeopathic general practitioner, first in England and then in Perth, Australia. He has also studied and practises counselling and psychotherapy, and has worked in the Danish Health Service with Youth Psychiatry. He is author of the well-known Homeopathic textbook 'Homeopathic Psychology', as well as 'Carcinosinum - A Clinical Materia Medica'. Philip is about to publish his third book, about the Lac remedies. He lectures internationally on homeopathy, and also gives seminars on family constellations.

Iris R. Bell, MD PhD MD(H) is Professor of Family and Community Medicine, Psychiatry, Psychology, Medicine (Center for Integrative Medicine), and Public Health at the University of Arizona in Tucson, Arizona. She has published over 100 scientific papers and two dozen book chapters on her work, which has addressed mainly interdisciplinary studies in areas of complementary and alternative medicine. In the past decade, much of her effort has focused on clinical and basic science research, as well as developing a nonlinear dynamical complex systems model for understanding homeopathic healing in the person as a whole. She is also a licensed homeopath in the state of Arizona..

Daniel J. Benor, MD ABIHM, is a wholistic psychiatric psychotherapist who includes body-mind approaches, spiritual awareness and healing in his practice. Dr. Benor has taught this spectrum of methods internationally for 25 years to people involved in wholistic, intuitive, and spiritual approaches to caring, health and personal development. He founded The Doctor-Healer Network in England and North America. Dr. Benor is the author of Healing Research, Volumes I-IV and many articles on wholistic, spiritual healing. He appears internationally on radio and TV. He is a Founding Diplomate of the American Board of Holistic Medicine and for many years on the advisory boards of the journals, Alternative Therapies in Health and Medicine, Explore, Subtle Energies (ISSSEEM), Frontier Sciences, and the Advisory Council of the Association for Comprehensive Energy Psychotherapy (ACEP). He is editor and producer of the International Journal of Healing and Caring

Dr Manish Bhatia is the Founder-Director of Hpathy.com, the world's leading homeopathy portal. He is the Editor-in-Chief of the monthly e-journal, *Homeopathy 4 Everyone*. He practises at Asha Homeopathy Medical Centre, Jaipur and is also a lecturer of homeopathic philosophy at Jaipur, India.

Kate Chatfield, MSc RSHom is Senior lecturer in Homeopathy, University of Central Lancashire. Kate is the course leader for MSc Homeopathy (e-learning) at UClan. Her first degree was in philosophy but she retrained as a homeopath in 1990. Since 1999 she has taught homeopathy at UCLan and has been involved with homeopathic research in the UK since 2000. She is also co-director of the Galway College of Homeopathy in Ireland.

Jane Tara Cicchetti, RSHom(NA) CCH has been practising homeopathy since 1984. After ten years of supervision with a Jungian analyst, she began teaching post-graduate courses on the integration of Jungian dream analysis into the practice of homeopathy. Jane is the author of 'Dreams, Symbols, and Homeopathy, Archetypal Dimensions of Healing'. She is currently working on a book on the relationship between psyche and matter.

Joy Duxbury, PhD is Reader in Mental Health Nursing, University of Central Lancashire. Joy is Divisional Leader for Mental Health at UCLan and has experience of working in acute inpatient and medium secure units. Joy's ongoing research has largely focused on the challenges associated with aggressive patients and how these are managed in the UK and in other European countries. Accordingly the bulk of her research work and publications has been on interventions that address the complexities of aggression and violence in inpatient services for both staff and patients.

Jane A. Ferris, PhD is a depth psychologist in private practice in San Francisco. She teaches and continues to explore the integration of energy medicine and depth psychotherapy. Her doctorate is from Pacifica Graduate Institute in Santa Barbara, CA. and her graduate internship was at the C. G. Jung Institute in San Francisco.

Corina Güthlin, PhD worked in the field of Evaluation Research of Complementary Medicine for more than ten years. She moved recently to the Institute of General Practice of the Goethe University Frankfurt, Germany, where she is still doing research on complementary medicine in general practice. Her research interests besides homeopathy and complementary medicine are research methodology and quality of life research. She earned her PhD in 2006 combining Quality of Life Research with Complementary Medicine Research.

Christopher Johannes, PhD DHM HD(RHom) MARH NCC LPC LMHC is a homeopath, counsellor, polarity therapist, and educator living in Kyoto, Japan. He holds Masters degrees in health psychology and education, a doctorate in transpersonal psychology, a doctorate in homeopathy, an honorary doctorate in complementary medicine, several professional qualifications in homeopathy, and is a Licensed Professional Counsellor, a Registered Polarity Therapist, and a registered homeopathic doctor (NUPATH, Canada). He serves as Tokunin Assistant Professor at Kansai Gaidai University and as the Program Director of the Integral Health Studies program at Akamai University.

Mary Koithan, RN PhD is Associate Professor of Nursing in the College of Nursing and Research Assistant Professor of Family and Community Medicine and Medicine (Center for Integrative Medicine) at the University of Arizona in Tucson, Arizona. She is a licensed nurse/clinical specialist in chronic illness and an interdisciplinary qualitative researcher focused on healing outcomes associated with complementary/integrative health promotion strategies. Her recent research has included characterizing unstuckness and transformation in persons treated with constitutional homeopathy and other whole systems of complementary and alternative medicine.

Peter Morrell, BSc MPhil PGCE graduated in Zoology from Leeds University in 1973. Following his first exposure to homeopathy in 1978 he became a self-taught homeopath practising in the UK on a part-time basis throughout the 1980s and to a diminishing extent since. He completed an MPhil thesis on the history of British homeopathy at Staffordshire University in 1999 and published a collection of his essays as *"Hahnemann and Homeopathy"* in 2004. His extensive and ongoing writings on the history of homeopathy and the life of Hahnemann have been published in a range of homeopathic journals in the UK, the USA, Australia, Sweden and Romania.

Judyth Reichenberg-Ullman, ND DHANP LCSW is a 1983 graduate of Bastyr University (Seattle. USA), and received a Master's in psychiatric social work from the University of Washington in 1976. She is the author of six books on homeopathy, including the bestselling *Ritalin-Free Kids, Rage-Free Kids, Prozac-Free*, and *A Drug-Free Approach to Asperger Syndrome and Autism*, and author of *Whole Woman Homeopathy*. She and her husband, **Robert Ullman, ND DHANP**, have taught internationally and practise at The Northwest Center for Homeopathic Medicine in Edmonds, Washington. They live on Whidbey Island, WA and in Pucon, Chile. Drs. Ullman jointly authored *Mystics, Masters, Saints, and Sages: Stories of Enlightenment*, with a foreword by His Holiness the Dalai Lama.

Dr Joseph Rozencwajg, MD PhD NMD graduated from medical school in Brussels in 1976 with a specialisation in general, thoracic and cardiovascular surgery. Since January 2001 after relinquishing the practice of conventional medicine, he uses only homeopathy, herbalism, homeobotanicals, acupuncture, TCM, nutrition, and naturopathy. He also holds doctorates in Natural Medicine, Naturopathy, and Homeopathy and is currently working towards an Oriental Medicine Doctorate (OMD) and a Doctorate in Osteopathy (DO Drugless). He has a full-time private practice in New Plymouth, New Zealand.

Dr Seema, BHMS MD Hom has been practicing homeopathy in Bangalore, India since 2003. She has a Bachelors degree and MD in homeopathy and is currently pursuing the diploma from IACH Greece. She has been trained under George Vithoulkas. She, along with her husband Dr. Mahesh and with another homeopath from London, Dr. Craig Talbot, founded the Centre For Classical Homeopathy in Bangalore in 2005. The centre has over 12,000 documented cases so far, ranging from allergies, dermatitis, vitiligo, asthma to diabetic gangrene, autism, psychiatric disorders, cancer, AIDS and so on. The centre caters to the urban as well as rural health needs in that part of the world. It conducts the Vithoulkas video course regularly along with clinical training. Many students from abroad have stayed at the centre to learn homeopathy and to have a rural as well as an urban clinical exposure of such variety. Dr. Seema is the education director of the centre and may be contacted for this purpose. She is also serving as a faculty member for Akamai University, USA.

Edward Shalts, MD DHt ABPN ABHT ABHM was born in Moscow, Russia in 1955. He graduated from medical school in Moscow in 1982 and worked as a family physician and a homeopath while also conducting research in neurophysiology. In 1988 he immigrated to the USA, initially working as a Research Fellow in the Neuroendocrinology lab at Columbia University from 1989 to 1993. Dr. Shalts has published papers in major journals in the field of neurophysiology. After passing the medical boards he became a Resident and eventually a Chief Resident at the Department of Psychiatry at the Beth Israel Medical Center, NY. Currently in private homeopathic and holistic psychiatric practice in Manhattan, Dr. Shalts worked as a homeopath at the Center for Health and Healing at the Beth Israel Medical Center, NY for over four years. He served as the Vice President of the National Center for Homeopathy and the Second Vice President of the American Institute of Homeopathy. Board Certified in Psychiatry, Homeopathy and Holistic Medicine, Dr. Shalts has been able to utilize his vast knowledge in treating various chronic and acute conditions in patients of various age groups. He has also been teaching homeopathy to professionals and has presented various homeopathy topics at numerous Grand Rounds and professional conferences. He is on the faculty of the Center for Health and Healing at the Beth Israel Medical Center, New York, the Institute for Complementary and Alternative Medicine, UMDNJ and the New York College of Osteopathic Medicine.

Dr. Shalts has authored numerous papers and book chapters on homeopathy, including a review paper "Homeopathy" published in The Medical Clinics of North America (vol.86, pp.47-62, Jan. 2002). He is also the author of two books: "The American Institute of Homeopathy Handbook for Parents" and "Easy Homeopathy".

Kenneth Silvestri, EdD CCH RSHom (NA) is a licensed family therapist and certified classical homeopath. He has a doctorate in anthropology and psychology from Columbia University. He studied with Luc De Schepper and David Little and has private practices in Green Village and Montclair, New Jersey, USA. He is also an active Black Belt student of Aikido, a martial art dedicated to peace and harmony.

Prof Dr Traian D. Stănciulescu (born in 1951, Romania) graduated from the Institute of Architecture and from the Faculty of Philosophy. He is currently a full professor at the Alexandru Ioan Cuza University of Iassy in Romania (where he teaches semiotics, hermeneutics, creatology, etc. and coordinates doctoral papers in these fields) and a senior scientific researcher (head of the Department of Synergetics & Biophotonics) at the National Inventics Institute in Iassy. He is the President of AROSS (the Romanian Association for Semiotic Studies), Vice-president of ANATECOR (the Romanian National Association for Complementary Therapies), F.R.C.P. – M.A. (Fellow of the Royal Complementary Practitioners of Sri-Lanka & Alma-Ata), Fellow of the International Communicology Institute (Illinois, USA), associate professor at AKAMAI University (USA) and member of many other (inter)national professional associations. He has published over 200 scientific studies and articles in Romanian and overseas publications and participated in over 250 (inter)national scientific meetings. He has written and co-written 32 books, including: Signs of Light, Semiotics of Light, The Vital Force, El Poder de la Luz (The power of light) which aim firstly to unify the perspective of human (spiritual) sciences with that of biophotonics, and secondly to make connections between allopathic and alternative holistic medicine for the benefit of human health. For his theoretical and practical research he has received many (inter)national awards, starting with the Romanian Academy prize and finishing with gold medals for papers including "Healthy synergetic clothing", "Eco-sane architecture" and "Biophotonic resonator".

Ian Townsend, MA RSHom (ret'd) is an educator, homeopath, person-centred counsellor and supervisor with over two decades experience teaching *'caring skills'* in private UK colleges of homeopathy. As part of a multi-disciplinary team of homeopaths, herbalists and massage therapists at the University of Central Lancashire, for the past ten years he has been involved with two undergraduate modules: *Communication and Caring in the Patient-Practitioner Relationship* and *Developing the Therapeutic Relationship*. He currently continues to develop that work with postgraduate students in UCLan's MSc Homeopathy in *Therapeutic Relationships and Supervision in Homeopathy modules*.
[See http://www.uclan.ac.uk/information/courses/msc_homeopathy_by_elearning.php]

Dana Ullman, MPH is "homeopathic.com" and is widely recognized as a foremost spokesperson for homeopathic medicine in the U.S. He has authored nine books, including his newest work, *The Homeopathic Revolution: Why Famous People and Cultural Heroes Choose Homeopathy* (North Atlantic Books/Random House, 2007). Dana also co-authored the best-selling *Everybody's Guide to Homeopathic Medicines* with Stephen Cummings, MD (Tarcher, 2004), Homeopathic Medicines for Children and Infants (Tarcher, 1992), and a regularly updated eBook entitled *Homeopathic Family Medicine: Evidence-Based Homeopathy*, which describes the most recent clinical research and primary care. He has served in an advisory and/or teaching capacity at alternative medicine institutes at Harvard, Columbia, University of Arizona, and University of Alaska schools of medicine. He has also authored chapters on homeopathic medicine in medical textbooks in the fields of oncology, pain management, and veterinary medicine.

Harald Walach, PhD is a research professor in psychology. He holds a PhD in Clinical Psychology (1990) and a PhD in the History and Theory of Science (1995). His background is in the evaluation of unconventional interventions, exceptional experiences and mindfulness research. He has conducted a variety of clinical, experimental and epidemiological studies and has published widely on homeopathy research. He is the editor-in-chief of the Karger journal "Research in Complementary Medicine – Forschende Komplementärmedizin" and of the Wiley Journal "Spirituality and Health International". Publications: 100 refereed journal articles, 48 book chapters, 5 edited books, 6 authored monographs, among them a German-language textbook on the philosophy and theory of science for psychology students.

Harry van der Zee, MD Hom, born in the Netherlands in 1953, has been working in private practice as a classical homeopathic physician since 1987. He has investigated the importance of the birth experience in homeopathic case-taking and published two books on the subject - 'Miasms in Labour' (2000) and 'Homeopathy for Birth Trauma' (2007) which provide a deeper understanding of the theory of miasms. Since 1996 he is editor-in-chief of Homœopathic Links, an international journal for classical homeopathy. He has published several articles, has been teaching homeopathy for many years around the globe, and is publisher (Homeolinks Publishers).
After investigating the efficacy of a homeopathic treatment for HIV/AIDS in Malawi in 2004, he decided to support this work and co-established the Amma Resonance Healing Foundation (2007) that focuses on providing sustainable homeopathic health care for the treatment of epidemics and trauma in Africa and other developing countries. In regard to this work in Africa he edited and published Peter Chappell's book 'The Second Simillimum', is author of the 'Amma4Africa Manual' and producer of a documentary on the treatment of AIDS, malaria and war trauma (www.ARHF.nl).

Index of remedies

Index

unipolar depression, 22

unstuck, unstuckness, 60, 61, 62, 63, 64, 65, 66, 67, 68, 69, 208, 272, 326

V

vaccination, 237, 239

vaccines, 24

vibrational, 81, 82, 84

vigilance, 132

vigor vitae, 206

violence, 89, 116, 139, 161, 164, 244, 286, 287, 326

violent behaviour / impulses, 139, 140, 237, 286, 287

vital force, dynamis, 92, 93, 94, 152, 164, 165, 170, 192, 202, 203, 204, 206, 207, 217, 225, 228, 248, 293, 294, 299, 300, 303, 305, 308, 310, 312, 313, 328

vital sensation, sensation method, 138, 139 159, 160, 197, 243

vitalist, 93, 94, 255, 263

voices, 112, 120, 121, 132

W

war, 52, 78, 79, 130, 131, 133, 135, 145, 148,149, 153, 154, 155, 156, 157, 160, 161, 162; 163, 166, 329

well-being, 21, 42, 43, 66, 67, 131, 209, 216

Whitmont, 72, 75, 76, 77, 83, 115, 186, 212

WHO (see World Health Organization)

wholistic (see holistic)

World Health Organization, WHO, 23, 24, 28, 149, 202, 310

World Health Report, 22, 23

Y

yin and yang, 245, 246

yoga, 63, 229